Basic and Advanced Laser Surgery in Gynecology

Basic and Advanced Laser Surgery in Gynecology

Michael S. Baggish, M.D.

Professor and Chairman
Department of Obstetrics and Gynecology
State University of New York, College of Medicine
Syracuse, New York

 APPLETON-CENTURY-CROFTS/Norwalk, Connecticut

0-8385-0520-1

85 86 87 88 89 / 10 9 8 7 6 5 4 3 2 1

Prentice-Hall of Australia, Pty. Ltd., Sydney
Prentice-Hall Canada, Inc.
Prentice-Hall Hispanoamericana, S.A., Mexico
Prentice-Hall of India Private Limited, New Delhi
Prentice-Hall International (UK) Limited, London
Prentice-Hall of Japan, Inc., Tokyo
Prentice-Hall of Southeast Asia (Pte.) Ltd., Singapore
Whitehall Books Ltd., Wellington, New Zealand
Editora Prentice-Hall do Brasil Ltda., Rio de Janeiro

Library of Congress Cataloging-in-Publication Data
Main entry under title:

Basic and advanced laser surgery in gynecology.

Includes index.
1. Lasers in surgery. 2. Gynecology, Operative.
I. Baggish, Michael S. [DNLM: 1. Genitalia, Female—
surgery. 2. Lasers—therapeutic use. WP 660 B311]
RG104.B33 1985   618.1′45   85-11135
ISBN 0-8385-0520-1

Design: Lynn M. Luchetti

Cover Illustration: J. A. Ruiz

To my children,
Cindy, Jeffrey, Mindy, and Stuart Baggish,
who have served as a source of pride and inspiration for their father
M.S.B.

Contributors

Michael S. Baggish, M.D.
Professor and Chairman
Department of Obstetrics and Gynecology
State University of New York, College of
    Medicine
Syracuse, New York

M. A. Bruhat, M.D.
Chef de Service
Polyclinique Philippe-Marcombes
Service de Gynecologie et d'Obstetrique
Centre Hospitalier Regional de Clermont-
    Ferrand
Clermont-Ferrand, Cedex, France

Louis Burke, M.D.
Associate Professor, Department of Obstetrics
    and Gynecology
Chief, Colposcopy/Laser Clinic
Harvard University Medical School
Beth Israel Hospital
Boston, Massachusetts

Augusto P. Chong, M.D.
Director, Reproductive Endocrinology and
    Infertility Division
Department of Obstetrics and Gynecology
Mount Sinai Hospital
Hartford, Connecticut
Associate Professor, Department of Obstetrics
    and Gynecology
University of Connecticut Health Science Center
Farmington, Connecticut

James F. Daniell, M.D.
Associate Professor, Department of Obstetrics
    and Gynecology
Vanderbilt Medical School
Nashville, Tennessee

James H. Dorsey, M.D.
Chief of Gynecology
Greater Baltimore Medical Center
Assistant Professor of Obstetrics and
    Gynecology
Johns Hopkins University School of Medicine
Baltimore, Maryland

Thomas J. Dougherty, Ph.D.
Head, Division of Radiation Biology
Department of Radiation Medicine
Roswell Park Memorial Institute
Buffalo, New York

John C. Fisher, Sc.D.
Visiting Associate Professor of Laser Medicine
    and Surgery
Department of Surgery
College of Medicine
University of Cincinnati
Cincinnati, Ohio

Terry A. Fuller, Ph.D.
President, Fuller Research Corporation
Vernon Hills, Illinois

Fred M. Gardner, Ph.D.
Professor of Physics, Department of Physics
University of Hartford
West Hartford, Connecticut

Milton H. Goldrath, M.D.
Chairman, Department of Obstetrics and
    Gynecology
Sinai Hospital of Detroit
Detroit, Michigan

Vernon W. Jobson, M.D.
Assistant Professor, Department of Obstetrics
    and Gynecology

Section on Gynecologic Oncology
Bowman Gray School of Medicine, Wake
  Forest University
Winston-Salem, North Carolina

Robert W. Kelly, M.D.
Associate Professor, Vice Chairman, and
  Director, Division of Reproductive
  Endocrinology
Department of Obstetrics and Gynecology
University of Kansas School of Medicine at
  Wesley Medical Center
Wichita, Kansas

Katherine Dexter Laakmann, Ph.D.
General Manager, Laakmann Electro-Optics,
  Inc.
Vice President, Xanar, Inc.
San Juan, California

G. Mage, M.D.
Adjoint Chef de Service
Polyclinique Philippe-Marcombes
Service de Gynecologie et d'Obstetrique
Centre Hospitalier Regional de Clermont-
  Ferrand
Clermont-Ferrand, Cedex, France

Daniel Clyde Martin, M.D.
Clinical Assistant Professor, Department of
  Obstetrics and Gynecology
University of Tennessee Center for the Health
  Sciences
Memphis, Tennessee

C. Kumar N. Patel, Ph.D.
Executive Director of Research, Physics
  Division
AT&T Bell Laboratories
Murray Hill, New Jersey

J. L. Pouly, M.D.
Chef de Clinique-Assistant
Polyclinique Philippe-Marcombes
Service de Gynecologie et d'Obstetrique

Centre Hospitalier Regional de Clermont-
  Ferrand
Clermont-Ferrand, Cedex, France

Ralph M. Richart, M.D.
Professor of Pathology
Columbia University College of Physicians and
  Surgeons
Director of the Division of Obstetric and
  Gynecologic Pathology and Cytology
The Sloane Hospital for Women
New York, New York

Helmut F. Schellhas, M.D.
Professor, Department of Obstetrics and
  Gynecology
Director, Gynecologic Oncology
Professor, Radiation Oncology
University of Cincinnati College of Medicine
Cincinnati, Ohio

Duane E. Townsend, M.D.
Consultant, Gynecologic Oncology
Sutter Memorial Hospital Cancer Center
Sacramento, California

Barbara Winkler, M.D.
Assistant Professor of Pathology
State University of New York at Stony Brook
Staff Pathologist, Long Island Jewish Hillside
  Medical Center
Stony Brook, New York

Obert R. Wood II, Ph.D.
Member of Technical Staff
AT&T Bell Laboratories
Holmdel, New Jersey

V. Cecil Wright, M.D.
Associate Clinical Professor
Department of Obstetrics and Gynecology
St. Joseph's Hospital
The University of Western Ontario
London, Ontario, Canada

Contents

Preface

The impetus leading to the publication of this book was a perceived need for a comprehensive and practical presentation of laser surgery for the gynecologist. This treatise will serve as a basic text, a concise atlas, and a ready reference source. The format for *Basic and Advanced Laser Surgery in Gynecology* follows the structure of a teaching seminar and begins with a thorough history of laser technology appropriately co-authored by C. K. N. Patel, the world famous inventor of the carbon dioxide laser. The subjects of laser physics, laser–tissue interaction, and laser safety are covered by four of the most renowned physicists in the medical laser field. Three key chapters detailing the pathology of lower genital tract neoplasia, colposcopy as a method for diagnosis, and laser instrumentation complete the basic foundation section.

A "how to" section of lower genital tract laser surgery contains chapters covering cervical, vaginal, and vulvar techniques. These chapters provide both the basis and specifications for the treatment of invasive cancer, intraepithelial neoplasia, and viral venereal infections.

The third section covers advanced laser surgery and specifically the subjects of photoradiation therapy, intraabdominal laser surgery, and laser endoscopy. Chapters on complications of laser surgery and the implementation of a laser program complete this section. The profuse number of line drawings, halftone illustrations, black and white photographs, and color plates offer the reader the best method for combining full text explanations with practical visual learning aids.

Finally, the contributors to the clinical sections of this book were selected on the basis of their recognized intellect, skill, and scientific veracity within the area of laser surgery.

Michael S. Baggish

Acknowledgments

Many individuals have, by their hard work, patience, and support rendered this book possible. I would like to thank my staff in Syracuse, particularly Emilie, Gwen, and Paula; those in Hartford, Marge and Caryl; my artist, Mr. Ruiz; and Nancy McSherry-Collins, Jane Licht, Susan Neitlich, and the staff at Appleton-Century-Crofts.

1

History of the Laser

C. Kumar N. Patel
Obert R. Wood II

INTRODUCTION

The word "laser" is now common in everyday usage. Lasers are used routinely in a variety of applications from the lightwave systems of the communications industry to the welders of the automotive industry. Yet few realize that the invention of the laser took place only 25 years ago and that its acceptance as a useful tool has taken place only recently, much of it in the last ten years. The era of lasers may be traced from the beginning of the twentieth century.

In 1900, Max Planck proposed a theory, now referred to as the *quantum theory*, which described energy as traveling in packets rather than by wave phenomenon.[1] Planck predicted that the energy of an oscillator was equal to the frequency of radiation expressed in cycles per second (c/s) times a constant. The constant, called Planck's constant, is given as 6.6262×10^{-27} erg seconds.[2] In 1913, Niels Bohr[3] postulated that the hydrogen atom had a number of orbits or shells in which electrons could rotate around the nucleus. The orbits farther out corresponded to higher energy states and those closer to the proton, to lower energy states. When the electron dropped from an outer orbit to an inner orbit, it emitted photons; when the electron moved from an inner orbit to an outer orbit, a quantum of energy was absorbed.[3]

LASER PHYSICS

A laser is a device that produces a highly directional beam of a special kind of light that can be focused to a very small spot. Laser light behaves as one single wave (coherent light) because of its single frequency nature. In contrast, ordinary light consists of many individual waves which combine in a random fashion (incoherent light).

1

The Active Medium

A schematic diagram of a laser is shown in Figure 1–1. Central to the device is the light amplifier (or active medium) that provides amplification by the process of stimulated emission of radiation. Until 1917, it was inconceivable that light could be amplified. The process of stimulated emission of radiation was first described by Albert Einstein in 1917.[4] In order to explain thermal equilibrium in a gas that was both absorbing and emitting radiation, he showed that three processes were involved: (1) absorption, (2) spontaneous emission, and (3) stimulated emission. Under normal circumstances, the first two processes are dominant. Energy can be transferred to atoms from a source (Fig. 1–1) in several ways: (1) by thermal heating, (2) via the absorption of light, or (3) in collisions with electrons in an electric current. In each of these "pumping" processes, part of the energy increases the random motion of the atoms and part is absorbed causing electrons to move to the higher energy levels of the atoms. The former part is not useful in producing amplification, but the latter part (electronic excitation) turns out to be extremely useful.

Excited atoms radiate their energy in the form of light when the electrons fall back to their lowest energy state. The light that is emitted has a frequency that corresponds exactly to the energy the electrons gave up according to Einstein's formula $E = h\nu$, where E is energy, h is Planck's constant and ν is the frequency of the radiation. In single atoms the energy states of the electron, and thus the frequency of the emitted light, is precisely defined. Single atoms or molecules (such as those in a gas) therefore emit very pure frequencies. In liquids and solids the atoms are so closely packed that their energy levels are smeared out. Consequently, molecules in liquids and solids generally emit a spectrum of frequencies. In either case (narrow or broadband), stimulated emission can occur when light interacts with an atom that has energy stored in an excited state. The incident light must have the exact energy that the atom can give up when its electron falls to a lower state. If this requirement is satisfied, the atom will emit its light in the same direction as the incident light, and the emitted light will be in phase with the incident light. In other words, light can be amplified by stimulating atoms to emit radiation. A competing process, known as absorption, can remove light from the beam by raising electrons from the lower energy state to higher ones. Thus, in order to have net amplification (instead of absorption) when the light passes through the active medium, there must be more atoms with electrons at the higher

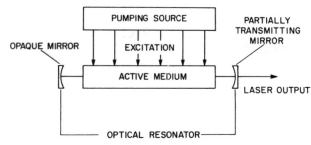

Figure 1–1. Schematic diagram of a laser illustrating the terminology.

energy state than at the lower energy state. This condition is called a population inversion.

In most lasers, amplification takes place within a long narrow region. If the light that passes through the length of the amplifier is increased by say 5 percent (typical of many lasers), the active medium is said to have a gain of 5 percent. If light from an ordinary source such as a flashlight were shown through such an amplifier, it would not look much different from the original flashlight beam. If mirrors however are placed at opposite ends of the amplifier in such a way that nearly 100 percent of the light leaving the amplifier is reflected back into it (Fig. 1–1), this light would grow by about 5 percent every time it passed through the amplifier. After 100 passes, the initial light intensity would be increased approximately 130 times, and after 200 passes it would be increased over 17,000 times. In any case, only a portion of the beam (that which was reflected by one mirror in such a way that it would arrive at the other mirror after having passed through the amplifier) is preserved in the multiple reflection process. Thus, a few hundred passes would provide a very precise direction to the beam of light. Some of this light could be made available (coupled out) by making one of the resonator mirrors partially transmitting (1 or 2 percent is typical). The number of times the beam can pass through the active medium before it ceases to grow is limited by the amount of energy stored in the amplifier. When this limit is reached, the amplifier is said to be saturated.

Optical Resonators

Charles Townes became interested in microwave spectroscopy while working on radar technology during World War II. In 1953, Townes and coworkers used a strong electrostatic field to force a beam of excited ammonia molecules through a small hole into a cavity tuned to 23,870 megacycles per second (Mc/s).[5] By concentrating the excited ammonia molecules into a cavity, Townes hoped to achieve a population inversion or a surplus of excited molecules. After achieving the latter condition, the excited molecule would slip back to the ground state and could trigger the rest of the molecules into emitting coherent radiation at 23,870 Mc/s. By continuing to squirt the beam of excited molecules into the small hole in the cavity, coherent oscillation could be sustained indefinitely. The new device was called a maser or *m*icrowave *a*mplification by *s*timulated *e*mission of *r*adiation.

In 1957, Townes and his brother-in-law Arthur Schawlow investigated the possibilities for making an optical maser.[6] They suggested using two parallel flat mirrors between which was a collection of atoms, most in an excited energy state. A single quantum of energy from one atom would trigger or stimulate emission from others. If the stimulated emission was directed perpendicular to the two parallel mirrors, light would be reflected back and forth between the mirrors. If the total amount of light emitted from the atoms was greater than the losses incurred by reflection from the mirrors, the light wave would gain in intensity during the process. Ultimately the wave would sap the energy of all the excited atoms in the space between the mirrors and it would not grow further. At this point steady oscillation would be attained. The oscillator would be coherent in space with all photons in phase and it would be pure in frequency. This 1958 hypothesis, published by Schawlow and Townes,[6] proposed the use of an optical resonator with a relatively long cylindric geometry bounded, as previously noted, at the two ends of the cylinder by flat mirrors and with the remaining walls of the cylinder left open. At that time, it was not entirely clear what modes would be supported in such a resonator or, in fact, if such a resonator would support modes with sufficiently low loss. The computer calculations of Fox and Li[7] and analytic calculations of Boyd and Gordon[8] showed very clearly that the losses for the fundamental modes of a plane parallel mirror (or a spheric mirror) resonator would be much lower than what would be expected from simple considerations and that, in fact, such a resonator would provide a small number of very low loss modes which could be used to obtain laser action. By "modes" we refer to a particular set of electromagnetic field configurations, propagating back and forth along the laser axis, whose pattern over the surface of the mirrors is maintained upon completion of each round trip. Because of the relatively long cylindric geometry of a laser resonator, these electromagnetic field configurations can be separated into transverse and longitudinal modes which are nearly independent of one another. Laser oscillation is only possible in those modes for which the amplification of the active medium makes up for the total round trip diffraction and transmission losses. A complete understanding of the modes inside resonators with curved mirrors was obtained by Boyd and Kogelnik[9] in 1962 and later generalized by Kogelnik.[10]

Boyd and Gordon[8] found that the fundamental transverse mode of a spheric mirror resonator, usually designated with the notation TEM_{00} (transverse electromagnetic wave), has a Gaussian distribution with an intensity which is maximum along the laser axis gradually diminishing in the radial direction. Higher order transverse modes have a more complex intensity distribution described mathematically by a product of Hermite and Gaussian functions (exhibiting a number of maxima and minima in the radial direction) and occupy a larger area than the fundamental transverse mode. For the confocal resonator illustrated in Figure 1–2 (two spheric mirrors separated by a distance, d, equal to their radii of curvature, R), the beam radii of the fundamental Gaussian mode, w_0 in the center of the resonator and w_1 on the surface of the curved mirrors, are given by[10]

$$w_0 = (\lambda d/2\pi)^{1/2} \tag{1-1}$$

and

$$w_1 = (\lambda d/\pi)^{1/2} \tag{1-2}$$

In addition to limiting oscillation to a small number of transverse modes, the optical resonator also determines the exact frequencies at which the laser operates. Laser oscillation is only possible at those frequencies for which the total phase shift after a complete round trip is an integral multiple of 2π. This condition, to a good approximation, leads to oscillating frequencies equal to $nc/2d$ where n is a positive integer and c is the velocity of light in the medium. The different integers n correspond to the longitudinal modes of the resonator. In general, each transverse mode has associated with it a number of longitudinal modes separated in frequency by $c/2d$.

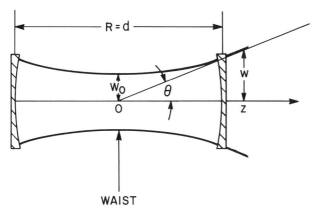

Figure 1–2. Gaussian beam propagation starting from the waist of a confocal resonator.

TYPES OF LASERS

Laser action or amplified spontaneous emission has now been observed at wavelengths that range from the vacuum ultraviolet at around 100 nm to beyond 1000 μm in the submillimeter region of the spectrum. Stimulated emission has been reported on more than 1000 electronic transitions in the atomic species of over 40 elements and on numerous vibrational-rotational transitions in a wide variety of molecular compounds as well as in a number of liquids and solids. Peak power outputs have been increased to gigawatt power levels in several systems.

Lasers can be classified according to whether their active medium is a gas, a liquid, or a solid. Some of the more prominent members of each type of laser together with their operating wavelengths are listed in Figure 1–3. The active medium of a gas laser, a low pressure gas, is usually excited with an electric discharge either radio frequency (RF) or direct current (DC). The active medium of the most important class of liquid lasers, organic dyes dissolved in various solvents, is usually excited by optical pumping with flashlamps or the output from other fixed frequency lasers. The active medium of solid state lasers, ions doped into crystal or glass hosts, is usually excited by a flashlamp.

Lasers are generally operated in one of the following modes: (1) continuous wave (CW), (2) pulsed, (3) Q-switched, or (4) mode-locked. In the CW mode, a continuous beam of constant power is emitted by the laser. In pulsed operation, pulsed pumping of the active medium results in relatively high energy pulses at repetition rates from one to hundreds of pulses per second. The techniques of Q-switching and mode-locking are often employed when pulses of extremely short duration are required (see the Neodymium: YAG Laser and the Organic Dye Laser in this chapter). The power output attainable in these short pulses greatly exceeds that which can be achieved during CW or pulsed operation. Typical pulse durations range from hundreds of femtoseconds (10^{-15} seconds) to hundreds of nanoseconds (10^{-9} seconds) depending on the particular laser system and mode of operation.

This section briefly surveys the operation and the general properties of several of the most important lasers used in medicine and surgery.

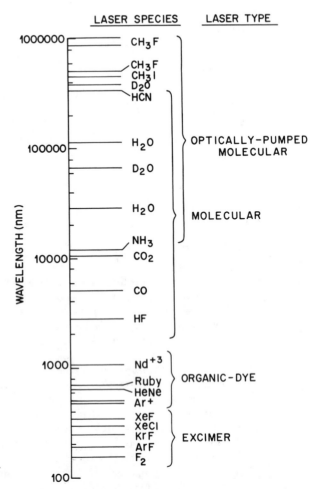

Figure 1-3. Chart of commercially available lasers.

The first experimental demonstration of laser oscillation was made by Theodore H. Maiman in 1960[11] while working at Hughes Research Laboratories. Maiman constructed a laser from a ruby crystal pumped with light from a xenon flash lamp. This produced a fine beam of coherent, monochromatic deep red light. The device remained unsatisfactory for most surgical procedures because it operated at high power levels and only in pulses.

The Helium-Neon Laser

In 1961, a Bell Laboratories group consisting of Ali Javan, William R. Bennett, and Donald R. Herriott invented the gaseous laser.[12] Javan used a small radio transmitter to excite an electric discharge in a quartz tube filled with a mixture of helium and neon gases. The discharge excited the helium atoms which then transferred their energy to neon atoms making the number of neon atoms in the upper excited state larger than the number of neon atoms in intermediate energy states. The gas laser oscillated continuously and could be precisely controlled to give a high frequency purity. It was also highly efficient. The first device was operated in the infrared and produced a power output of the order of 15 mW on several wavelengths near 1 μ. White and Rigden[13] soon found that the same gas mixture could operate on a red transition at a wavelength of 632.8 nm. Because the visible emission is generally more useful, virtually all commercial He-Ne lasers are now designed to emit only in the red.

The active medium in a He-Ne laser is a mixture of helium and neon gases at total pressures between a fraction of a torr and several torr. The gas mixture (5:1, helium to neon) is excited with a few milliamps of DC current at a voltage of a few kilovolts. Electrons passing through the gas collide with both helium and neon atoms, raising them to excited levels. Most of the energy is collected by the helium atoms, which can transfer that energy to neon atoms readily because the two have excited states at about the same energy. Emission is possible on several transitions, as shown in Figure 1–4. Mirrors on each end of the discharge tube form an optical resonator. The choice of mirror coating usually limits laser oscillation to one wavelength.

Virtually all commercially available He-Ne lasers are characterized by output powers of 0.5 to 10 mW at 632.8 nm. The overall efficiency of a He-Ne laser (defined as the ratio of optical power divided by the electric power input) is low,

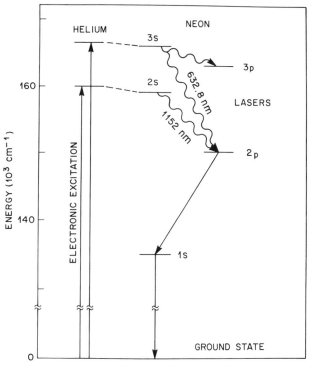

Figure 1–4. Energy level diagram for the He-Ne laser.

typically, in the range of 0.01 to 0.1 percent. Even so, it is the least expensive visible wavelength laser by about an order of magnitude. He-Ne lasers are used for a broad range of applications, the most common being alignment and positioning.

The Argon-Ion Laser

This second type of gas laser operates on transitions in the ions of the noble gases,[14] argon, krypton, xenon, and neon. In this type of laser, fast-moving electrons within the gas discharge excite gas atoms to very high energy states and ionize (remove an electron from) many of them. The most useful laser in this class is the argon-ion laser first operated in CW by Bridges and his colleagues.[15]

The active medium of the CW argon-ion laser is an ionized plasma of argon at a fraction of a torr pressure. The pertinent energy level scheme is shown in Figure 1–5. A high current DC or RF discharge produces electrons with an average energy of 4 to 5 electron volts (eV).[15] Since the upper laser levels of the argon-ion laser

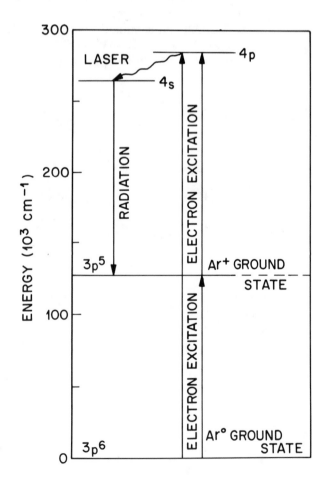

Figure 1–5. Energy level diagram for the argon-ion laser.

are about 20 eV above the ground state of the ion, more than one electron collision is required to excite an argon ion to one of these levels. Large population inversions can be produced because the lower laser levels, which lie approximately 17 eV above the ion ground state, have a negligible population. Furthermore, a population inversion can be produced either on a transient or CW basis because the lower laser levels have very short lifetimes, quickly decaying to the ion ground state.

Noble gas ion lasers require high input powers, necessitating expensive discharge tubes and water cooling to dissipate large amounts of heat. Even so, commercial units providing tens of watts of power are now available. The dominant emission lines in the argon-ion laser lie in the blue and green spectral region at 488.0 and 514.5 nm, whereas the dominant emission lines in the krypton-ion lasers lie in the red and yellow spectral region at 647.1 and 568.2 nm. Argon-ion lasers find extensive use in ophthalmology and as pumping sources for other types of lasers.

The Carbon Dioxide Laser

CW laser operation at 10.6 μm in CO_2 was first announced by Patel[16] in 1964. Since that time, CO_2 lasers have remained of great interest because they give a higher CW output with higher efficiency than any other laser. Commercially available CO_2 lasers can be made to emit radiation at a number of discrete wavelengths between 9 and 11 μm, can produce CW powers ranging from under 1 W for scientific applications to many tens of kilowatts for material working, and can also produce short, intense pulses. Custom-made CO_2 lasers can emit CW powers of hundreds of kilowatts for military applications or single nanosecond pulses with more than 40 kilojoules of energy for fusion research applications.

The active medium of a conventional CO_2 laser is an electrically excited mixture of carbon dioxide, nitrogen, and helium. An energy level diagram illustrating the population inversion mechanism in a CO_2 laser is shown in Figure 1–6. Laser action occurs on a vibrational-rotational transition of the ground electronic state of CO_2. The v = 1 level of N_2 is in close coincidence with the upper laser level ν_3

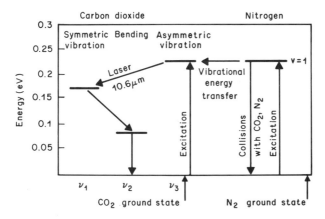

Figure 1–6. Energy level diagram for the CO_2 laser.

of CO_2, and rapid energy exchange between the two takes place. The N_2 level, which is readily excited by electron collisions, is metastable and thus provides a reservoir of stored energy for selective and efficient excitation of the ν_3 level of CO_2. The lower laser level decays to the ground state by means of ν_2, and the rate of depopulation of this level can be the rate-limiting process in the laser. Since the ν_2 level lies close to the ground state, the gas temperature must be kept low to prevent this level from becoming thermally populated. The presence of helium in the gas mixture helps to cool the gas and, in addition, increases the relaxation rate of the lower laser level.

Two versions of this laser have recently been developed: the transversely excited atmospheric (TEA) CO_2 laser[17,18] and the waveguide CO_2 laser.[19] The output energy from a given laser volume depends on the gas pressure. The pulse duration is inversely proportional to the gas pressure. Thus, higher peak powers are obtainable from a smaller laser when the gas is at higher pressure. Because they operate at high pressures, TEA CO_2 lasers are capable of peak powers comparable to those of solid-state lasers. The waveguide laser is so-called because its discharge tube, whose inner diameter is only a few millimeters, not only confines the discharge but functions as a dielectric waveguide for the laser light as well. The resulting laser is small, inexpensive, sealed-off, and, thus, attractive for applications requiring continuous powers in the range from under 1 W to about 50 W.

The CO_2 laser is the most versatile industrial laser. The most common applications of CO_2 lasers are in material processing, cutting, welding, drilling, and heat-treating various metals.

The Organic Dye Laser

The most useful liquid lasers are the organic dye lasers invented by Sorokin and Lankard[20] in 1966. Tunable dye lasers now are available which cover the spectrum from the near ultraviolet to the near infrared. A second important feature of dye lasers is their broad emission bandwidth which permits the generation of ultrashort optical pulses.

An energy level diagram for a dye laser is shown in Figure 1–7. Each electronic level is a band composed of a continuum of vibrational and rotational levels. The

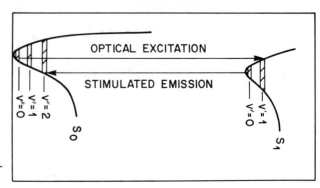

Figure 1–7. Energy level diagram for an organic dye laser.

upper laser levels are populated by optically pumping dye molecules from the singlet ground state, S_0, to the first excited singlet, S_1, with light from a flashlamp or with the output from another laser. Both the ground and excited states thermalize separately resulting in a Boltzmann distribution of occupied levels within each band. Because the Franck-Condon effect shifts the emission band to longer wavelengths, a population inversion between levels at the bottom of the excited singlet state (the upper laser level) and any of the continuum of unoccupied vibrational and rotational levels in the ground state (the lower laser level) can be established. After emission of a photon, rapid thermalization of the singlet ground state takes place, emptying the lower laser level.

A dye laser with a broadband optical resonator usually oscillates with a bandwidth of 50 to 100 angstroms (Å). Soffer and McFarland[21] discovered that with the insertion of a frequency selective element into the resonator, the broadband emission could be reduced to a small fraction of an angstrom without an appreciable loss in power and that a simple rotation of a grating (a plane diffraction grating functions as one resonator mirror) resulted in tuning of the dye laser.

The technique of generating ultrashort pulses with a laser is called "mode-locking."[22] In an ordinary laser, if no special precautions are taken, a number of longitudinal modes (see Optical Resonators in this chapter) will usually oscillate simultaneously. The process of mode-locking involves the establishment of a definite phase and amplitude relationship between these modes by active or passive means. Under the right conditions, constructive and destructive interference between these discrete frequencies can lead to a train of very narrow pulses. The uncertainty principle between frequency and time variables limits the width of such pulses to $\Delta t \sim 1/\Delta v$ where Δt is a pulse length and Δv is bandwidth. The broadband emission of a dye laser permits the locking of thousands of longitudinal modes, and the generation of pulses as short as 30 femtoseconds. Mode-locking also leads to an n-fold increase in the peak power of the pulses where n is the number of coupled modes.

Dye laser systems are available with a wide variety of optical pumping sources and resonator geometries. Pulse energies from a few millijoules for laser-pumped systems to many joules for flashlamp-pumped systems are readily available. Systems producing a high repetition rate train of picosecond pulses are also available commercially. Even though these systems are expensive, they have found extensive use in high resolution spectroscopy and in the study of ultrafast phenomena in biologic as well as other systems.

The Neodymium:YAG Laser

Though the first laser would operate only under high power pulsed excitation,[11] it was clear from the outset that a solid-state laser capable of CW operation should be possible. A number of different ion-host combinations were studied in detail and many have been found to operate in a CW mode, however, the only really satisfactory solid-state CW laser is the neodymium:YAG (Nd:YAG) laser developed by Geusic and his colleagues[23] in 1964. The active medium of this laser is the trivalent rare-earth ion Nd^{+3} in a host material of yttrium-aluminum-garnet (YAG). An energy level diagram for neodymium ions in a crystalline host is shown in Figure 1–8. Nd^{+3} ions are optically pumped using a broadband incoherent

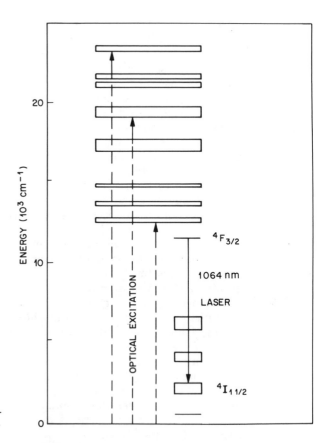

Figure 1-8. Energy level diagram for the Nd:YAG Laser.

source, such as a flashlamp or a tungsten lamp, from the $^4I_{9/2}$ ground level to high lying levels. These excited ions decay nonradiatively with nearly unity quantum efficiency into the $^4F_{3/2}$ level, which serves as the upper laser level for a 1.06 μm laser transition between the $^4F_{3/2}$ and the $^4I_{11/2}$ levels. Since the lower laser level, $^4I_{11/2}$, lies well above the ground level, its population is negligible. This leads to the creation of a population inversion with only modest pumping powers.

In addition to CW operation, where powers up to 250 W have been achieved, it is also possible to repetitively Q-switch these devices. In order to Q-switch a laser,[24] the resonator losses must initially be large enough to prevent the build-up of laser oscillation. Then, at some later time, the resonator losses are suddenly reduced (preferably to zero). Because the pumping process continues to create a large population inversion even when the cavity losses are high, the gain will greatly exceed the resonator losses (after they have been reduced) and all of the energy accumulated in the active medium will be discharged in one giant pulse. In a Nd:YAG laser this technique can lead to 10 to 100 nsec duration pulses containing a few hundred millijoules of energy at repetition rates from 10 to 100 p/s. In applications requiring higher powers, an oscillator-amplifier configuration may be used to increase the output above that available from the oscillator alone.

Nd:YAG lasers are used extensively in material processing applications and as pumping sources for dye lasers.

SELECTED MEDICAL APPLICATIONS OF LASERS

Lasers have been used in ophthalmology, gynecology, gastroenterology, dermatology, oncology, orthopedics, otolaryngology, burn therapy, plastic and reconstructive surgery, thoracic surgery, neurosurgery, and urology. A list of all reported circumstances in which lasers have been applied in medicine and surgery would require a bibliography the size of this book. Instead, this section briefly describes four specific medical applications of lasers chosen because they illustrate some of the characteristics of lasers that make them especially well suited for medical applications.

Retinal Photocoagulation

In the early 1950s, Meyer-Schwickerath[25] collaborated on the design of the first xenon arc photocoagulator and successfully used it in the treatment of retinal detachments. In the early 1960s, Koester[26] and others introduced the ruby laser photocoagulator, transforming this treatment from an operating room procedure to one that could be performed on an outpatient basis. In the late 1960s, L'Esperance[27] introduced the argon-ion laser photocoagulator which is now the instrument of choice for a number of ophthalmic procedures.

Cornea, aqueous humor, lens, and vitreous are all transparent to light in the visible spectrum, whereas the iris, the pigment epithelium of the retina and the choroid, all of which are pigmented, are not. Since light will be selectively absorbed in pigmented tissues, such tissues can be selectively heated and, thus, coagulated. This process can be used to form a scar, which can bridge, for example, the pigmented epithelium and the sensory epithelium of the retina, for the repair of a retinal detachment. This process can also be used to occlude retinal or choroidal vessels formed as a result of diabetic retinopathy. A curve showing the transmission of the transparent structures of the eye as a function of wavelength together with the absorption of a 100 μm thick film of oxygenated blood[28] is shown in Figure 1–9. As shown, light from the argon-ion laser, while not precisely in the most effective wavelength region, is nearly so.

Because light from a xenon arc is not absorbed well by hemoglobin or melanin pigment, more energy is required to produce a retinal lesion. This can lead to larger coagulation spot sizes and excessive heating of the vitreous. Because there is not sufficient time for heat to be conducted from the center of a lesion produced by a Q-switched ruby laser, these lesions have a higher incidence of hemorrhage than do lesions made by argon lasers or xenon arc photocoagulators. For these reasons, the argon-ion laser photocoagulator (even though it is more complex and costly than either xenon arc or ruby laser photocoagulators) is now used extensively for panretinal photocoagulation in the treatment of diabetic retinopathy[29] and for exposure around the trabecular meshwork for the treatment of glaucoma.[30]

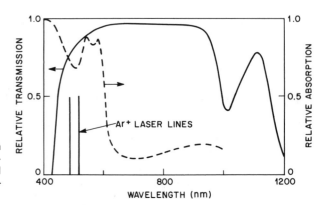

Figure 1-9.   Transmission spectra of the transparent structures of the eye and oxygenated blood. *(Adapted from Hochheimer BF.[28])*

Excision, Incision, and Vaporization of Tissue

Because of an ability to coagulate, ablate, or vaporize tissue, argon, CO_2, and Nd:YAG lasers have been applied extensively in surgery. Yahr and Strully[31] were apparently the first to use radiation from a CO_2 laser for this purpose.

Approximately 90 percent of the composition of all cells in the body is water. A measurement of the absorption coefficient α, of deionized water[32] in the wavelength region from 2.5 to 25 μm is shown in Figure 1-10. Here α is defined by the absorption law $I = I_0 \exp(-\alpha t)$ where I_0 is the incident light intensity, I is the transmitted intensity, and t is thickness. For reference, the normal operating wavelengths of the three most important infrared molecular lasers (CO_2, CO, and HF) are also shown in Figure 1-10. The absorption coefficient at the emission wavelength of a CO_2 laser is approximately 950 cm^{-1}. This means that the beam from a CO_2 laser will be intensely absorbed by water and it explains why the CO_2 laser is so effective at vaporizing and cutting tissue. In addition, it implies that, at lower power levels and short exposure times, a CO_2 laser could be used to remove

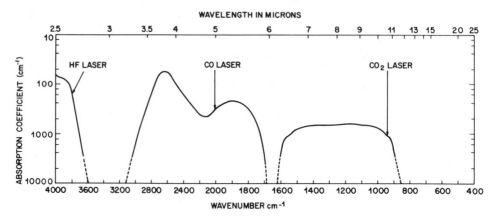

Figure 1-10. Absorption coefficient of deionized water in the infrared. *(From Karlin et al.[32])*

tissue to a depth of 25 to 50 μm with great precision. The small penetration depth also means that the application of CO_2 laser radiation should result in very little undesirable diffusion of light into surrounding tissue.

In practice it has been found that the CO_2 laser, used at or near focus, can incise all soft tissues at power densities of 2000 to 20,000 W/cm^2 (20 to 80 W at spot sizes from ⅛ to 2 mm).[33] The predictions of a theoretic model for CO_2 laser surgery,[34] shown in Figure 1–11, are in reasonable agreement with these experimental data and indicate that power densities in the range of 1000 to 10,000 W/cm^2 should be suitable for CO_2 laser surgery. Since the rate of energy input from the laser is high compared to the rate of heat conduction to adjacent areas, the temperature of the tissue in the focal region will rise rapidly, quickly leading to steam and vapor formation, which can then be sucked away. A simple calculation shows that the energy required to transform 1 mm^3 of water (initially at 37°C) into steam at 100°C is about 2.5 joules (J). This would require the application of at least 25 W for 0.1 seconds—a value in reasonable agreement with experiment.

The CO_2 laser is used extensively in gynecology (where the laser is usually coupled to a colposcope) to treat various premalignant and malignant conditions involving the cervix and vagina and in otorhinolaryngology (where the laser is coupled to an operating microscope) to treat stenosis and tumors of the trachea or vocal cords. The chief advantages attributed to the laser technique are an ease and precision of application, the absence of bleeding, and a considerably shorter period of convalescence and healing following treatment.[35]

Posterior Capsulotomy

The mode-locked or Q-switched output from a Nd:YAG laser is now being used to break up the opacified membrane that often forms in the eye after cataract surgery and intraocular lens implantation. This procedure, initially devleoped by

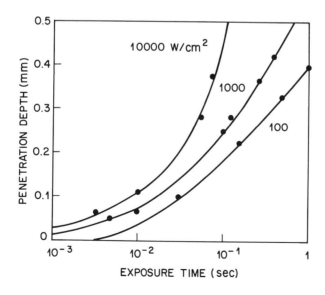

Figure 1–11. Depth of penetration of CO_2 laser radiation into tissue predicted by computer model.

Aron-Rosa[36] in 1980 and Fankhauser[37] in 1981, in most cases eliminates the need for reoperations, is noninvasive, eliminates the risk of intraocular lens dislocation, and in some cases allows cutting of other intraocular tissues (e.g., iris, trabecula, and vitreous strands) as well.

The implantation of an intraocular lens at the time of cataract surgery is an increasingly common procedure. Typically, a patient receives a two-loop iridocapsular or a four-loop iris clip lens (Binkhorst styles) immediately following extracapsular cataract extraction and a careful polishing of the posterior lens capsule,[37] a procedure that leaves the vitreous cavity undisturbed. In an uncomfortably high percentage of cases, however, a membrane begins to form on the posterior capsule very soon after the surgery.

Secondary opacification of the posterior capsule can be treated, without any anesthesia, by focusing the output from a mode-locked or Q-switched Nd:YAG laser through the intraocular lens to an approximately 50 μm diameter spot on the posterior capsule. Using an incident pulse energy at the surface of the cornea of 3 to 4.5 millijoules (mJ), a power density of approximately 10^{12} W/cm^2 can be produced at the beam waist. The plasma produced by this high power density serves two functions: (1) it blocks further energy transmission (a dense plasma can reflect as well as absorb laser light) and thus reduces the risk of injury to underlying tissue; (2) its rapid expansion results in the formation of a hydrodynamic shock wave in the focal region.[37] This shock wave, with shock front pressures of 10^7 mm Hg at a distance of 0.1 mm and 10 mm Hg at a distance of 10 mm, is used to rupture mechanically the opacified membrane and clear the visual axis. The use of a highly converging incident beam (20 degrees or more cone angle) reduces the risk of damage to the plastic implant or the cornea. Both the shielding effect of the plasma and the large cone angle beyond the focus reduce the risk of damage to the retina.

Initially there was some uncertainty as to whether a mode-locked pulse (30 psec) or a Q-switched pulse (10 nsec) was best suited for this procedure. It now appears that either can be used, and that the Q-switched laser with its high output energy capabilities can also be used to create holes in the iris for the treatment of open-angle glaucoma.

Photodynamic Therapy

The use of hematoporphyrin derivative (HpD) as both a diagnostic and a therapeutic tool in the treatment of cancer is being extensively investigated.[38] To date, more than 1500 patients, with cancer of the skin (primary and metastatic), lung, trachea, esophagus, bladder, brain, eye, and peritoneal cavity have been treated with an overall positive response in nearly 70 percent of the cases.

Endogenous porphyrins (constituents of hemoglobin) have long been suspected as being the cause of the red-orange fluorescence given off by some tumors when exposed to near ultraviolet light. This fact has recently been used for the early detection of lung cancer with laser fluorescence bronchoscopy.[39] Fluorescence excitation and emission spectra for HpD in human serum is shown in Figure 1–12. Excitation is provided by a CW krypton-ion laser operating at 406.7, 413.1 and 415.4 nm, well within the Soret absorption band of HpD. The excitation is delivered to the bronchial mucosa via a single 400 μm diameter core quartz fiber

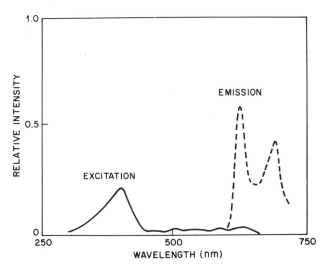

Figure 1–12. Excitation and emission spectra of hematopor-phyrin in human serum at 27°C.

inserted into the biopsy channel of a fiberbronchoscope. Under these conditions, emission from malignant tissue appears brighter than the surrounding tissue.

After injection, HpD disseminates throughout the body. HpD rapidly moves out of normal tissue, but remains longer in neoplasic tissue,[38] as shown in Figure 1–13. After 3 to 6 days, a peak differential exists between the concentrations of HpD in the tumor cells and the normal cells. When such a tumor is exposed to light, a photochemical reaction takes place that produces singlet oxygen affecting the cell membrane through a photooxidation process. Since there is less photosensitivity in normal tissue, a much less severe (or in some cases no) reaction occurs in this tissue, although following injection, patients must be kept out of sunlight (or any bright light) for approximately 30 days.

Dougherty and coworkers[40] have been successful in treating cancer patients with

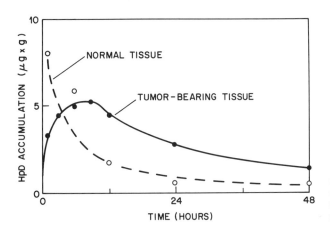

Figure 1–13. Time dependence of HpD accumulation in the liver of tumor and nontumor bearing rats. *(From Tomio L et al.[38])*

HpD and red light from an argon-ion laser-pumped Rhodamine-B dye laser tuned to 620 +/− 10 nm. The absorption spectrum for HpD (Fig. 1–12) is greater in the 405 nm range than at 631 nm, but red light penetrates tissue better than does blue-green light (the penetration depth at 631 nm is about 2 cm). The output of the dye laser is coupled to as many as four 400 μm diameter quartz fibers for simultaneous interstitial implantation. The power output from the dye laser is of the order of 3 W and the overall efficiency (dye laser output through the fiber compared to argon laser output) is approximately 10 percent. The delivery end of the fiber provides a beam with a divergence angle of approximately 20 degrees. Exposure times of tens of minutes are generally required for the procedure.

This new form of therapy has opened an entirely new field, but many questions remain. Why does HpD remain in the malignant tissue longer than in healthy tissue? Can the treatment procedure be quantified? Can it be made better? Clearly, there is much more work to be done.

FUTURE DIRECTION

It is now 25 years since the advent of the laser, yet laser technology continues to evolve rapidly. New developments are being made in at least two areas of relevance to medicine and surgery: (1) in the size, cost, and availability of lasers, and (2) in the performance of laser systems.

Lasers

With the possible exception of a large medical center, the size and cost of a new medical instrument are important considerations. The theater in which laser-surgical systems are applied is frequently cramped and crowded, with space at a premium. Consequently these systems must be portable and relatively indestructible. Systems currently on the market range in price from about $25,000 for small argon laser systems to more than $80,000 for large Nd:YAG laser systems. An important recent development in this area is the increasing availability of low cost waveguide CO_2 lasers (see The Carbon Dioxide Laser in this chapter). These devices are considerably smaller than the conventional CO_2 laser (providing a 10.6 μm power output of nearly 1 W/cm of length), can be supplied, sealed-off, and air-cooled, and are operated at low supply voltages. Because laser-surgical equipment based on waveguide CO_2 lasers is now (or shortly will be) offered by a number of different companies, these systems will become more competitively priced, more widely available, and could eventually find their way into the offices of individual doctors.

A second important advance in this area is the recent development of phase-locked gallium-aluminum-arsenide diode laser arrays producing CW output powers up to 2.6 W.[41] Because phase-locking can lead to a coherent combination of the power from a number of semiconductor lasers (i.e., a high output power device) and to a narrower far field pattern (i.e., a smaller beam waist), these very efficient laser devices may eventually replace much larger and more costly water-cooled krypton and argon-ion lasers in some medical applications.

A third important advance in this area is the recent development of more powerful, more reliable, and lower cost pumping sources for dye lasers. Given the greatly increased interest in the selective absorption of molecules (or tissues of the body) at different wavelengths, and in photochemical processes in general (see Photodynamic Therapy in this chapter), the wider availability of tunable dye lasers is expected to lead to a number of exciting new applications in medicine and surgery.

Delivery Systems

Delivery systems, the devices that bring light from the laser to the operating site, have tended (with a few notable exceptions) to be inconvenient, to say the least. The articulating arms currently used in the delivery systems of CO_2 lasers, are frequently so bulky and awkward that they prevent the surgeon from gaining a feel for the interaction between the instrument and tissue, something that is essential for delicate procedures. In addition, unless the input beam is launched precisely on axis and the mechanism of the arm is precisely correct, the output beam will wander in a complicated manner as the arm is manipulated. Two recent developments in delivery systems promise to alleviate these problems. First, several manufacturers of CO_2 medical lasers are (or will be shortly) offering miniature articulating arms containing hollow dielectric waveguides.[42] A photograph of a CO_2 laser delivery system incorporating such an arm[43] is shown in Figure 1–14. The 40 cm long arm (shown in Fig. 1–14) has a transmission of 80 percent and can access any point in an 80 cm diameter sphere. The 1.55 mm diameter output beam is substantially single mode and can be focused to a near diffraction limited spot. This arm has the advantages over previous articulating arms of compactness and superior pointing accuracy.

Another important advance, which is just now on the horizon, is the development of a flexible infrared transmitting waveguide that can be passed through endoscopes and, thus, utilized in the cavities of the body. For wavelengths longer than about 5 μm, there are, as yet, no entirely satisfactory waveguides. Flexible metal hollow waveguides,[44] polycrystalline and single crystalline fibers of the thallium,[45] and silver halides[46] have been extensively studied. A low transmission loss (0.4 dB/m) and a high power handling capability (100 W CW) has been achieved in extruded polycrystalline KRS-5 fibers,[47] however, fibers of this material are toxic, have a short shelf life and may be photosensitive. A difficulty with both metal waveguides and infrared fibers (in presently developed form) is the multimode nature of the guide. In such a guide, single mode radiation from a laser is rapidly degraded into a multiple mode pattern which changes in form as the guide is moved around. This degradation reduces considerably the maximum intensity that can be obtained at the output of the fiber.

There is a growing consensus that fluoride glasses[48] may be the most promising materials for infrared fibers,[49] although the exact glass composition for drawing a good fiber has yet to be determined. While these materials transmit well in the 2 to 7 μm wavelength region, it is now thought that their performance will probably be optimized at wavelengths between 3 and 4 μm. Laser radiation in this spectral region will be intensely absorbed by water (see Fig. 1–11) and, hence, should be just as effective as CO_2 laser radiation at vaporizing and cutting tissue. The development of a practical surgical system, however, will not only depend on the success to be achieved with fluoride fibers but also on the development of a suitable

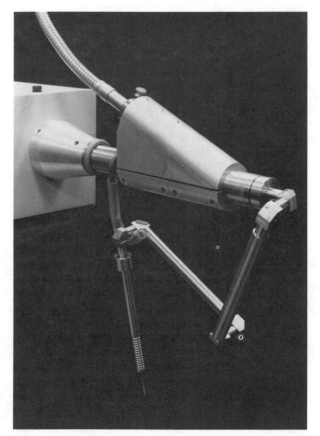

Figure 1–14. Photograph of waveguiding articulating arm for CO_2 laser radiation. *(From Bridges TJ, Strnad AR.[43])*

laser source. Possible laser sources in this spectral region include the HF laser at 2.8 μm, the DF laser at 3.8 μm, and optically-pumped color-center lasers (0.8 to 3.3 μm).[50]

REFERENCES

1. Planck M: Uber eine Verbesserung der Wien' schen Spektralgleichung. Ver Deutsch Phys Ges 2:202, 1900; Ann physik 4:553, 1901
2. Allen CW: Astrophysical Quantities. London, Athlone, 1973, p 13
3. Bohr N: On the constitution of atoms and molecules. Phil Mag 26:476, 1913
4. Einstein A: Zur Quanten Theorie der Strahlung. Phys Zeit 18:121, 1917
5. Gordon JP, Zeiger, HJ, Townes, CH: Phys Rev 99:1264, 1955
6. Schawlow AL, Townes CH: Infrared and optical masers. Phys Rev 112:1940, 1958
7. Fox AG, Li T: Proc Institute of Radio Engineers (Correspondence) 48:1904, 1960; Bell Sys Tech J 40:453, 1961
8. Boyd GD, Gordon JP: Bell Sys Tech J 40:489, 1961
9. Boyd GD, Kogelnik H: Bell Sys Tech J 41:1347, 1962

10. Kogelnik H: Bell Sys Tech J 40:455, 1965; Appl Opt 4:1562, 1965
11. Maiman TH: Stimulated optical radiation in ruby masers. Nature 187:493, 1960
12. Javan A, Bennett WB Jr, Herriott DR: Phys Rev Lett 6:106, 1961
13. White AD, Rigden JD: Proc Institute of Radio Engineers (Correspondence) 50:1967, 1962
14. Bridges WB: Appl Phys Lett 4:128, 1964
15. Bridges WB, Chester AN: Appl Opt 4:573, 1965
16. Patel CKN: Phys Rev 136:A1187, 1964; Appl Phys Lett 7:15, 1965
17. Dumanchin R, Rocca-Serra J: CR Acad Sci Paris 269:916, 1969
18. Beaulieu AJ: Appl Phys Lett 16:504, 1970
19. Bridges TJ, Burkhardt EG, Smith PW: Appl Phys Lett 20:403, 1972
20. Sorokin PP, Lankard JR: IBM J Res Dev 10:162, 1966; 11:148, 1967
21. Soffer BH, McFarland BB: Appl Phys Lett 10:266, 1967
22. Hargrove LE, Fork RL, Pollack MA: Appl Phys Lett 5:4, 1964
23. Geusic JE, Marcos HM, Van Uitert LG: Appl Phys Lett 4:182, 1964
24. Hellwarth RW: Advances in Quantum Electronics. New York, Columbia University Press, 1961
25. Meyer-Schwickerath G: Light Coagulation. St. Louis, CV Mosby, 1960
26. Koester CJ, Switzer E, Campbell CJ, Ritter MC: J Opt Soc Am 52:607, 1962
27. L'Esperance FA: Trans Am Ophthalmol Soc 66:827, 1968
28. Hochheimer BF: In Wolbarsht ML (ed): Laser Applications in Medicine and Biology, Vol. 2. New York, Plenum, 1974, p 70
29. Zweng HC, Little HL, Vassiliadis A: Argon Laser Photo Coagulation. St. Louis, CV Mosby, 1969, p 193
30. Podos SM, Kels BD, Moss A, Ritch R: Am J Ophthal 88:836, 1979
31. Yahr WZ, Strully KT: JJAAMI 1:1, 1966
32. Karlin DB, Patel CKN, Wood OR II, Llovera I: Ophthalmology 86:290, 1979
33. Stellar S, Polanyi TG, Bredemeier HC: In Wolbarsht ML (ed): Laser Applications in Medicine and Biology, Vol. 2. New York, Plenum, 1974, p 270
34. Webb R: Tech, Digest of First International Congress on Applications of Lasers and Electro-Optics, Boston, Mass. Sept. 20–23, 1982, p 6
35. Dixon JA: Proc of the Institute of Electrical and Electronics Engineers 70:579, 1982
36. Aron-Rosa D, Aron JJ, Griesemann M, Thyzel R: Am Intra-Ocular Implant Soc J 6:352, 1980
37. Van Der Zypen E, Fankhauser F, Bebie H, Marshall J: Adv Ophthalmol 39:59, 1979
38. Tomio L, Reddi E, Jori G, et al: In Pratesi R, Sacchi CA (eds): Lasers in Photomedicine and Photobiology. Berlin, Springer-Verlag, 1980, p 76
39. Dorion DR, Profio AE: In Pratesi R, Sacchi LA (eds): Lasers in Photomedicine and Photobiology. Berlin, Springer-Verlag, 1980, p 92
40. Dougherty TJ, Thoma RE, Boyle DG, Weishaupt KR: In Pratesi R, Sacchi CA (eds): Lasers in Photomedicine and Photobiology. Berlin, Springer-Verlag, 1980, p 67
41. Scifres DR, Lindstrom C, Burnham RD, et al: Electron Lett 19:169, 1983
42. Marcatili EAJ, Schmeltzer RA: Bell Sys Tech J 43:1783, 1964
43. Bridges TJ, Strnad AR: Tech Digest First International Congress on Applications of Lasers and Electro-Optics, Boston, Mass, Sept. 20–23, 1982, p 25; Lin C, Beni G, Hackwood S, Bridges TJ: Bell Sys Tech J 62:2479, 1983
44. Garmire E, McMahon T, Bass M: Appl Phys Lett 31:92, 1977
45. Pinnow DA, Gentile AL, Standlee AG, et al: Appl Phys Lett 33:28, 1978
46. Bridges TJ, Hasiak JS, Strnad AR: Opt Lett 5:85, 1980
47. Sakuragi S: Society of Photo-optical Instrumentation and Engineers 320:2, 1982
48. Poulain M, Chanthanasinh M, Lucas J: Mater Res Bull 12:151, 1977
49. Matachi S, Manabe T: Jap J Appl Phys 19L:313, 1980
50. Mollenauer LF: In Tang CL (ed): Quantum Electronics, Part B—Color Center Lasers. New York, Academic Press, 1979, Chapter 6

2

Laser Physics I

Fred M. Gardner

INTRODUCTION

Laser is an acronym for *l*ight *a*mplification by *s*timulated *e*mission of *r*adiation. A wide variety of lasers have been developed which have output wavelengths ranging from the ultraviolet to the infrared (Fig. 2–1, see Color Plate I*).[1]

Today, nearly 30 years after the development of the first stimulated emission device, the laser has many uses in basic science, engineering, and medicine. Twenty years of laser application to the field of medicine has led to ever increasing experimentation and use in gynecology, ophthalmology, dermatology, neurosurgery, and general surgery. The laser is becoming an important modality for medical treatment. Applications in the allied areas of photobiology and photochemistry will eventually expand the effect of the laser on the field of medicine.[2,3]

Of all the lasers that have been developed to date, the carbon dioxide (CO_2) laser with the 10.6 μm output, has been found to be the most useful in the practice of gynecology. Many features of the CO_2 laser, however, are common to all lasers and much of the qualitative material which follows pertains to lasers in general.

ELECTROMAGNETIC RADIATION

The output of any laser is an electromagnetic wave. These waves consist of time-varying electric and magnetic fields which travel at a characteristic velocity of 3 $\times$ 10^8 m/s in a vacuum. Figure 2–2 shows the orthogonal arrangement of the electric and magnetic fields for a plane-polarized wave. The waves are characterized by the frequency (f) of oscillation of the electric and magnetic fields and the wavelength (λ), the distance between successive peaks. The frequency and wavelength are related by the velocity equation $c = f\lambda$, where c is the velocity of electromagnetic waves in a vacuum.

In addition to its wave characteristics, an electromagnetic wave also has a particle-like nature. In some phenomena, radiation acts as if it consists of particle-like quanta of energy called *photons*.† Each photon possesses a discrete amount

---

*Color Plate I appears following p. 177.
†See the Glossary at the end of this volume for physics terminology.

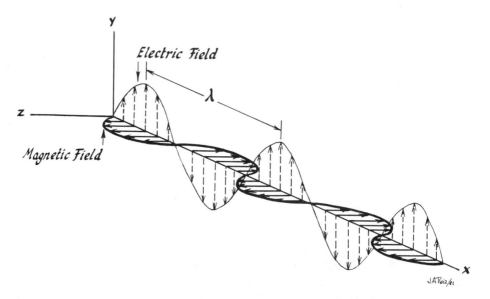

Figure 2–2. The schematic of a plane polarized electromagnetic wave traveling in the x direction, viewed at a particular time.

of energy given by $E = hf = hc/\lambda$, where E is the photon energy in joules and h is Planck's constant, 6.63×10^{-34} joule seconds.

Without examining all the complexities of the interaction of radiation with atomic and molecular systems, it is instructive to calculate some photon energies and compare these with typical energies found in molecular systems. The energy of an ultraviolet photon having $\lambda = 200$ nm is

$$E = \frac{hc}{\lambda} = \frac{(6.6 \times 10^{-34}\,\text{J}\cdot\text{S})(3.0 \times 10^8\,\text{m/s})}{200 \times 10^{-9}\,\text{m}}$$

$$E = 9.0 \times 10^{-20}\,\text{J} = 6.2 \text{ electron volts (eV)}.$$

(2–1)

This energy is clearly greater than many bond energies in organic molecules. For example, the C—C single bond has an energy of approximately 3.5 eV. On the other hand, a 10.6 μm photon has an energy of 0.12 eV. This energy is sufficient to excite rotational and vibrational energy levels in molecules, but is well below the value of primary bond energies and electronic energy levels.[4]

PROPERTIES OF LASER RADIATION

The usefulness of the laser in medicine is related to the properties of monochromaticity, directionality, brightness, and coherency possessed by the output radiation. The laser possesses these properties to a far greater degree than conventional sources of radiation.

The word *monochromatic* applied to electromagnetic radiation means single frequency or single wavelength. No radiation source, however, not even the laser, is absolutely monochromatic. There must always be some spread in frequency and a corresponding spread in wavelength. The most nearly monochromatic radiation is produced by a laser oscillating with a single longitudinal mode. Without elaborate measures, a laser can be brought to a frequency stability of about 1 part in 10^9.[4]

Another important characteristic of laser radiation is the highly directional or collimated nature of the beam. *Directionality* is a measure of the divergence of the beam and is expressed in terms of the angle in radians made by the outer edge of the beam, as shown in Figure 2–3. Typical full angle beam divergence for a laser is of the order of a few milliradians. The lower limit of beam divergence is set by a wave interference phenomenon called diffraction, and not by any engineering design feature. The diffraction in turn is related to the monochromaticity and to the beam coherence.

The *brightness* of a source of radiation is defined as the power emitted per unit area per unit solid angle. Lasers can emit high power in highly collimated beams and are the brightest sources of radiation known.

Coherence in a radiation source implies a fixed time relationship for amplitude and phase between any two points on the wave. Most sources of radiation, such as an incandescent bulb, emit radiation in a random and uncorrelated manner, and consequently the radiation is incoherent. Complete coherence is never attained, even in a laser, but one can define intervals of space and time over which the radiation is effectively coherent. Lasers typically have coherence times of milliseconds or longer, which implies coherence lengths of centimeters to hundreds of kilometers. For single transverse mode continuous wave (CW) lasers, the spatial coherence is nearly the width of the beam.[3]

EMISSION OF RADIATION FROM MOLECULAR SYSTEMS

The vibrational and rotational energy states in molecular systems such as CO_2 are quantized according to rules of quantum mechanics. The change of an energy state with the simultaneous absorption or emission of radiation is referred to as a *transition*. Transitions between energy states are described in terms of transition probabilities. Associated with any given pair of energy levels are three transition probabilities, the spontaneous emission probability (Fig. 2–4A), the absorption probability (Fig. 2–4B), and the stimulated emission probability. The latter is illustrated in Figure 2–4C, using the 001 and 100 vibrational energy levels for CO_2.

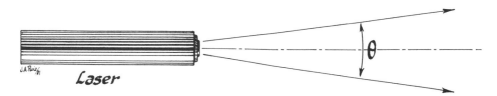

Figure 2–3. The beam divergence of a laser; θ (in radians), is twice the angle from the center to the outer edge of the beam.

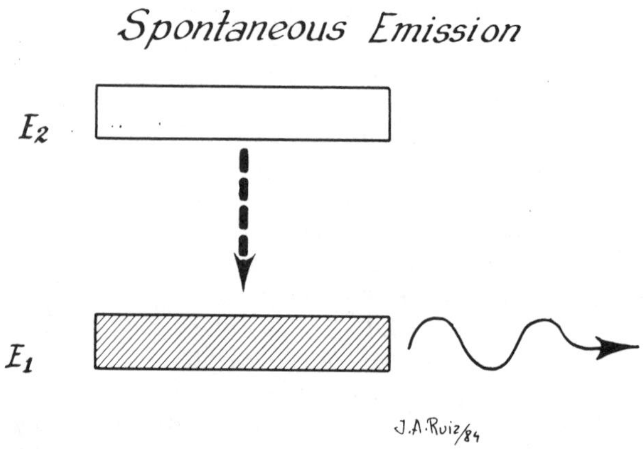

Spontaneous Emission

Figure 2–4A. An atomic or molecular system in an excited state, E_2, spontaneously reverts to a lower energy state, E_1, with the simultaneous emission of a photon.

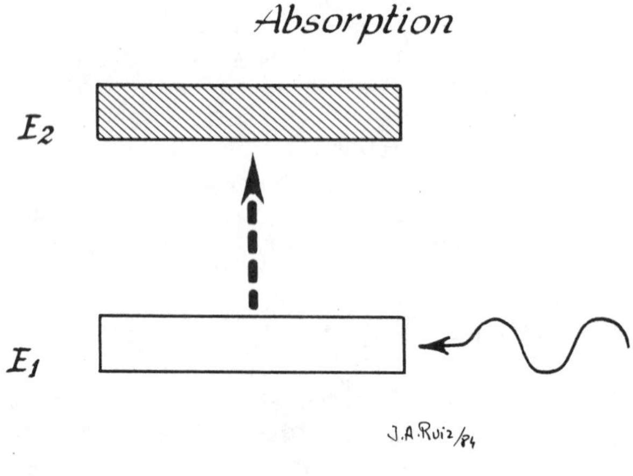

Absorption

Figure 2–4B. An atomic or molecular system making a transition from a lower energy state, E_1, to a higher energy state, E_2, by the absorption of a photon.

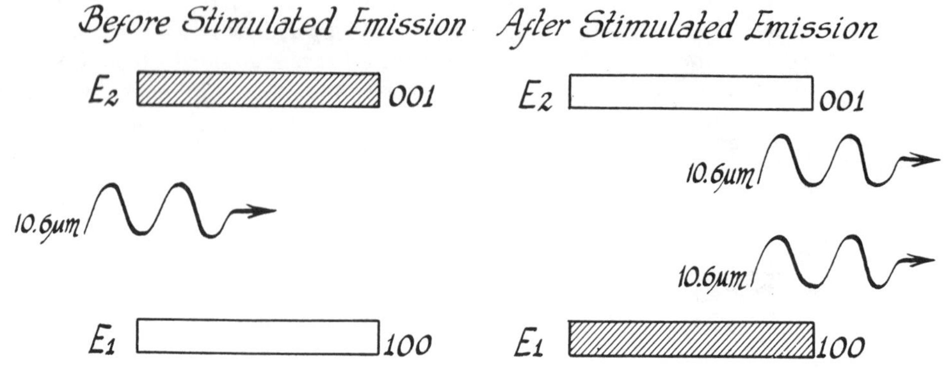

Before Stimulated Emission   After Stimulated Emission

Figure 2–4C. An illustration of a stimulated emission. The photon on the left stimulates a transition from energy state E_2 to E_1, producing a second photon identical to the stimulating photon.

Before stimulated emission, the CO_2 is in an excited vibrational state with energy E_2. The 10.6 μm incident photon has exactly the energy E_2-E_1 and stimulates the molecule to make a transition from E_2 to E_1 and to emit an identical photon. The stimulated and the stimulating photon are identical in all respects; they have the same energy, the same frequency, the same phase, the same direction of travel, and the same polarization. Consequently, the generations of photons produced by the first stimulting photon add constructively to produce an amplified wave.

The stimulated emission and absorption are competing processes. In order for the former to predominate over the latter process, there must be an inverted population between the two states, i.e., E_2 must have a higher population than E_1. The stimulated emission process is an essential part of every laser and serves as the origin for the third and fourth letters of the acronym laser.

THE DC EXCITED AXIAL FLOW CO_2 LASER

Numerous materials have been used to generate laser radiation but the basic requirements or conditions necessary to produce radiation are essentially the same for all lasers. These requirements are (1) an active medium which may be a collection of atoms, molecules, or ions in a solid, liquid, or gaseous form, (2) a population inversion in the allowed energy states of the active medium, and (3) an optical resonant cavity.

The active medium in the CO_2 laser is the CO_2 molecule. The laser, however, is normally operated by a continuous electric discharge through a mixture of CO_2, N_2, and He gas at pressures of about 10 to 50 torr. The relative concentrations of the three gases vary and are usually chosen to optimize the operation of a particular laser.

CO_2 is a triatomic linear molecule. The three atoms lie in a straight line with the smaller carbon atom in the middle. Three distinct modes of vibration are possible as shown on the energy level diagram in Figure 2–5: the symmetric stretching mode, the bending mode, and the antisymmetric stretching mode. The fundamental frequencies of these vibrational modes are ν_1, ν_2, and ν_3, respectively, (Fig. 2–5). These frequencies, and hence the energies, are quantized according to the rules of quantum theory. In addition, each vibrational level is split into sublevels of energy (not shown in Fig. 2–5) by the quantized rotational states associated with the rotation of the CO_2 molecule about its center of mass.

Pumping of the CO_2 molecule into the antisymmetric vibrational level (the population inversion) occurs directly by electron impact, by resonant energy transfer from vibrationally excited N_2, and other processes of excitation. The pumping of the antisymmetric vibrational level is very efficient and accounts for the high efficiency of the CO_2 laser.[5]

The amount of laser radiation amplification provided by the stimulated emission process in most active media is not sufficient to make a useful single pass device. More amplification is provided by the placement of mirrors at both ends of the cavity containing the active medium. If the mirrors are properly aligned, the radiation can pass back and forth many times through the active medium, effectively increasing the length of the laser. The multiple passes increase the amount of stimulated emission and the total amplification of the laser.

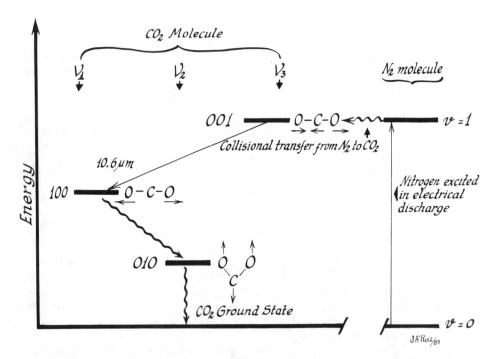

Figure 2–5. Schematic energy level diagram for the important vibrational energy levels in CO_2 and N_2 which are active in producing 10.6 μm radiation.

Some lasers take a relatively long time to build up a sufficient radiation field and can only be operated in a pulsed mode. Other lasers, however, such as the CO_2 laser, can be operated either in a pulsed or CW mode.

A schematic of a DC-excited axial-flow laser is shown in Figure 2–6. The gas mixture of CO_2, N_2, and He flows through the discharge tube and is continuously excited by the applied DC voltage. The discharge tube is terminated by two mirrors, one fully reflective and one partially reflective, which provide the optical feedback for the 10.6 μm radiation. The mirrors form an optical resonator in which the 10.6 μm radiation is amplified to an intense collimated beam, a fraction of which is coupled out of the laser through the partially reflective mirror.

Modern multi-purpose surgical CO_2 lasers are shown in Figures 2–7 and 2–8. Typically the instrument consists of a roll-away cabinet containing the gas supply and electrical instrumentation, the CO_2 laser tube, usually outside the cabinet, and a 10.6 m delivery system. Since there is no practical and approved fiber optics available for 10.6 μm radiation, the delivery system is a balanced mirror-type articulated arm which usually terminates in a hand piece (Fig. 2–8) containing the focusing lenses. The 10.6 μm radiation may also be delivered through the articulated arm to a micromanipulator coupled to an operating microscope (colposcope), as shown in Figure 2–7, or the articulated arm may be coupled to a laparoscope. The 10.6 μm radiation is invisible and requires an auxillary visible light source to

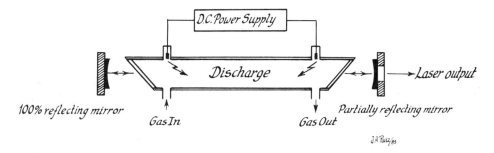

Figure 2–6. Schematic of a DC excited axial flow CO_2 laser.

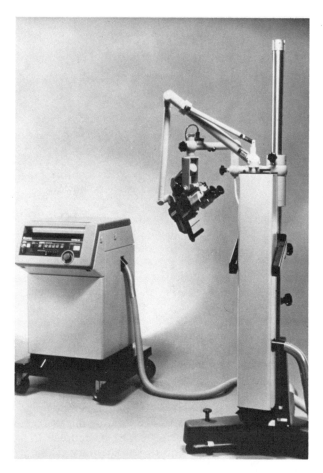

Figure 2–7. The coherent 451 laser system.

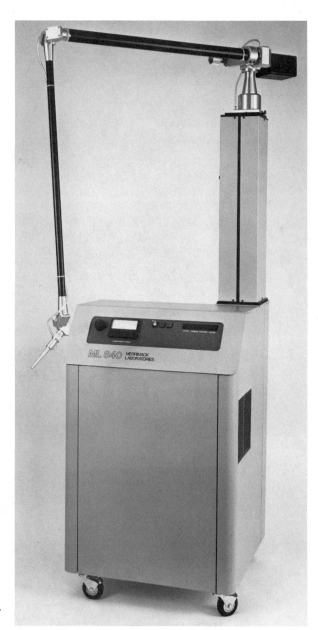

Figure 2–8. The Merrimack ML 840 CO_2 laser system.

provide an aiming spot at the work site. In most cases a He-Ne laser beam coincident with the 10.6 μm radiation is used as an aiming device.

Figure 2-9 shows a typical operating console on the cabinet of a laser system. The available control options vary with the manufacturer, but all units provide a read-out of the radiant flux in watts, controls for operating the laser in a pulsed or CW mode, and various safety switches, such as an emergency shut down.

THE CO_2 LASER OUTPUT

Longitudinal or Axial Resonant Modes

A number of possible mirror configurations can be used to successfully enclose the active medium in a resonant or optical cavity. The spheric mirrors used are at a separation that is many times the average wavelength of the radiation in the cavity. The resonant condition for such a cavity is that the separation between the mirrors must be equal to an integral number of half wavelengths of the radiation, i.e., $L = n \lambda/2$, where L is the distance between the mirrors and n is an integer. The laser transition is usually broad enough in frequency so that the radiation in the cavity will contain a number of wavelengths and hence, a number of frequencies which satisfy the above resonant condition. Thus, there can be many axial or

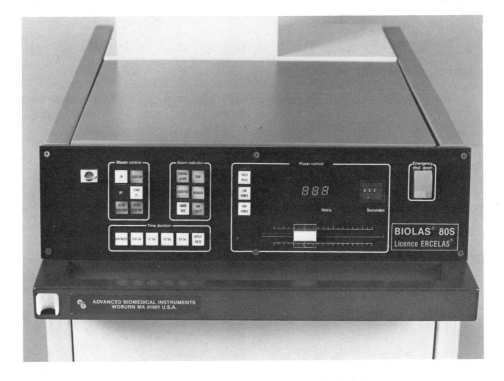

Figure 2-9. The operating console on the Biolas 80S CO_2 laser system.

longitudinal mode frequencies contained in the typical broadened stimulated emission line width. The frequency difference between the axial modes, however, is very small compared to the operating frequency of the laser, consequently, the output of the laser is still highly monochromatic. By constructing the laser so that only one frequency has low loss and high amplification in the resonant cavity, one frequency will predominate over the others which are suppressed. The laser will then operate in a single axial mode and is the closest approximation to a monochromatic source of radiation known.

Transverse Modes

The spatial patterns of the radiation perpendicular to the axis of the laser cavity are called the transverse modes. The resonant conditions which determine the spatial profiles are set by the geometry of the laser cavity. The transverse modes are characterized by two integers (m and n) which can be interpreted as the numbers of nulls in the radiation pattern in the two orthogonal directions transverse to the cavity axis. The TEM_{00} is the mode of highest symmetry for both cylindric and rectangular cavity geometries. The TEM_{00} and some higher order modes are shown in Figure 2–10. A laser may operate in a number of modes simultaneously. The TEM_{01*}, for example, sometimes called the donut mode, represents a superposition of the TEM_{01} and the TEM_{10}.[4]

The TEM_{00} Gaussian Mode

The TEM_{00} is frequently called the Gaussian mode because the spatial profile of the beam is approximately Gaussian or bell shaped, as shown in Figure 2–11. The

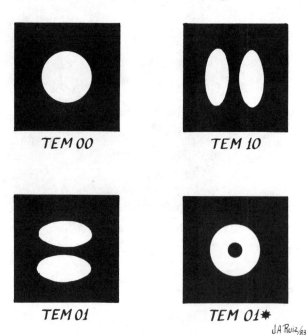

Figure 2–10. Some typical transverse mode patterns. The light regions represent areas of radiation, however, the distribution of radiation intensity is not uniform over these areas.

TEM 00

TEM 10

TEM 01

TEM 01✳

JA Ruiz/83

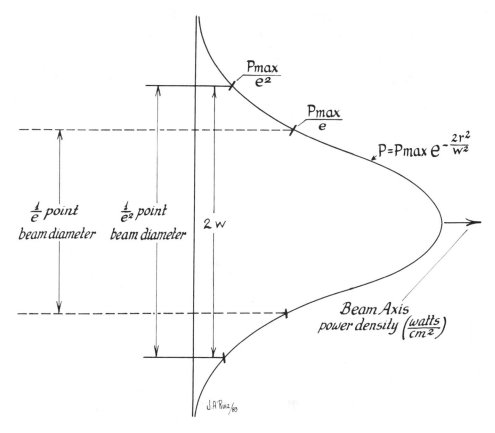

Figure 2–11. The Gaussian cross-section of a TEM$_{00}$ mode. The equation $p = p_{max}e^{-2(r/w)^2}$ gives the power density as a function of r, the radial distance from the beam axis.

Gaussian beam is usually preferred for medical purposes because of its symmetry and because the beam retains its spatial profile as it is transmitted through external optics. It should be noted that a higher order mode cannot be focused into a TEM$_{00}$. The mode structure is determined by complex boundary conditions within the laser cavity and not by external optics.

The Gaussian Beam Diameter

The distribution of the power density in an ideal Gaussian beam is given by

$$p = p_m e^{-2(r/w)^2}, \tag{2-2}$$

where p_m is the power density on the beam axis, r is the radial distance from the beam axis, and w is the radial distance from the beam axis at which the power density is p_m/e^2. The factor e is the base of the natural logarithm, 2.718. The ideal Gaussian beam profile is shown in Figure 2–11.

The Gaussian profile permits an infinite number of definitions of the beam diameter. The most commonly accepted diameter, however, is defined as 2w. It is obvious from examining Figure 2–11 that radiation falls outside the defined 2w diameter. In fact, 13.5 percent of the radiation falls outside the diameter 2w and 86.5 percent of the beam power passes through the defined diameter.[5] An important parameter to the surgeon is the average power density within the defined beam diameter. Since 86.5 percent of the total beam power, p_0, passes through the circle of diameter 2w, the average power density across the Gaussian beam is obtained by dividing $0.865\,p_0$ by the cross-sectional area, πw^2,

$$p_{av} = \frac{0.865 p_0}{\pi w^2} = \frac{0.275}{w^2}\, p_0 \text{ W/cm}^2. \qquad (2-3)$$

If the beam diameter is defined as the distance between the p_m/e points on the power density curve, the total beam power divided by the area of the beam defined gives an average beam power density equal to the peak power density of the beam, p_m. From the viewpoint of safety, the latter definition of beam diameter represents a more realistic estimate of the actual exposure.[3] The diameters defined at the p_m/e^2 and the p_m/e points on the Gaussian curve differ by a factor of 1.414.[6]

Delivery of the 10.6 μm Radiation

The laser beam is not ready for use as it emerges from the cavity. The beam must be focused by lenses to the appropriate spot size and must be delivered to the work site. To date there is no flexible fiberoptic on the market that will carry 10.6 μm radiation to a lasing site at sufficiently high power densities for general surgical use. Consequently, the laser beam is brought to the work site via an articulated arm (see Fig. 2–8) and handpiece. The handpieces are interchangeable and provide a choice of beam diameters and focal lengths. For microsurgery the handpiece is placed into an operating microscope. The laser beam is focused at the object plane of the microscope and can be moved continuously to various lasing sites by means of a mirror attached to a joystick control. The operator turns the laser beam on and off by means of a foot switch which activates a shutter system on the laser beam. If the laser runs continuously, the closed shutter reflects the radiation into a heat sink. The open shutter allows the beam to impinge on the work site. The beam may also be turned off and on by gating the electric energy to the active medium.[7]

SUMMARY

In a period of twenty years the CO_2 laser has developed into a well-understood and reliable instrument with many applications in industry and medicine. Within the field of gynecology it has become an important instrument for photovaporization and photocoagulation. Future developments of fiber-optic delivery systems, size reduction and total system control and flexibility will undoubtedly occur resulting in increased applications in medicine and surgery.

REFERENCES

1. Klauminzer GK: Twenty years of commercial lasers—A capsule history. Laser Focus 20 (12):54, 1984
2. Hillenkamp F, Pratesi R, Sacchi CA (eds): Lasers in Biology and Medicine. New York, Plenum, 1980
3. Pratesi R, Sacchi CA (eds): Lasers in Photomedicine and Photobiology. New York, Springer-Verlag, 1980
4. O'Shea DC, Callen WR, Rhodes WT: An Introduction to Lasers and Their Applications. Reading, Addison-Wesley, 1977
5. Duley WW: Laser Processing and Analysis of Materials. New York, Plenum, 1983
6. Mallow A, Chabot L: Laser Safety Handbook. New York, Van Nostrand, 1978
7. Fuller TA: The physics of surgical lasers. Lasers in Sur and Med 1, 5, 1980

3

Laser Physics II

Katherine Dexter Laakmann

Laser devices emit narrow, highly directional beams of monochromatic light. The highly directional nature of the laser beam allows it to be focused to very small spots and hence permits the achievement of intensities many orders of magnitude higher than that possible with conventional light sources. More generally, masers and lasers are devices that amplify or generate radiation by the stimulated emission process. The word "maser" originates from the acronym *m*icrowave *a*mplification by *s*timulated *e*mission of *r*adiation. The acronym *maser* was changed to *laser* as the technology shifted from microwaves to light.[1]

REVIEW OF THE PHYSICS OF LIGHT

X-rays, visible light, infrared light, and radio waves all belong to what is known as the electromagnetic spectrum. All electromagnetic waves are subject to the same laws of physics and travel at the speed of light. They sometimes exhibit particle-like behavior while on other occasions show wave-like (i.e., diffraction) activities. Generally, the electromagnetic spectrum is classified by wavelength, λ, although at times physicists may prefer frequency, denoted generally by ν. The wavelength and frequency are inversely proportional and are expressed by the formula

$$\lambda\nu = c, \qquad \text{(3–1)}$$

where c is the speed of light.[2]

The visible portion of the electromagnetic spectrum is very narrow, with the typical eye response ranging from about 0.4 μm in the violet to about 0.7 μm in the red. The peak eye response is in the blue-green ($\sim$.510 μm) range. Beyond the red lies the infrared portion of the spectrum, which extends from about 0.7 to 300 μm. Beyond the infrared are the millimeter wave region and the radio wave region ranging from about 10 mm and higher. On the other side of the visible is the ultraviolet, which has wavelengths from about 0.03 to about 0.4 μm. X-rays extend beyond the ultraviolet rays, but the shortest wavelengths lie in the gamma ray region, which typically includes wavelengths of 10^{-5} μm and less.

Conventional light sources tend to emit a broad spectrum of light, frequently spanning from the mid-infrared through the visible. White light, of course, is light which spans the entire visible spectrum. Lasers, on the other hand, tend to emit in a narrow spectrum and hence appear to have a very pure color. The property of high spectral purity is often referred to as *monochromaticity*. The spectral purity of lasers ranges from 10 nm on the high end to less than 10^{-4} nm on the low end. In medicine, high spectral purity is important because it allows for the possibility of specific damage (i.e., only certain tissues absorb the light and hence are heated).

In laser surgery, the primary focus centers on the infrared and visible portions of the electromagnetic spectrum. The units most commonly used for expressing wavelengths are angstroms, micrometers or microns, or nanometers. The conversion relationships are

$$1 \ \mu m = 10^{-6} \ m \ = 10^{-4} \ cm = 10^4 \ \text{Å} \quad = 10^3 \ nm,$$
$$1 \ \text{Å} = 10^{-8} \ cm = 10^{-10} \ m \ = 10^{-1} \ nm = 10^{-4} \ \mu m, \qquad \textbf{(3--2)}$$
$$1 \ nm = 10^{-3} \ \mu m = 10^{-9} \ m \ = 10^{-7} \ cm = 10 \ \text{Å}.$$

The most useful laser for gynecologic surgery is the carbon dioxide (CO_2) laser, which emits at 10.6 μm. The CO_2 laser has an extremely short penetration depth in water and hence in human tissue. For other specialties, sundry lasers are applied when tissue transparency, specific damage, or greater penetration depth by the laser beam is desired.

Nd:YAG (neodymium: YAG)	1.06 μm (near infrared)
Argon-ion	Blue-green
Dye	Visible
He-Ne	0.6328 μm (red)

All lasers used for medical purposes with the exception of the He-Ne laser produce tissue ablation or some other form of tissue modification. The He-Ne laser emission is very low in power and is used only as an aiming device.[3,4]

Laser Characterization

Besides wavelength, laser beams are most generally specified or described by such qualities as power, pulse energy, peak power, pulse repetition rate, divergence, and intensity. If the laser light remains on target quasi-continuously, we refer to that laser as being *continuous wave (CW)*. The CW laser may indeed be gated on and off by a mechanical shutter or electronically. On the other hand, if the laser is operated in a burst mode, the laser is referred to as a *pulsed laser*. Many CW lasers can be operated in a "super pulsed" mode, in which the peak power is greater than the CW power. Output power, peak or average, is generally measured in watts. Figure 3–1 shows the output power of a 20 W CW laser versus time, Trace a. Trace b shows the output power of the same laser but operated in *super pulsed* mode. Note that the peak power initially spikes to about 40 W but decays to about 20 W towards the end of the pulse. Trace c shows the average output power of the same super pulsed laser. Note that the average power is only 2 W.

Using the above example, it is useful to define several other quantities. The *pulse width*, T, refers to how wide the pulse is, and the period, T, refers to the

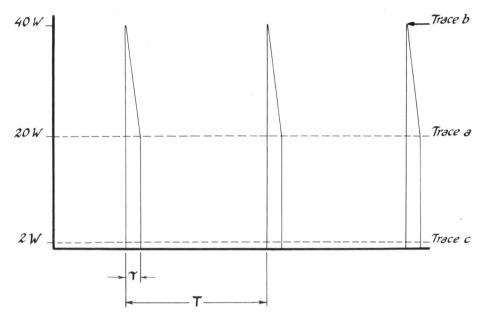

Figure 3–1. Output power trace of a 20 W CO_2 laser in CW mode and in super pulsed mode.

time duration between the start of one pulse and the next. The *pulse repetition rate* (PRR) is the reciprocal of the period *1/T*. The *pulse energy, E_p*, is, of course, the energy in a particular pulse. The product of (average) peak power and pulse width is the *energy per pulse*. In the example, the average peak power is 30 W, and hence the pulse energy E_p is

$$E_p = \overline{P_p} \cdot T = 30 \text{ T (W·sec).}$$ (3–3)

The energy unit most commonly used is the joule (J), which is equal to 1 watt· second. The average power in the pulse train is simply computed by multiplying the energy per pulse by the PRR, i.e.,

$$\overline{P} = E_p \cdot (PRR) = \frac{E_p}{T}.$$ (3–4)

PRINCIPLES OF LASER ACTION

Maser action is based on the quantum theory, which dictates that all atoms (molecules or ions) exhibit discrete modes of excitation. The interaction of light with matter depends upon the type of matter, the wavelength of the light, and the intensity of the light. Three basic processes are to be considered: (1) absorption, (2) stimulated emission, and (3) spontaneous emission. All three processes play a role in laser surgery, with the laser, of course, based on stimulated emission.

Absorption is the process by which light is absorbed by matter. Typically, matter releases this energy in the form of heat, causing such matter to rise in temperature. Without absorption there would be no laser surgery. Spontaneous emission is the process on which all conventional light sources are based.

Absorption

Consider an atom with two levels. Let E_1 be the energy of the lower level and E_2 the energy of the upper level. When the atom is sitting in the rest state E_1 and irradiated by a beam of light of frequency ν, the probability per unit time that the atom will be excited from Level 1 to Level 2 is given by

$$P = \begin{cases} W_{1,2} \text{ when } \nu = \dfrac{E_2 - E_1}{h} \\[2ex] 0 \text{ when } \nu \neq \dfrac{E_2 - E_1}{h}, \end{cases} \tag{3-5}$$

where $W_{1,2}$ is called the absorption transition probability and h is Planck's constant. Note that the probabiliity of the absorptive transition is zero when the energy of the photon $h\nu$ is not equal to the energy difference between the two atomic levels. This is, of course, just a statement of conservation of energy. It should also be pointed out that the atom can be excited in a nonradiative way. The absorptive transition probability is proportional to the photon flux of the incident wave, with the proportionality constant having the dimensions of area. Algebraically, this can be expressed as

$$W_{1,2} = \sigma_{1,2}(I/h\nu), \tag{3-6}$$

where $\sigma_{1,2}$ is the cross-section, I is the intensity of the wave in W/cm^2, and $I/h\nu$ is therefore the photon flux.

Now, the rate of excitation of these atoms to the upper Level 2 will obviously be proportional to the number of atoms in the lower level. That is, if there are N_1 atoms per unit volume in the lower level and N_2 atoms per unit volume in the upper level, the excitation rate due to this process (in units of atoms per unit volume per unit time) is given by

$$\left(\frac{dN_1}{dt}\right)_{a,b} = -\sigma_{1,2}(I/h\nu)N_1,$$
$$\left(\frac{dN_2}{dt}\right)_{a,b} = -\left(\frac{dN_1}{dt}\right)_{a,b}. \tag{3-7}$$

In the model just presented, the reader may infer that matter is translucent at most all wavelengths, except for certain discrete wavelengths. In the real world, however, matter rarely behaves as a two-level system. To further complicate the picture, real matter is made up of a variety of molecules and atoms, each with different energy levels. Because of the sheer number of possible absorptive transitions, human tissues tend to be at least partially opaque throughout the visible and infrared portions of the spectrum.

Stimulated Emission

Stimulated emission (see Fig. 2–4A) is just the reverse process of absorption; however, instead of the atom lying in the ground State E_1, it is found in the upper Level E_2. When an atom lying in Level E_2 is irradiated with light of frequency ν, there is a finite probability the atom will emit another photon of frequency ν and will simultaneously relax from the upper state to the lower state. Just as in the absorption case, however, the incident radiation must be in resonance with the energy difference between the upper and lower states such that

$$h\nu = E_2 - E_1. \tag{3–8}$$

The stimulated transition probability $W_{2,1}$ is also proportional to the photon flux and is expressed by the formula

$$W_{2,1} = \sigma_{2,1}(I/h\nu), \tag{3–9}$$

where $\sigma_{2,1}$ is the stimulated emission cross-section. Einstein showed that the stimulated emission cross-section is equal to the absorptive cross-section; hence, $\sigma_{1,2}$ equals $\sigma_{2,1}$. For convenience, we will drop the subscripts and denote the cross-section as simply σ.

Following along the same lines as we did in the absorptive case, the relaxation rate, $(dN_2/dt)_{st}$ (in units of number of atoms per unit time per unit volume) due to this process is given by

$$\left(\frac{dN_2}{dt}\right)_{st} = -\left(\frac{dN_1}{dt}\right)_{st} = -\sigma(I/h\nu)N_2. \tag{3–10}$$

Perhaps the most important feature of stimulated emission has yet to be discussed. In stimulated emission, the atom emits a wave which has a definite phase relationship to that of the incident wave. Since the emitted wave is of the same frequency, phase, direction, and polarization as the incident wave, it is possible to develop a highly intense unidirectional beam. This property is known as *coherence,* and it is precisely this property which makes the laser such a useful instrument in medicine as well as in a number of other fields.

Spontaneous Emission

Just as in the stimulated emission case, let us again consider an atom which is lying in the excited state Level 2. There is a finite probability that the atom will spontaneously relax from Level 2 to Level 1 and in the process give off a photon of energy equal to the difference in energy between the upper and lower levels, i.e.,

$$h\nu = E_2 - E_1. \tag{3–11}$$

The probability per unit time for an atom in Level 2 to relax spontaneously to Level 1 is given by the coefficient A, known as the *Einstein A coefficient*. The rate of decay of atoms due to spontaneous emission is again proportional to the number of atoms in the upper level and is therefore given by

$$\left(\frac{dN_2}{dt}\right)_{sp} = -\left(\frac{dN_1}{dt}\right)_{sp} = -AN_2. \tag{3-12}$$

The reciprocal of the Einstein A coefficient is known as the *spontaneous lifetime*.

THE LASER AMPLIFIER AND OSCILLATOR

In the previous section it was shown that photon emission (stimulated emission) can occur when an atom is lying in the upper state, and photon absorption can occur when the atom is lying in the lower state. Whether there is net amplification or net attenuation depends upon whether there are more atoms lying in the upper state than in the lower state. Consider now a medium made up of our two-level atom and of width dz. If we irradiate that medium with light of frequency $h\nu$ and intensity I, the change in intensity dI is given by

$$dI = -h\nu \left(\frac{dN_1}{dt}\right)_{a,b} \cdot dz + h\nu \left(\frac{dN_2}{dt}\right)_{st} dz. \tag{3-13}$$

This equation follows since with each absorptive or emissive transition there is either absorption or emission of a photon. Substitution of Equations 3.7 and 3.10 in Equation 3.13 yields the following equation for the change in intensity per unit length

$$dI/I = -\sigma(N_1 - N_2)dz. \tag{3-14}$$

Hence, under normal thermoequilibrium conditions, since there are more atoms in the lower state than in the upper state, the net response will always be absorptive. If, however, the population difference can be inverted so that there are more atoms in the upper state than the lower state, then the net response will be emissive, i.e., the medium will give net energy to the optical signal and amplify it. The challenge researchers faced in trying to make a laser (and indeed still face with many laser media) is in achieving a *population inversion*.

All lasers, independent of the type, behave in essence much the same as just described. Atomic lasers, or ion lasers, rely on transitions between the electronic levels. Typically, these lasers emit in the visible, and are exemplified by the helium-neon (He-Ne) and the argon-ion lasers.

The means of attaining a population inversion is frequently referred to as "pumping." Lasers may be optically pumped, chemically pumped, or electrically discharge pumped, with the exact method depending upon the type of laser. Carbon dioxide lasers and argon-ion lasers are electrically discharge pumped, where electrons or ions in the gaseous discharge transfer their kinetic energy, either directly or indirectly, to the lasing species. A YAG laser, on the other hand, is an example of an optically pumped laser where photons from a flashlamp excite higher energy levels within a crystal.

The Laser Oscillator

To make a laser amplifier into a laser oscillator, one needs to add some form of positive feedback. Typically, this feedback consists of two highly reflective mirrors. Consider a wave packet of intensity I_0 starting out at mirror 1 as shown in Figure 3–2. As it transverses through the active medium, it will be amplified by the active medium by a factor G, with a resultant intensity I' given by

$$I'/I_0 = e^{g\ell} = G, \tag{3-15}$$

where $g = \sigma(N_1 - N_2)$ for our two-level system. After striking mirror 2 with reflectivity R_2, the resultant flux is $R_2 I'$. This wave packet is in turn amplified again by the active medium on the return trip. The intensity at this point is given by

$$I'' = R_2 I_0 e^{2g\ell}, \tag{3-16}$$

where R_2 is the reflectivity of mirror 2. Finally, this wave packet is reflected by mirror 1, and the intensity after this is expressed by the formula

$$I''' = R_1 I'' = R_1 R_2 I_0 e^{2g\ell}. \tag{3-17}$$

Oscillation now will occur only if the gain is equal to or greater than the losses. From Equation 3–17, oscillation implies that $I''' \geq I_0$ or $R_1 R_2 e^{2g\ell} \geq 1$. Defining

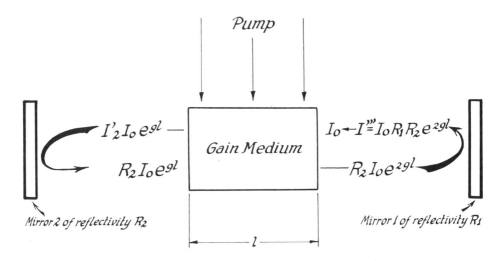

Figure 3–2. The intensity of a laser beam inside a resonator.

the threshold condition as when the inequality becomes an equality, the threshold gain is given by

$$g_{th} = \frac{\ln(R_1 R_2)}{2\ell}.$$

(3–18)

The gain must be equal to or exceed this quantity for oscillation to take place.

In most lasers, the original photon flux, which is eventually amplified, are photons spontaneously emitted in some narrow acceptance angle along the cavity axis. If the gain of the laser now exceeds the threshold gain, then there will be net amplification of this noise as it makes a round trip pass through the cavity. On each successive round trip, this amplified noise grows in intensity. This amplification process, however, is eventually quenched as the power in the optical beam becomes of the order of the stored optical power. This process is known as saturation. In a steady-state situation, the saturated gain is clamped to the threshold gain such that there is no net round trip cavity gain.

So far in our treatment of a laser resonator, we have only considered the photon nature of light and not the wave nature of the light. In the steady-state condition, the optical beam, phase, and amplitude must be invariant after a round trip pass through the laser resonator. Let us now consider the implications of the optical phase invariancy. The phase shift an optical beam makes after transversing a round trip through the cavity of length L is given by

$$\Delta\phi = 2\pi/\lambda \cdot (2L),$$

(3–19)

where λ is the wavelength. Optical phase invariancy implies that the phase shift must be some integral multiple of 2π. Since $\Delta\phi$ must be equal to $M2\pi$ where M is integer, the wavelength of any resonating mode must therefore have an integral

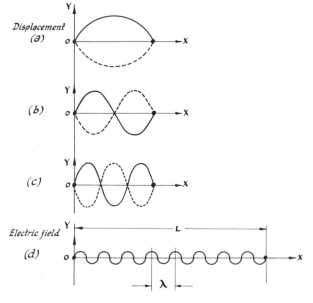

Figure 3–3. Illustrations of the resonant mode condition of a vibrating guitar string and a laser. Parts a, b, and c show displacement of the guitar string's first three modes. Part d shows the electrical field amplitude in a resonant laser cavity. Note that in all cases nodes occur at the ends.

number of wavelengths in twice the cavity length. Alternately $M\lambda = 2L$. Hence, the resonator itself only supports certain discrete wavelengths where the wavelengths are, of course, given by the above equation.

The resonant condition of allowing only an integral number of wavelengths is a phenomenon found much throughout nature. A vibrating guitar string, for example, will only resonate at frequencies such that there are nodes in the standing wave pattern at the end of the string. Figure 3–3 shows a comparative sketch of the standing wave pattern on a string versus that in a laser resonator.

COMPARISON OF LASER LIGHT TO THERMAL LIGHT

As stated earlier in these discussions, laser light compared to light emitted by other sources tends to have a far greater degree of directionality, monochromaticity, coherence, and brightness. Some of these characteristics are, of course, interrelated or highly dependent on one another.

Any material (solid, liquid, or gas) of finite temperature will radiate light over a spectrally broadband range and in all directions. This tendency to radiate is known as blackbody radiation and is a consequence of spontaneous emission. For an ideal blackbody, the spectral energy density (i.e., the amount of light per unit area of radiator per unit spectral width) is given by Planck's law[5] and is shown in Figure 3–4. As can be seen from these curves, the emissive properties of an ideal

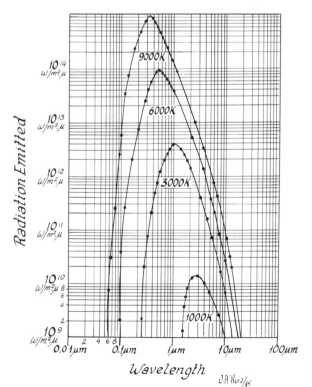

Figure 3–4. Planck's spectral emittance curves of a blackbody.

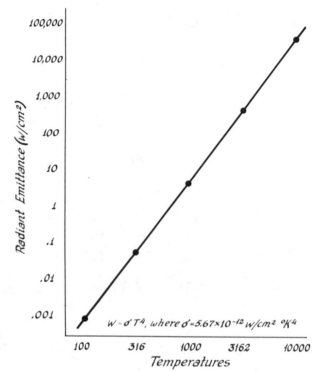

Figure 3–5. Radiant emittance according to the Stefan-Boltzmann law.

blackbody is a function of temperature only. The total amount of radiation over all wavelengths is given by the Stefan-Boltzmann equation and is shown in Figure 3–5. No real material looks like a perfect blackbody but radiates somewhat less by a factor ε than that predicted by the Planck curves. The factor ε is known as the emissivity and is usually a function of wavelength. For a perfect blackbody, ε is unity.

Any incoherent or conventional (i.e., nonlaser) light source shows much the same behavior. For most gases, however, the gas is essentially transparent (i.e., ε → 0), except for discrete wavelengths in which the gas is almost opaque (ε → 1). The light from these sources is, of course, emitted in all directions.

Brightness

Although an incoherent light source can emit at least as much power as a laser and with greater efficiency, this power is generally quite broadband spectrally and, in addition, is omnidirectional. Some xenon arc lamps, for example, can deliver over 100 W; however, their brightness (defined as power per unit area of radiation emitted per unit solid angle) is actually much less than that of even a low power laser. The brightness of a 100 W xenon lamp with an effective area of 2 mm² is

$$\frac{1}{2\pi \text{ster}} \frac{10^2 \text{ W}}{\pi/4(0.2 \text{ cm})^2} \approx 500 \text{ W/cm}^2/\text{steradian}. \qquad \textbf{(3–20)}$$

A 1 W diffraction limited CO_2 laser with a radius W_ω, on the other hand, has a brightness of

$$\frac{1 \text{ W}}{\pi/4 \cdot \left(\frac{\lambda}{\pi \text{ W}_\omega}\right)^2 \cdot \pi \text{ W}_\omega^2}. \tag{3-21}$$

Hence, a 1 W CO_2 laser has brightness of over 1000 times a 100 W xenon lamp!

Directionality

Because only discrete transverse modes are allowed to oscillate in a laser resonator, any laser will have a high degree of spatial coherence. "Spatial coherence" means that at any given time there is a definite phase relationship between the wave at any two points over which the wave is coherent. Figure 3–6 shows a wave with coherence length ℓ_c. An incoherent (i.e., conventional) light source will typically have a coherence length of several λ, whereas a laser will have a coherence length generally of the order of its aperture diameter. The angular spread of a beam is given by

$$\theta = \alpha \frac{\lambda}{\ell_c}, \tag{3-22}$$

where α is a proportionality constant of the order of unity and depends upon the exact amplitude distribution of the wave. Since the coherence length of a laser is much larger than that of incoherent light, the angular spread or divergence is much less. Figure 3–7 gives a comparative sketch of the constant spread of a laser versus thermal source. A CO_2 laser with a 1 mm TEM$_{00}$ beam has an angular spread of roughly 1/300 of that of an incoherent source.

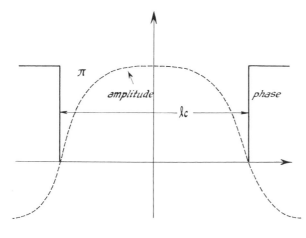

Figure 3–6. The amplitude and phase profile of electric field of coherence length "ℓc".

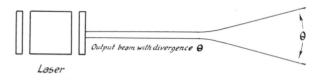

Laser

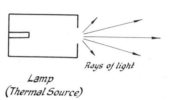

Figure 3-7. A comparative sketch of the behavior of light output from a thermal source versus a laser source.

Lamp
(Thermal Source)

Behavior of Laser Beams in Optical Systems

A laser beam can be focused with a lens to a very small spot, as shown in Figure 3–8A. Since the laser is so directional, it can collect virtually 100 percent of the laser energy. By contrast, it is not possible to efficiently focus incoherent light down to a small point. The best that can be done is to image and demagnify the source. As one moves the source further and further away from the lens, the spot size can be made smaller, but only at the expense of having the lenses collect less and less of the thermal source. Figure 3–8B shows this schematically.

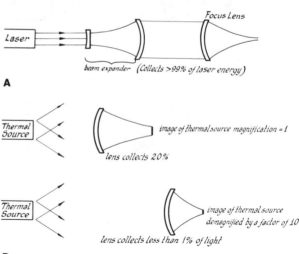

Figure 3-8. A laser beam focussed to a small spot **(A)**, and a thermal source focused **(B)**.

THE CO₂ LASER

A conventional CO_2 laser is basically quite simple, consisting of a glass tube, typically with an inner diameter of about 7 mm. A high voltage applied to each end of the tube ignites and sustains a gas discharge. The laser gas is a mixture of helium to aid thermal conductivity, nitrogen to enhance the "pumping efficiency," and CO_2 to serve as the lasing medium. Because of the dissociation of the CO_2 molecule in the discharge as well as impurities released by the glass tube, the gas is flowed through the tube. Flowing the gas requires a high-pressure gas tank on one end to serve as a source and a vacuum pump on the other end to suck the gas out. The laser mirrors are typically attached to an optical rail which is also shared by the laser tube. Cooling of the laser is accomplished by flowing water through a glass jacket which surrounds the tube.

A newer technology in CO_2 is the radio frequency (RF) sealed-off waveguide technology (Fig. 3–9). Sealed-off means that the gas fill is static and quasi-permanent. Here, the tube walls are a metal/ceramic composite instead of glass, and the bore cross-section is much smaller. The smaller bore permits a more stable optical alignment. An RF voltage applied to the electrodes creates a gas discharge, just as in the conventional CO_2 laser case. However, since the discharge runs transversely to the laser walls rather than longitudinally, the voltage is much lower (i.e., 300 V with RF versus 15,000 V with DC). The power supplies are therefore substantially smaller and safer. The RF laser has a somewhat cooler discharge, thereby permitting long tube lifetimes (greater than 1 year on a single fill) in a

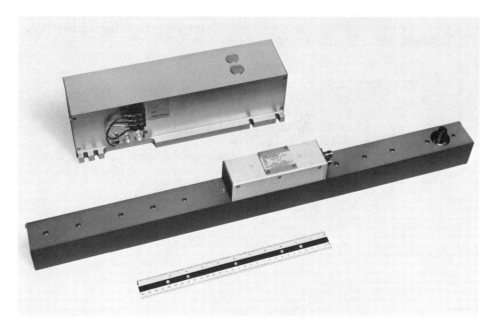

Figure 3–9. Xanar waveguide laser.

sealed-off configuration. The sealed-off nature of the tube is advantageous to the user because it not only allows the reduction in system bulk but is also more convenient and less prone to trouble because of the elimination of the gas supply and concomitant difficulties. Finally, these lasers are typically air-cooled, permitting even greater flexibility and portability.

A highly transmissive fiber for CO_2 wavelength does not exist as yet, although many researchers are making substantial attempts to this end. Hence, the beam is more generally directed by a series of mirrors, sometimes attached to an articulating arm and/or sometimes with lenses interspersed. A microscope or colinear He-Ne beam is used for viewing. Because focused CO_2 laser beams diffract so rapidly, generally the beam is manipulated only when it is large ($\sim$1 cm) and then focused just prior to the target.

The lenses used with CO_2 lasers are of different materials from what one is accustomed to in the visible. Glass is opaque in the infrared, while ZnSe and Ge are highly transmissive in the infrared and most often used for lens material. ZnSe has a yellowish hue, while Ge looks gray-black and is opaque in the visible. Because of the high refractive index of these materials, left untreated they are highly reflective and hence can cause substantial power loss (34 percent with ZnSe and 65 percent with Ge). Generally, these materials are coated with what is known as an antireflective coating. These coatings allow optical transmission to exceed 98 percent. The drawbacks to these coatings are cost and subjectivity to coating damage. Coating damage can occur very easily, as any sort of debris landing on the optics will be burned off, causing the coating to be burned simultaneously. In spite of such drawbacks, antireflective coatings are used routinely. Mirrors in the infrared are almost always front-surface mirrors, coated with silver and most generally a protective layer. Just as with the antireflective coatings, these mirrors are subject to damage by debris burns.

REFERENCES

1. Svelto O: Principles of Lasers. New York, Plenum Press, 1982
2. Bennett Jr WR: The Physics of Gas Lasers. New York, Gordon & Breach, 1977
3. Lengyel BA: Lasers, 2nd ed. New York, Wiley, 1971
4. Siegman AE: An Introduction to Lasers and Masers. New York, McGraw-Hill, 1971
5. Wolfe WL (ed): Handbook of Military Infrared Technology, Office of Naval Research, Department of the Navy, Washington DC, 1965
6. Laakmann KD: US patent No. 4,169,251, September 25, 1979
7. Laakmann KD: Transverse RF Excited Waveguide Lasers. Lasers '79, December 1979, Orlando, Fla.

4

Laser Tissue Interaction: The Influence of Power Density

Terry A. Fuller

INTRODUCTION

The use of the surgical laser has been complicated by the confusing and often conflicting use of terms and definitions. The ability to duplicate the works of others has been hampered by this confusion. In this chapter we shall investigate the variables that influence the effect of the interaction of laser light and tissue and define the terms needed for communication of these results. The physical parameters of power, power density, wavelength, and duration will be explored. Emphasis will be placed on the definition and utilization of the concept of *power density*.

Lasers are sources of radiant energy which, like conventional light sources, can interact with tissue to cause biologic, photochemical, or thermal reactions.[1] A narrow band of radiant energy from the electromagnetic spectrum is capable of stimulating the retina and thus inducing the response of vision, yet this same radiant energy is unobservable as an independent entity. To help visualize the characteristics of this and other sources of optical radiation we can consider the *photon*. A photon is a quantum or packet of light energy of a particular frequency or wavelength. Laser surgery is performed by utilizing large populations of photons that interact with tissue to cut, vaporize, coagulate, or stimulate individual or groups of cells. The energy of the photon is directly proportional to its frequency.

What separates laser sources from other conventional sources of energy are principally three characteristics: (1) monochromaticity, (2) coherence, and (3) intensity, which have been described in Chapters 1, 2, and 3. Perhaps the most important characteristic of the radiant energy emitted from a laser for surgery is its monochromaticity or color purity. The importance of a highly monochromatic beam of light in surgery is exemplified by its selective absorption by chromagens or pigments in tissue as well as other absorbing substances. This selective absorption of tissue by various wavelengths is one of the most unique characteristics of surgery with a laser. The carbon dioxide (CO_2) laser's emission at 10.6 μ is heavily absorbed by water. The absorption is so great that radiant energy is instantaneously converted to heat resulting in vaporization of the fluid and solid cellular components. The net result is surgical ablation.

As a result of coherence, radiant energy can be effectively captured and focused to an extremely small spot. This concentration of power increases the effectiveness of the laser beam as a cutting tool. The intensity of the laser beam, measured in watts, is one of two primary variables controlled by the surgeon to alter the effect of the laser on tissue. Movement of this beam over tissue results in a surgical incision.

The diameter of the beam emitted from a laser oscillator is typically too large for most surgical applications. In addition the power contained in a large beam is usually not of sufficient intensity to vaporize or even coagulate tissue. Thus a lens must be introduced to focus the laser beam to an appropriate spot size. This will not only provide a beam small enough to limit the size of the surgical incision (zone of vaporization) but will also increase the effective use of the power of the laser. It is this concentration of power or the power density that is of principal

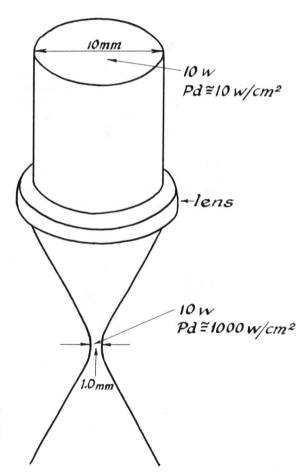

Figure 4–1. Changes in power density as a result of focusing a 10 W laser beam from 10 mm diameter (PD = 10 W/cm²) to 1 mm (PD = 1000 W/cm²).

importance to the surgeon desiring to predict and control the effectiveness of the laser beam. The power density is a measure of the power contained in a unit area, i.e., the number of watts absorbed by tissue per square centimeter (W/cm^2).[2]

The importance of increasing or decreasing the power density by altering either the power or the spot size cannot be overstated. Such changes determine the depth of penetration and thus the cutting properties of the laser beam. To begin to appreciate the importance of the power density consider an unfocused CO_2 laser. A typical unfocused beam (Fig. 4–1), such as the output of an articulated arm without a lens, is just under 1 cm in diameter. If the laser were set to deliver 10 W of power, the power density would be approximately 10 W/cm^2; this power density is not sufficient to vaporize tissue. Focusing the same 10 W laser beam to a 1.0 mm spot size would provide a power density of approximately 1000 W/cm^2 or enough to remove tissue rapidly by vaporization. Changes in the cutting properties of the laser beam therefore can be made by changing the power density. Such changes can be accomplished by increasing or decreasing the power of the delivered laser beam or altering the focused spot size.

ENERGY

To conceptualize fully the effects and importance of changes in power density, the effects of changes of another parameter, *duration,* must be understood. The time or duration of exposure of the tissue to the laser emission is typically controlled by a shutter system or other such device which can rapidly and reliably turn the laser beam on and off. This permits a precise dose of energy to be delivered to the patient. As it is the primary goal when using the CO_2 laser to remove tissue, the relationship of power density and duration of exposure must be understood. The unit of energy, the joule, is the product of that delivered power and time. One joule (J) equals 1 watt (W) times 1 second (s). The principle parameter defining the *volume* of tissue removed by the laser is energy. The *rate* at which the tissue is being removed (volume per unit time) is primarily the power density.

TRANSVERSE ELECTROMAGNETIC MODE (TEM) AND TISSUE INTERACTION

The directional distribution or divergence of energy outside the laser cavity is characteristic of the *transverse electromagnetic (TEM_{00}) mode.* In the fundamental mode, energy is traveling along the laser axis and is thus the most parallel beam of light. This central, parallel beam can be focused to a much smaller spot than the higher order, off-axis modes. For most surgical applications, the significance of the TEM mode is academic; it is of little clinical significance. In applications where very small spot sizes are required, however, a fundamental TEM_{00} mode can be important. These applications include cases in which limited power is available from the laser and high power densities are needed, e.g., some microsurgical procedures where small spot sizes are required to limit the volume of tissue removed. An example in which a small spot size would be of value is in fertility surgery where the surgeon cuts adhesions or dissects the fallopian tube. In such instances both a high power density and small spot size will yield less tissue damage and thus better surgical results. In applications such as vaporization of a cervical neoplasia, where bulk tissue removal is required, a large spot size with high power density is desired to facilitate the rapid removal of tissue. In this type of situation, any mode of laser with sufficient power will suffice.

CALCULATION OF THE POWER DENSITY

The calculation of the power density is complicated by the laser beam's TEM mode. Consider two lasers delivering the same power but operating in different modes. The result will be two different focused spot sizes and thus different power densities. To frustrate matters further, the mode of many surgical lasers is not specified. The mode changes with time, temperature, and power, and is altered by diffraction upon beam delivery. The result is a beam of undefined mode structure and size. All of these variables make an accurate determination of the power density difficult. Although accurate techniques for quantifying the power density are available, fortunately, they are not required by the laser surgeon. Almost every surgical application of the CO_2 laser can tolerate a significant degree of variance in the specification of the power density. This permits shortcuts and approximations to be used with confidence when determining the power density and when setting the power and spot size in preparation for a procedure.

The central problem we are confronted with is determining the *optical spot size* or *optical beam diameter* of the focused laser beam. The optical spot size is the diameter of the beam measured at a percent (86 percent) of the peak beam intensity (Fig. 4–2) and does not change with alterations in delivered power. Although precise techniques to measure this parameter exist, they do not lend themselves easily to the surgical arena. In practice we take shortcuts or use approximations. There is a tendency, by users of surgical lasers, to observe the size of a laser cut or burn and use the resultant damaged area as the size of the beam. Changes in the delivered power or the use of different materials on which the laser is focused will cause changes in the diameter of the damage even though the actual optical spot size has not changed. These changes can be understood by considering a Gaussian laser beam. Figure 4–2 (curve A) illustrates a Gaussian profile laser beam focused onto tissue. An intensity less than the vaporization threshold will not cut or remove tissue. The tails of the intensity distribution are not of sufficient intensity to vaporize tissue. The volume of tissue vaporized is illustrated by the line A'. Curve B illustrates the same laser, i.e., same optical spot size (radius) with the intensity decreased. As expected, a smaller volume of tissue has been removed. The intensity in the tails of the Gaussian distribution has also been decreased resulting in a smaller damaged area, illustrated as line B', even though the optical spot size has not changed.

To avoid gross errors in determining the focused spot size and to provide a uniform way of reporting power density, the industry has arbitrarily and unofficially adopted the idea of measuring the diameter of the resulting burn on a wooden

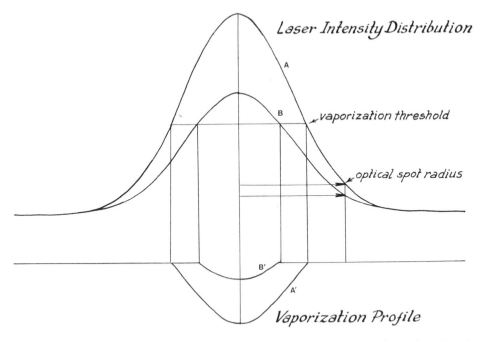

Laser Intensity Distribution

A

vaporization threshold

B

optical spot radius

B'

A'

Vaporization Profile

Figure 4–2. Two laser beam power profiles of the same optical spot size. Curve A represents higher power than B. The effect is shown in A' and B'. Note the change in both width and depth of the vaporization profile caused by tissues vaporization threshold of the tissue.

tongue blade exposed to a 10 W, 0.1 second CO_2 laser burst. Although this technique is filled with inaccuracy and pitfalls and should be used only for spot diameters less than 3 mm, it is useful for the degree of accuracy needed in laser surgery to approximate the spot size and power density. A much more accurate and reproducible—but more cumbersome—technique is the use of a fluorescent infrared phosphor as a target material. When using a phosphor, the beam diameter will not significantly change with power. Any power setting thus can be used as long as the power density (PD) of the phosphor is not exceeded.

$$PD_1 = \left(\frac{\text{power in watts}}{\pi r^2 \text{ (in cm}^2)} \right) \times 0.86 = W/cm^2 \qquad \textbf{(4–1)}$$

To calculate the power density we simply divide the power of the laser by the area of the focused beam area and multiply the quotient 86 percent (to assume a Gaussian beam). This can be approximated as

$$PD = \frac{(\text{power in watts}) \times 100}{(\text{spot diameter in mm})^2} W/cm^2. \qquad \textbf{(4–2)}$$

MODEL PARAMETERS

We have seen that altering the power density will change the *rate of vaporization* of tissue and that altering the energy, i.e., changing the duration of exposure at constant power, will change the *volume of tissue removed*. It has also been suggested that different wavelength lasers will have differing effects due to the absorption characteristics of tissue. Other parameters important to the development of a model predictive of the nature of the damage produced by a laser beam are the degree of energy *scatter* within the tissue, the *density* of the tissue, and the *thermal conductivity*. The thermal conductivity is a function of the water content of the tissue and the degree of local circulation.[3] Table 4–1 summarizes the major variables that determine the effect a laser will have on tissue.

The relationship between the depth of vaporization (penetration) and coagulation necrosis in terms of power, spot size, and duration can be seen in Figures 4–3A and 4–3B. When a beam of CO_2 laser energy moves across the tissue, the duration of exposure can be described in terms of the velocity of that moving beam. Figure 4–3A illustrates the depth of vaporization of the laser as a function of the power (optical spot size = 2.0 mm) for three different velocities. It is apparent from this figure that the depth of penetration is dependent on both the power and the velocity of the beam. The same tissue has been studied histologically to determine the average depth of the zone of coagulation necrosis. Figure 4–3B illustrates the zone of coagulation necrosis as a function of power (optical spot size = 2.0 mm) at the same three velocities. It can be seen that unlike the depth of vaporization, the zone of coagulation necrosis is principally a function of velocity (duration) only. These two graphs together suggest that if we wish to cut tissue with little surrounding damage, we must use high power densities and sufficiently rapid velocities (short duration) to decrease the resulting coagulation necrosis. In contrast, when more hemostasis is required, greater coagulation necrosis will be an undesired offshoot. In such cases, it is necessary to diminish power density and slow the velocity of the cut. The net result will be an incision of similar depth to that previously described but with more hemostasis. Illustrated in a different way, Figure 4–4 is a plot of the power (optical spot size = 2.0 mm) versus duration. Points A, B, and C represent a curve of constant depth of penetration. Point A will result in a cut to depth 0.5 mm as will point C; however, at A the power is sufficiently high and the duration sufficiently short to result in little conducted heat and resulting thermal damage when compared to C. In contrast, at C the laser

TABLE 4–1. PRINCIPLE PARAMETERS DEFINING THE EFFECT OF AN IMPACT OF A LASER ON TISSUE

Laser-Defined Variables	Tissue-Defined Variables
Wavelength (frequency)	Absorption coefficient
Duration of exposure	Scatter coefficient
Power ⎫	Density
⎬ power density	Thermal conductivity
Spot size ⎭	

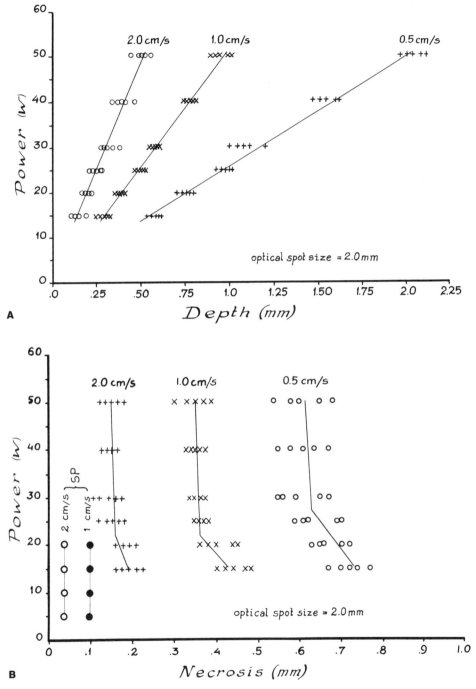

Figure 4–3. (A) Delivered power (W) vs. the depth of penetration in soft tissue, plotted as a function of the rate of movement of the beam over the tissue. The depth of penetration is thus determined by both the rate of cut and the power. **(B)** The power (W) vs. the degree of coagulation necrosis plotted as a function of rate of movement of the beam over the tissue. Super pulsed delivery results in significantly less necrosis than the continuous wave (unlabeled) curves (see text).

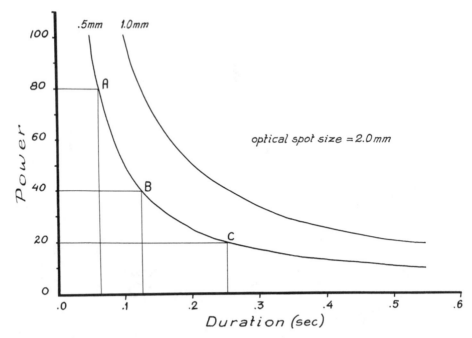

Figure 4–4. The depth dependency on delivered energy. The energy (power × time) is the principle variable effecting depth of vaporization.

is on for a longer time and with lower power resulting in a cut to the same depth but with much more coagulation necrosis. Point B represents a compromise and a good starting point for most surgical applications.

SUPER PULSE

Many surgical applications exist where it is desired to operate very slowly and precisely but with little coagulation necrosis. Such applications require characteristics of point A in Figure 4–4, i.e., minimal coagulation necrosis, and point C, i.e., slow rate of cut. These two seemingly conflicting requirements can be met by a technique developed by this author in 1975. The technique involved what is referred to as *super pulsing* (SP).[4]

The lasers presented thus far in this chapter run continuously and are referred to as continuous wave (CW) lasers. This means the laser is in contact with the tissue for a period set or controlled by the surgeon. The time "on tissue" is typically measured in seconds. Control is accomplished by a foot pedal. A CW laser can be automatically gated on and off electronically or mechanically; the important point being that the power is set and remains uniform throughout the lasing period. The typical maximum average power out of a CW surgical CO_2 laser ranges from 20 to 80 W. In contrast to CW operation, the super pulse (SP) laser has a maximum peak power ranging from 500 to 5000 W. The power is intermittently produced at a precise but rapid repetition rate and pulse duration. The result, as shown in Figure 4–5, is a train of pulses that delivers an average power ranging from less than 1 W to typically greater than 20 W. The primary importance of SP is the ability to cut tissue at a rate comparable to a CW laser and yet leave a zone of coagulation necrosis no greater than one third the zone created by a CW laser. Stated in a different manner, SP operation permits cutting at much slower velocities and thus with more precision than with a CW laser while causing at most one third the zone of necrosis. Referring back to Figure 4–3B, the two curves labeled SP illustrate the coagulation necrosis compared to a CW laser. The SP laser used in this illustration had a maximum average power of 20 W. Note that the change of slope seen in CW operation at low power is not present in the SP mode.

Not all "pulsed" CO_2 lasers are SP CO_2 lasers. To achieve the above described definition of SP, an appropriate combination of factors must be considered. The variables include the peak power, repetition rate, and pulse duration. An example of one possible configuration, the one used in Figure 4–3B, is a peak power of 1000

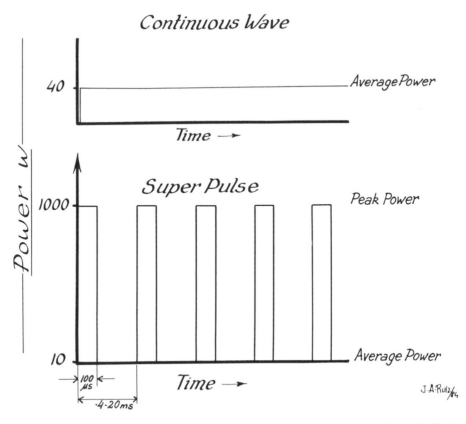

Figure 4–5. Continuous wave vs. super pulsed laser energy delivered (all variables typical), see text.

W, with a pulse duration of 100 microseconds (μsec) and a repetition rate variable from 50 to 250 pps. In general if the repetition rate increases significantly (in this example to >500 pps) so does the coagulation necrosis.

SUMMARY

There are many variables that define the extent of damage created by a laser. The variables include power, spot size, duration, wavelength, absorption characteristics, thermal conductivity, density, and scatter. This chapter concentrated on the power density, i.e., power and spot size, and the duration of exposure. The power density is the principle parameter defining the rate of vaporization by a CO_2 laser. The total energy delivered, i.e., the power-time product, describes the volume of tissue removed. We have explored the thermal effects of the duration of exposure and have seen that the depth of penetration is a function of the delivered power and duration (velocity of the beam). We have seen that the coagulation necrosis is caused by conducted heat away from the laser impact site. Thus the coagulation necrosis is principally a function of the duration of exposure.

There are instances in which it is desirable to vaporize tissue slowly and where little necrosis can be tolerated. In such instances where conventional techniques fail, due to the conflict of power and time, super pulsing is a solution. We have seen how high power, rapidly pulsed laser energy can vaporize tissue rapidly and leave a zone of necrosis one-third the zone created by a CW laser. Conversely, we have seen how the SP laser can be used to vaporize tissue slowly and precisely with little resultant thermal damage.

REFERENCES

1. Parrish JA: Photomedicine: Potentials for Lasers—An Overview in Lasers in Photomedicine and Photobiology. New York, Springer-Verlag, 1979, pp 2–22
2. Ramo S, Whinney JR, VanDozer T: Fields and Waves in Communication Electronics. New York, Wiley, 1965
3. Fuller TA: Fundamentals of lasers in surgery and medicine. In Dixon J (ed): Surgical Applications of Lasers. New York, Year Book Med Pub, 1983, pp 11–28
4. Fuller TA, Beckman H: Carbon dioxide laser surgery of the eye. Laser Surgery. Jerusalem, Jerusalem Acad Press, 1976, pp 214–226

5

Laser Instrumentation

Michael S. Baggish

THE CARBON DIOXIDE LASER

By far the most important and most frequently used laser in gynecologic surgery is the carbon dioxide (CO_2) laser. The reasons for the CO_2 laser's popularity relate to a multiplicity of factors. First, this laser produces a wide range of power output at reasonably low cost because of its relatively high efficiency. Second, since it emits at 10.6 μm, its beam is almost totally absorbed by cell water and is not color dependent. Finally, the continuous wave (CW) output of laser energy further adds to its attractiveness. The CO_2 laser is highly mobile and can be rolled from one operating room to another because it does not require complicated electric or plumbing installations.

The Perfect CO_2 Laser

The perfect CO_2 laser would have the following characteristics:

1. Stable TEM_{00} beam
2. Variable spot feature
3. Readout of power delivered at tissue
4. Accurate power output equally incorporating low and high ranges
5. Compact power source
6. Sealed tube
7. Flexible delivery system
8. Low cost
9. High quality variable magnification microscope
10. Maintenance free.

Obviously no such apparatus is currently available. Tremendous strides, however, have been made toward this ideal system by contemporary laser manufacturers. When one compares the equipment available today with the heavy, unwieldy instruments of the early 1970s, much credit is due to the laser industry for their research and development. Without the latter, little progress would be made; obviously at the same time research and development is expensive and adds to the costs of the production of lasers.

General Aspects

Since the CO_2 laser operates in the far infrared portion of the electromagnetic spectrum, the beam is invisible and must be aimed at the target by means of a visible coincidentally operating helium-neon (He-Ne) laser (Fig. 5–1A*). The major external components of the CO_2 laser consist of a console, a laser head, and a delivery system (Fig. 5–1B). A power readout and adjustment dial (watts), time gating mechanism (seconds), keyed off and on switch, power switch, stand-by and on lights, fault indicators comprise the console controls (Fig. 5–1C). The laser tube is mounted on the laser console in various configurations or it may be mounted to a colposcope (Fig. 5–1D).

At the writing of this book, no practical flexible fiber system has been developed. Several research endeavors, however, are well under way to produce a functional flexible delivery system. Currently, the CO_2 laser beam is delivered to the tissue site by an articulated arm and handpiece (Figs. 5–2, 5–3) or by means of a micromanipulator coupled to a colposcope or operating microscope (Figs. 5–4, 5–5). The articulated arm consists of rigid metal tubes connected at knuckled mirrors. These mirrors guide the laser beam along a tubular light path and direct it through a terminal lens to the tissue (Fig. 5–6). A shutter mechanism controls the laser output from the laser head or tube to the final delivery system. Most manufacturers control the shutter mechanism by means of a shielded foot pedal as well as a manual shutter located at the laser head. Some manufacturers also provide an additional safety feature, i.e., a foot pedal inactivation switch. This mechanism prevents an accidental laser discharge should the foot switch be depressed inadvertently.

Articulated arms vary in their weight, ease of movement, and counterbalance mechanism. The best arms are lightweight, easily manipulated to the tissue site, and have a wide range of movement. The handpieces are comfortably delicate and are fitted with various lenses usually ranging from 50 to 100 mm. Most manufacturers provide a measuring device at the terminus of the handpiece which indicates the point where the beam is in focus. Usually a N_2 blower is attached via plastic tubing to the laser handpiece. This prevents vapor from condensing on the handpiece lens (Figs. 5–7, 5–8). Dirty lenses tend to diminished power and changing modes.

Various designs of micromanipulators are currently available (Fig. 5–9). The key features include variable or fixed mirrors (Fig. 5–10). The variable spot micromanipulator is advantageous from the standpoint of delivering spots from 0.2 to 2 mm in diameter (Fig. 5–11). The excursion radius of the micromanipulator should encompass the lowest power microscopic field to offer the greatest flexibility. Several systems incorporate a handrest to diminish operator fatigue and add to the steadiness of manipulation. A few systems incorporate an automatic He-Ne

---

*All figures for this chapter appear following the text.

off/on function. When the laser discharges, the red He-Ne beam automatically shuts off. When the laser shutter is closed, the He-Ne aiming beam reappears. This function is highly advantageous in dark areas where the He-Ne beam renders vision difficult. The laser lens is focused between a 250 to 400 mm focal length range when coupled to the colposcope or microscope, therefore a blower is unnecessary. To be in focus the laser must be adjusted at the same focal distance as the microscope objective, e.g., at 300 mm, the laser lens should correspondingly be set at 300 mm.

For convenience, we can divide CO_2 lasers into office and hospital models. Before describing these two large categories, it would be convenient to mention two other subcategories: (1) sealed tube, and (2) flowing gas systems. The sealed tube laser essentially continuously reuses the same CO_2 gas within the laser tube. The flowing gas system requires external renewable sources of gas to be delivered by tanks mounted externally on the power console. Typically, three gases are contained in the laser tube: CO_2, N_2, and He.

Office Lasers

An office laser system must be compact and highly mobile to fit into the limited space requirements of a private office or clinic examining room (Fig. 5–12). Most of these systems include an attached colposcope. This equipment is meant to be utilized in a private office, clinic, or outpatient surgery unit. Such a unit need not deliver more than 20 W of power. This power level is clearly adequate for virtually all lower genital tract indications in gynecology. Several machines are currently available for office use in the $20,000 to $30,000 price range (Figs. 5–12, 5–13). Most frequently the office laser system is not the initial physician exposure to the laser.

The Hospital Laser System

Most physicians and nurses will be initiated into laser surgery by a hospital system. This equipment usually comprises intermediate and high-powered units, i.e., ranging from 30 to 50 W (Fig. 5–14) and upwards to 100 W (Figs. 5–15, 5–16). These instruments are always equipped with articulating arms which allow laser energy to be delivered either via free handpiece or micromanipulator. They are usually more costly systems, ranging in price from $50,000 to $100,000 and are meant for multispecialty applications. Although these lasers are equipped with wheels to allow some mobility, they are meant to be located in one—or at the most two—operating rooms. Some of these systems require dedicated circuits for proper functioning. These machines are fairly fragile units, e.g., if articulated arms are bumped or traumatized, the mirrors may be knocked out of alignment requiring a service call. Clearly, high-powered units, particularly those equipped with super pulse features must be carefully used by the inexperienced laser surgeon (Fig. 5–17). Many of these larger units have sophisticated control panels incorporating microprocessors (Fig. 5–18) and pulsed time sequence patterns. Virtually every one of these lasers is equipped with variable spot attachments and coupled to variable magnification microscopes equipped with beam splitters.

Accessories

Since the laser is a light beam and since this energy is converted to heat at the tissue site, certain precautions are necessary when the laser is used at various locations and with various instruments. Since the laser beam may be reflected from flat, shiny surfaces, accessory instruments must be light absorbing as well as heat absorbing. Additionally, as the tissue absorbs the CO_2 laser beam and vaporization occurs, smoke is produced. A smoke evacuator (Fig. 5–19) equipped with an odor-absorbing filter is an essential accessory. This device must produce a reasonable vacuum, but more importantly it must be able to move large volumes of air. Current units incorporate a vacuum cleaner motor with a filter constructed of activated charcoal. Fine, particulate components of the vapor are trapped in the filter at the same time the smoke is cleared from the operative field. In the past, these systems were very noisy, however, recently sound-deadening materials have made them less offensive to both physicians and patients.

A specially constructed laser speculum incorporates a smoke evacuation tube into its anterior blade (Fig. 5–20). This speculum allows vapor to be simultaneously evacuated from the vagina during laser vaporization. The interior aspect of the blades are constructed of a nonreflective, light absorbing material. Additionally, the speculum is hinged on one side only to allow angulation of the laser beam in order to be targeted between the instrument's blades (Fig. 5–21).

Backstop rods and spatulas absorb laser energy as tissue is transected. These items have found their major application within the abdomen (Fig. 5–22A). The best absorbing materials are constructed of titanium or anodized aluminum. An irregular surface promotes dispersion rather than reflection of the laser beam. Spheric design also promotes dispersion of the laser beam. Recently, we have constructed hollow manipulating rods which irrigate while simultaneously backstopping. The irrigating water serves to disperse absorbed heat and can be used with very high power density beams even when they are highly focused on the rods for long periods of time. Various angled rods provided with detachable handles furnish useful backstops for virtually every clinical situation.

Fine iris hooks mounted on long handles are ideal for manipulating the cervix when performing laser excisional cones and are indispensable for moving the cervix to treat vaginal fornix lesions (Fig. 5–22A). Additionally, these hooks are ideal to retract intraabdominal structures for delicate laser surgery.

Long-handled, thin-coated (gold) mirrors are very useful for reflecting the laser beam to reach otherwise inaccessible lesions (Fig. 5–22B). Lateral vaginal wall lesions may be hit perpendicularly by this technique. Also, foci of endometriosis on the posterior aspect of the cervix or ovary may be viewed in the mirror, then the laser is aimed at the image in mirror. Whatever is visualized can be vaporized accurately.

ARGON LASER

The argon gas laser emits in the visible, blue-green spectrum (488 to 514.5 nm). This laser is far less efficient than the CO_2 laser, i.e., requires substantial power input to obtain practical output power (0.1%). One advantage of the argon laser resides in its ability to be transmitted by a flexible fiber. Therefore, this laser's light can be delivered via an endoscope to the target tissue. Additionally, the argon laser can be used to drive a dye laser for photoradiation therapy. The argon laser alone has found little application in gynecology. Its major use to date centers around its preferential absorption by red, i.e., blood. Endometriotic foci absorb the beam while nonred tissue allows passage or reflects the beam. Limited experiences with the dye laser pumping rhodamine B dye at 630 nm and delivered via fibers have been reported for treating gynecologic malignancies. The system pictured incorporates two 7½ W argon lasers to drive a dye laser (Fig. 5–23). When using this system, goggles are required to protect the eyes of all people in the operating theater.

NEODYMIUM:YAG LASER

This solid-state laser emits in the near visible infrared portion of the electromagnetic spectrum at 1.06 μm. The advantage of this apparatus relates to its ability to deliver high power output laser energy via fine quartz fibers. This allows for convenient laser light transmission to the operative site. It specifically allows for endoscopic delivery. The major use of this laser in gynecology to date has been for intrauterine surgery via the hysteroscope.

The principal disadvantages of the Nd:YAG laser are its poor absorption in water and its rather deep and at times unpredictable tissue penetration.

This system can create short pulses with peak powers exceeding 100 W or deliver continuous outputs ranging between 50 and 100 W. Several of these machines require plumbing and 60 ampere, three phase electric current. The equipment illustrated delivers lower peak continuous power (50 to 60 W) but requires neither plumbing nor three phase electric circuitry (Fig. 5–24).

FREQUENCY DOUBLED ND:YAG LASER

The laserscope is a new laser system which is a frequency-doubled neodymium-doped, yttrium-aluminum-garnet laser producing all of its output at 532 nm (close to the output of the argon laser) (Fig. 5–25). The output is a train of light pulses running at a frequency of 25,000 Hz with a pulse duration of approximately 200 nanoseconds. The Nd:YAG rod is continuously pumped with a krypton arc lamp. The Nd:YAG wavelength (1064 nm) is frequency doubled to produce the 532 nm output. This laser is cooled by a water to water heat exchanger (plumbed). The laser is powered by a switching power supply operating at 208 volts AC, single phase.

The advantage of this system is that it emits in the argon range and is high powered enough to vaporize tissue. It can pass through liquid media and be transmitted by a fiber. The beam is preferentially absorbed by red pigment.

The disadvantages are similar to the argon laser—goggles are necessary to protect the operator's eyes.

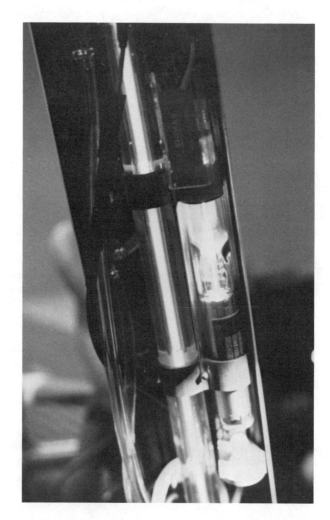

Figure 5–1A. CO_2 laser head (tube) exposed showing the CO_2 laser tube and a coincident He-Ne laser. *(Courtesy of Coherent Lasers.)*

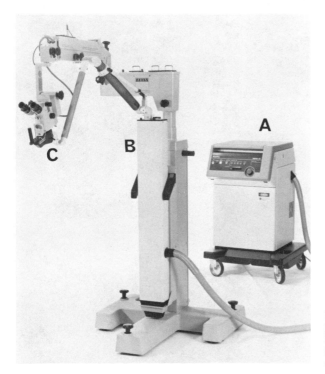

Figure 5–1B. The major components of a CO_2 laser system include: (A) console, (B) tube (head), (C) delivery apparatus. *(Courtesy of Carl Zeiss, Inc.)*

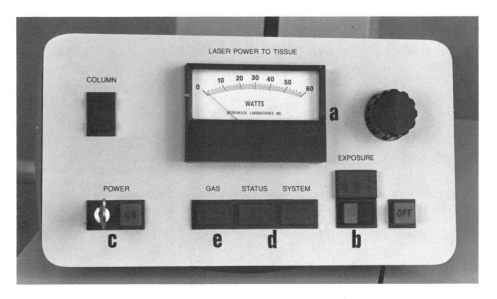

Figure 5–1C. Close-up of a laser control panel: (a) power panel and adjustment dial, (b) time exposure mechanism, (c) keyed off-on switch, (d) stand-by panel, (e) fault indicators. *(Courtesy of Merrimack Laboratories.)*

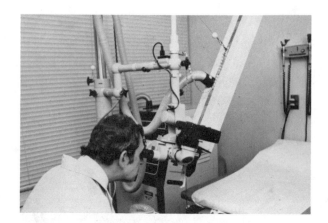

Figure 5–1D. The laser tube may be mounted to a colposcope.

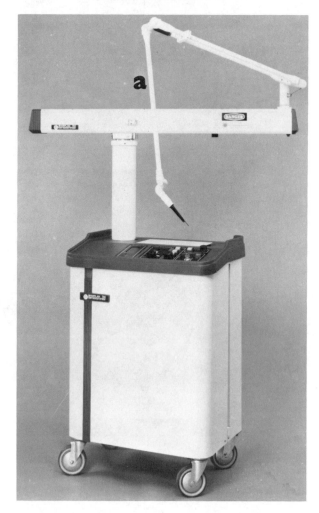

Figure 5–2. The laser beam may be delivered to tissue by means of an articulated arm (a). *(Courtesy of Advanced Surgical Technologies, Inc.)*

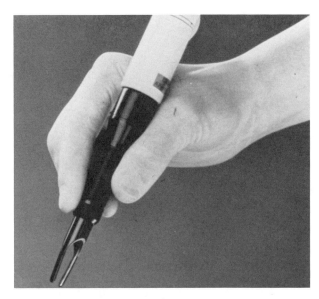

Figure 5–3. The final delivery system utilizes a ''pen-like'' laser handpiece which incorporates in its handle a focusing lens. *(Courtesy of Cooper Lasersonics.)*

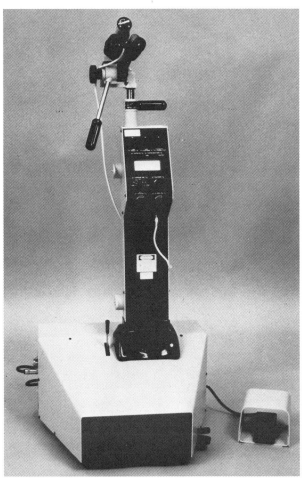

Figure 5–4. An alternative delivery method couples the laser's light path to the colposcope. *(Courtesy of Xanar Laser Systems.)*

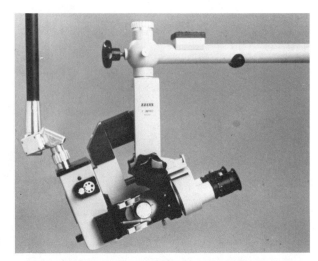

Figure 5–5. The laser's articulated arm may be attached to a micromanipulator which in turn is coupled to an operating microscope. *(Courtesy of Merrimack Laboratories.)*

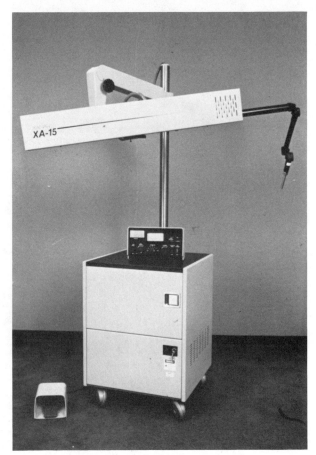

Figure 5–6. The laser beam is guided via metal tubes (articulated arm) connected at knuckles by mirrors which bend the light path according to the desired direction. *(Courtesy of Xanar Laser Systems.)*

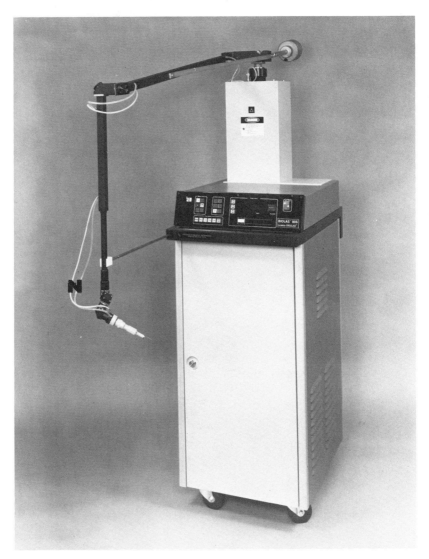

Figure 5–7. Nitrogen gas connected to the laser handpiece by plastic tubing (N) blows away laser vapor from the sensitive mirror and prevents deposition of debris. *(Courtesy of Advanced Biomedical Instruments.)*

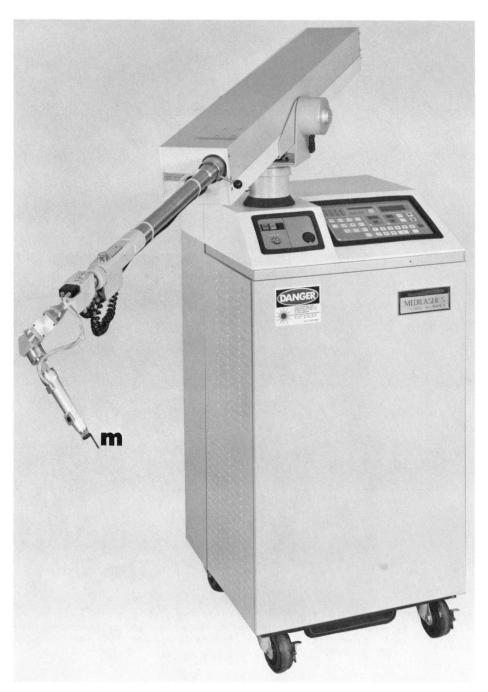

Figure 5–8. The laser handpiece is provided with a measuring device (m) which indicates the focal point of the laser beam. *(Courtesy of Cryomedics.)*

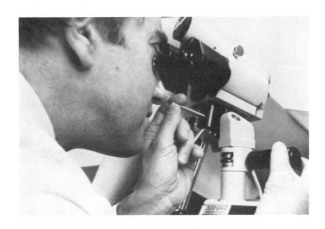

Figure 5–9. A micromanipulator directs the laser beam with great precision and a handrest diminishes operator fatigue. *(Courtesy of Xanar Laser Systems.)*

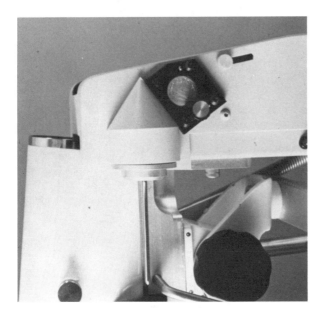

Figure 5–10. Several micromanipulators incorporate a variable spot feature into the design. *(Courtesy of Merrimack Laboratories.)*

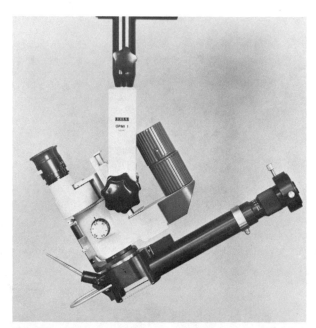

Figure 5–11. The variable spot feature permits movement of an internal mirror and allows the laser beam to be defocused. *(Courtesy of Xanar Laser Systems.)*

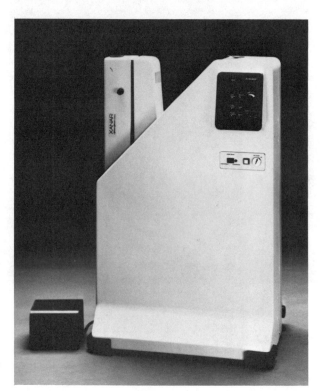

Figure 5–12. Office laser systems are designed to be compact, easily movable. A very compact mobile system showing a self-contained storage system for the laser tube. *(Courtesy of Xanar Laser Systems.)*

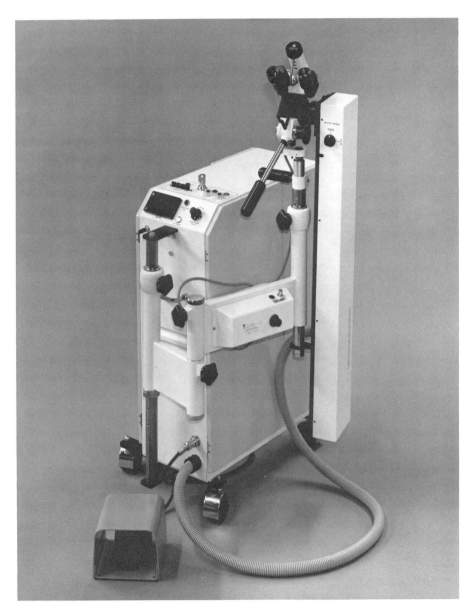

Figure 5–13. Several office lasers are available at lower price ranges than are inhospital units. *(Courtesy of Gyne-Tech Instruments Corp.)*

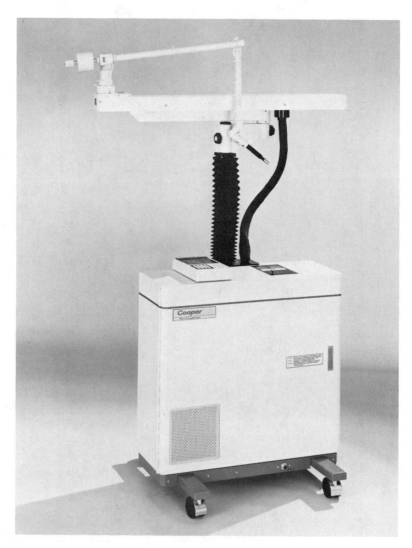

Figure 5–14. Intermediate hospital CO_2 lasers may produce from 30 to 40 W of power as illustrated here. *(Courtesy of Cooper Lasersonics.)*

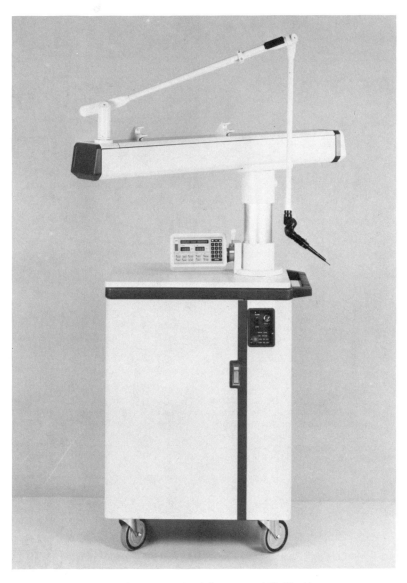

Figure 5–15. Multidiscipline high power units deliver up to 100 W of laser output energy to the tissue site. *(Courtesy of Advanced Surgical Technologies, Inc.)*

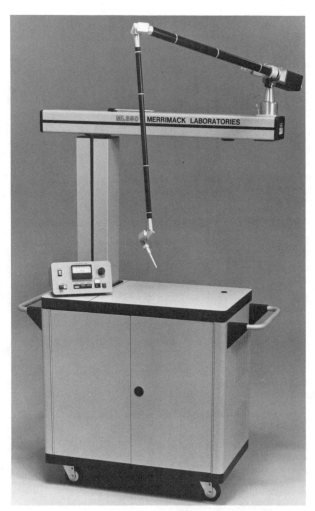

Figure 5–16. The high-powered lasers may be utilized in conjunction with the articulated arm/handpiece or by micromanipulator. *(Courtesy of Merrimack Laboratories.)*

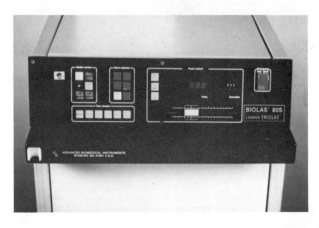

Figure 5–17. Several high power CO_2 lasers are equipped with a super pulse feature. This feature delivers very high power for very short periods of time. *(Courtesy of Advanced Biomedical Instruments.)*

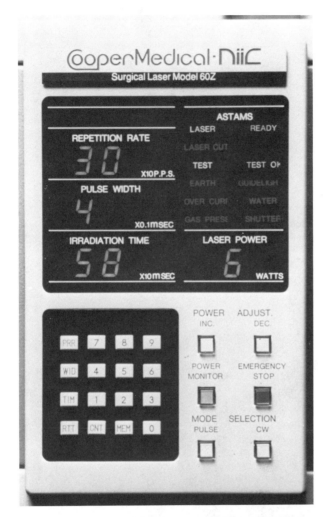

Figure 5–18. Microprocessor control panels allow for a multiplicity of power and time selections. The system illustrated here offers pulsed and continuous mode operation as well as super pulse variations. By varying the number of repetitions and pulse widths, the tissue action of the laser beam will likewise be altered. Memory capabilities are also possible. *(Courtesy of Cooper Lasersonics.)*

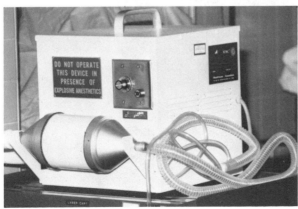

Figure 5–19. An efficient smoke evacuator equipped with odor and particulate matter absorbing filters are a required accessory for use in conjunction with the CO_2 laser. *(Courtesy of Stackhouse Associates.)*

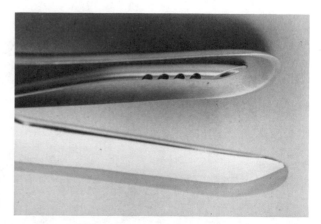

Figure 5–20. The anterior blade of the laser speculum has a built-in smoke evacuation channel. *(Courtesy of Codman Instrument Company.)*

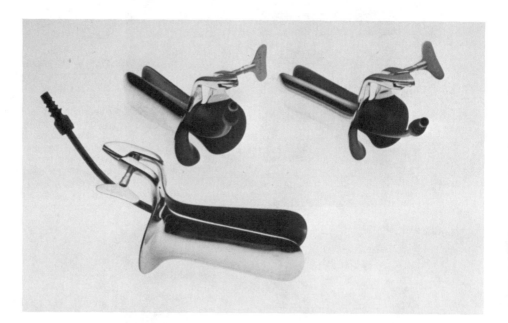

Figure 5–21. The laser specula illustrated here are hinged on one side only and are designed with light absorbing, nonreflective material on the inner aspect of the blades. *(Courtesy of Codman Instrument Company.)*

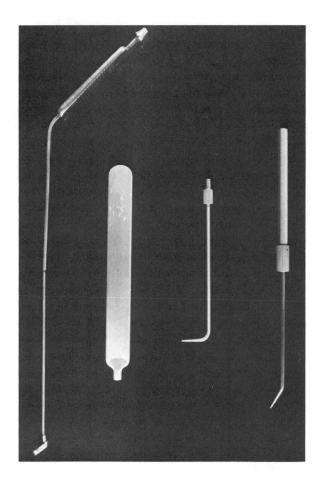

Figure 5–22A. A number of light and heat absorbing instruments are shown and include: (1) manipulating rods, (2) backstop spatula, (3) laser mirror. These are most frequently used in intraabdominal laser operations. *(Courtesy of Codman Instrument Company.)*

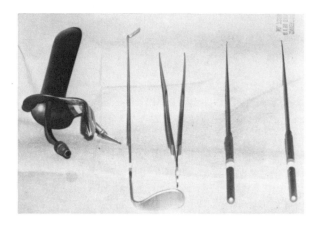

Figure 5–22B. Additional laser accessories include a measuring stick (mm), Bayonet forceps, and fine hooks.

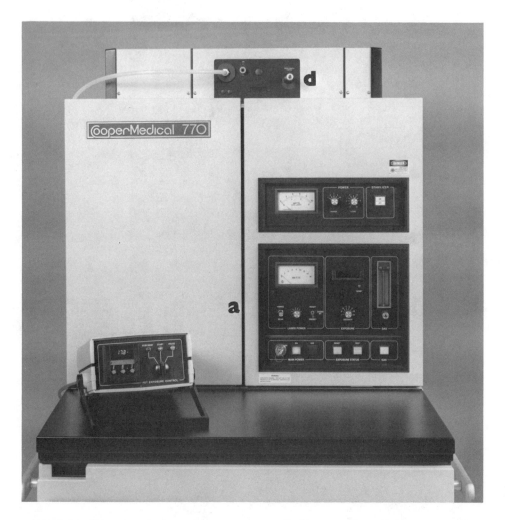

Figure 5–23. This argon-dye laser system couples two 7½ W argon lasers (a) to drive the dye laser (d). *(Courtesy of Cooper Lasersonics.)*

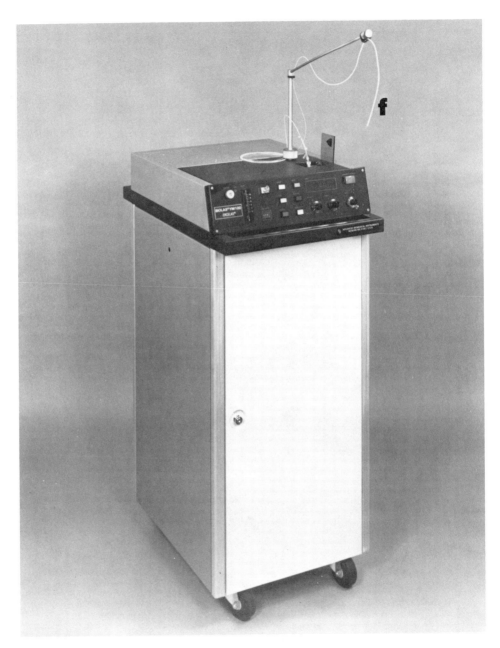

Figure 5–24. The neodymium:YAG laser pictured here does not require plumbing. Nd:YAG output can be transmitted by a quartz fiber (f) and is used via the hysteroscope for intrauterine surgical procedures. *(Courtesy of Advanced Biomedical Instruments.)*

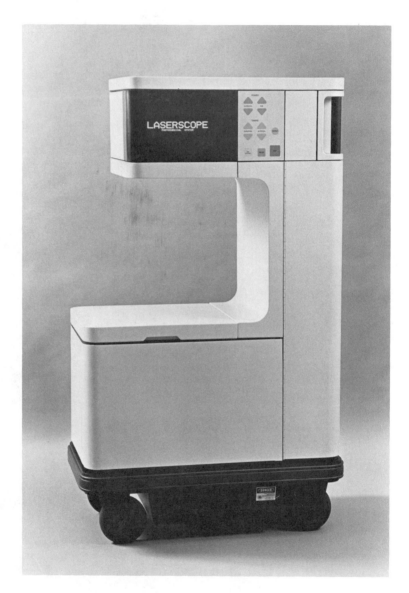

Figure 5–25. The laserscope is a new laser which produces 532 nm light by a frequency-doubling technology of a specially designed Nd:YAG system. Essentially this laser produces a powerful argon-like beam which can be transmitted via a variety of delivery systems including a flexible fiber. *(Courtesy of Laserscope.)*

6

Principles of Safety in Laser Surgery and Therapy

John C. Fisher

INTRODUCTION

Although voluminous literature has been published about the technical and biomedical aspects of lasers, most authors devote little or no discussion to the special safety problems of these instruments in medicine and surgery. This set of circumstances leaves the inquiring physician overwhelmed by extraneous information and bewildered about how to protect himself or herself and the patients. Such references are of little value to a busy medical doctor, nurse, or technician seeking practical knowledge about the dangers of lasers and means for averting hazards. It is with keen awareness of the pragmatic needs of those who deliver health care to patients that the author has written this chapter, which is a digest of an extensive experience in laser surgery and therapy over more than 8 years. The emphasis is practical; where theory is included, it is presented only to explain basic laser characteristics that the physician must understand to use lasers properly.

The first part of this chapter is devoted to operational problems in laser safety, with an emphasis on the causes and prevention of sundry laser accidents which have occurred in surgery and therapy with sufficient frequency so as to be regarded as realistic hazards. Although this book is dedicated to gynecology, a specialty which uses some, but not all, of the lasers now available for medical purposes, the hazards of all medical lasers are discussed. When a laser is acquired by a hospital at the request of one specialty, it usually finds increasing use by other specialists.

The author hopes that, by dealing in detail with the whole spectrum of laser hazards in surgery and therapy, this book may have a broader appeal than just to gynecologists. Practitioners in dermatology, oncology, general surgery, neurosurgery, orthopedic surgery, otolaryngology, thoracic surgery, gastroenterology, plastic and reconstructive surgery, and podiatry will find material herein which is quite pertinent to their uses of lasers. Furthermore, administrators, safety officers, institutional review boards, and engineering personnel of hospitals will be able to use this chapter as a reference manual in establishing the standards by which lasers are used and maintained, and under which accreditation of laser practitioners is conferred.

PREVALENT MISCONCEPTIONS

Many physicians and laymen are apprehensive about the popularly imagined dangers of lasers, but may not always be aware of the real ones. It is important to dispel false notions about laser hazards and to focus attention on the actual problems, without the distraction of unfounded fear.

Television, movies, and science fiction have created a false public image of the laser as a disintegrator which can cause people and inanimate objects to vanish in a cloud of vapor. Though there are military lasers which can be used as radiation cannon, the most powerful laser ever used in recorded[1] clinical applications delivered a maximum continuous wave (CW) power of 400 W. Given enough time, a 400 W carbon dioxide (CO_2) laser could vaporize a 100 kg (220 lb) patient, but this would require constant lasing of the patient for more than a week. Such a laser, though incredibly powerful by present medical standards, is clearly not an effective whole body evaporator. Presently there are no lasers used medically in the United States which can deliver more than 150 W, CW. This is sufficient to cause a serious, or even fatal, injury if used with gross ineptitude, but except for accidental irradiation of a critical part such as a major nerve or blood vessel, the human body is not highly vulnerable to a disabling or fatal injury by a medical laser.

Described in the simplest terms, a laser is a device which produces coherent, collimated, and monochromatic electromagnetic radiation. Electromagnetic radiation transmits energy through empty space or material media by coupled alternating electric and magnetic fields. The wavelength and frequency of this radiation are related by the simple equation:

$$f\lambda = v, \tag{6-1}$$

where f is frequency of alternation, expressed in cycles/time; λ is wavelength, expressed in units of (length); v is the speed of light, expressed in units of length/time. (In free space $v = c$, where $c = 2.998 \times 10^8$ m/s.)

The shortest wavelengths correspond to the highest photonic energies, and vice versa. Radiation becomes carcinogenic only when the photonic energy is high enough to cause ionization of atoms in living tissue. Among all the chemical elements, cesium has the lowest first ionization energy, 3.89 electron volts (eV) (1 eV $= 1.602 \times 10^{-19}$ J). In other words, a photon (a "particle" of radiation) having an energy of 3.9 eV will knock an electron out of orbit and ionize an atom of cesium if it strikes that atom. The longest wavelength at which the photonic energy equals or exceeds this value is 319 nm (a nanometer is one billionth of a meter). This wavelength is in the ultraviolet portion of the spectrum, beyond the blue edge of the visible spectrum, which is 400 nm. Since all the lasers presently being used for medical purposes have wavelengths longer than 319 nm, it can be stated that today's medical lasers do not cause oncogenic changes in living tissue.

At this point, it is appropriate to mention the physical fact that radiation of photonic energy lower than the first ionization energy of an atom can cause ionization of that atom if the power density of the radiation is high enough so that there is a high probability that the atom will absorb more than one photon simultaneously. Such power density, however, is far above the values attainable in medical lasers.

The Laser as a Disseminator of Viable Malignant Cells

Acoustic Shock Waves and Blast Effects

In the early years of the laser age, many investigators experimented with lasers on animals and humans. In that era, there was scant fundamental understanding of the interaction of laser light with living tissue. The experiments were often ill conceived and motivated by a let's-see-what-happens attitude. Not surprisingly, the results were frequently discouraging. Among the early units used for experimental surgery were the ruby and neodymium-glass lasers, each capable of operation only in a pulsed mode. When these lasers were used to irradiate malignant tumors in vivo, their ultrashort pulses (in the order of nanoseconds) of high radiant energy (many joules) produced enormous power densities which caused explosive disruption of tissue, hurling pieces of viable tumor about the operating room and into the surgeons' faces. One of the most vocal critics among the early laser surgeons was Dr. Alfred S. Ketcham, then at the National Institutes of Health in Washington, D.C. In a pair of papers,[2,3] he rightly criticized the pulsed lasers of that time, judging them unsuitable tools for cancer surgery. This stigma persisted until late in the decade of the 1960s, when the CW argon-ion (Ar), CO_2, and neodymium-yttrium-aluminum-garnet (Nd:YAG) lasers were first used successfully for surgery and therapy.

At power densities below 1,000,000 W/cm^2, CW CO_2, Nd:YAG, and Ar lasers do not produce blast effects. The Nd:YAG has a special problem, which will be discussed later, but when properly applied, it does not scatter viable tissue. Nearly any laser which can be operated in a CW fashion at a steady power output of P_0 will be capable of delivering a peak power of two to ten times P_0 when operated in pulsed fashion, or greater if the pulsing is achieved through Q-switching. With CO_2 and Nd:YAG lasers, pulsed operation is being increasingly used again, for minimization of thermal damage to tissue adjacent to the laser-impact site of the CO_2 laser, and for attaining the enormous power densities needed by the ophthalmic Nd:YAG laser for precise focal-point destruction of opacities in the eye. The pulsing is achieved by electronic techniques in the power supply of the CO_2 laser (the so-called super pulsed operation), and by either Q-switching or mode-locking in the ophthalmic Nd:YAG laser (ultra-short-pulsed operation). Electronic pulsing produces output pulses of many microseconds' duration, and does not drastically increase the maximum power density of the beam. Although the ultra-short-pulsed Nd:YAG lasers deliver single or sequential pulses having very short durations, picoseconds to nanoseconds (1 picosecond = 1×10^{-12} second) with peak powers of 10^{10} to 10^{14} W, the tissue damage they produce is of very small spatial extent and their shock waves are not deleterious, because the total energy per pulse is only a few millijoules. The damage mechanism is primarily that of photo-ionization of impacted atoms to produce an electric plasma at very high temperature. This ionization, achieved by the exceedingly high electric field of the laser rays, does not cause oncogenic mutation of cells because these cells suffer a total destruction of cytologic structure in the process of plasma formation and heating to 15,000°C or higher.

Smoke Plumes

Although today's medical lasers do not scatter intact fragments of malignant (or benign) tissue, they can produce a thick, malodorous smoke when used to vaporize tissue. This is particularly true of the CO_2 laser, which destroys tissue by rapid vaporization of the intra- and extracellular water, which ruptures the cells and ejects their nonliquid contents out into the incident laser beam, where, stripped of their aqueous protection, they are heated by the beam and burn in the ambient air. Many a laser surgeon has apprehensively wondered whether the smoke plume from a vaporized tumor contains viable cells. However, two well-designed and carefully executed studies[4,5] have demonstrated convincingly that the smoke plume created by a CO_2 laser does not contain any biologically viable cells, malignant or benign, although upon microscopic examination some of the plume-transported cells appear morphologically normal. The first of these studies attempted to grow cultures of cells from apparently normal cells retrieved out of the plume; the second analyzed, by means of radioactive tracers, the products of metabolism in cells collected from the plume, and the replication of DNA and transcription of RNA. Neither study showed any viability of the cells from the smoke plume of a CO_2 laser.

At this point, the reader may wonder whether the plume created by an Ar or Nd:YAG laser might contain viable cells. These lasers are not nearly so efficient as the CO_2 for vaporization of tissue, because scattering reduces the power density of the radiation within tissue. At points, however, where the histologic power density is sufficient to cause vaporization, the mechanism of cell destruction is the same as for the CO_2 laser: rapid boiling of histologic and cytologic water. As the cells rupture from internal formation of steam, their nonliquid contents are ejected outward. As these solid inclusions pass through the laser beam, the temperature to which they are heated depends upon the power density of the beam and the absorbance of the particles. Since, in general, reflectance increases for most solid particles as wavelength decreases from 10,600 nm (CO_2) to 488 nm (Ar), with wavelength-dependent variations according to the color of the particles, absorbance will decrease (absorbance + reflectance + transmittance = 1, and transmittance is small). Therefore, in a very general way, the solid particulate inclusions ejected from the ruptured cells will absorb less of the laser radiation in their trajectory through the beam of visible or near infrared lasers than through the beam of a CO_2 laser, if the power densities of the incident beams are equal. As a consequence, one might expect less denaturation of the organic compounds which constitute these particles. This is substantiated by the fact that, at comparable power levels and beam diameters, Ar and Nd:YAG lasers produce considerably less smoke than CO_2 lasers when vaporizing soft tissue. The author is not aware of any definitive studies done on the smoke plumes produced by Ar and

Nd:YAG lasers in surgery. The question of viability of cells from their plumes has not yet been answered. Both of these laser types however have been in clinical use for at least 15 years, and as yet the literature reports no evidence of oncogenesis in or on the bodies of surgical personnel using them. On the basis of more than 8 years of experience in laser surgery, the author believes that the hazard of viable malignant cells in the vapor plume of an Ar or Nd:YAG laser is probably quite small. There may be a small number of organic compounds in living tissue which do not suffer serious alteration of molecular structure when heated to 100°C, the temperature which all ejected cellular particles have already reached when they enter the vapor plume. Further study is necessary on this subject. Meanwhile, the surgeon using Ar or Nd:YAG lasers to treat malignancies is well advised, for the reasons set forth in the next section, to employ a good suction system to evacuate the vapors from the surgical site.

Intrinsic Carcinogenicity of Smoke

Irrespective of the absence of malignant cells in smoke plumes from lasers, the various combustion products which smoke contains can be chemically carcinogenic. A significant study of the smoke generated by CO_2 laser irradiation of animal tissue was done by Mihashi and his colleagues[6] in Japan at Kurume University in 1981. Using an excised canine tongue as the laser target, they collected the smoke and analyzed it for total particulates, particle size distribution, and mutagenicity of the condensates. The size distribution of particles showed that 77 percent of all particles were under 1.1 μm, the range in which accumulation of inhaled particles will be predominantly in the alveoli of the lungs. With no suction used, the weight of smoke condensates was 284 mg per gram of tissue vaporized (which indicates that the water content of the tongue in vitro was about 72 percent, somewhat lower than it would have been in vivo). A mutagenicity test was attempted, using the Ames microbial mutation test on *Salmonella typhimurium* (TA 98); though the results were not conclusive, they showed that there was measurable mutagenicity of the collected particulates. Most importantly, perhaps, the study showed that when a suction tip having a capacity of about 28 l/s was used to evacuate the smoke, nearly 99 percent of the smoke could be removed from the air with the tip 1.0 cm or less from the impact site, and only 51 percent at 2.0 cm from the site. A jet of cooling gas, such as is customarily used with surgical handpieces to keep the lens free of contamination, reduced the collection efficiency to only 62 percent with the suction tip 1 cm from the site.

These results suggest quite strongly that the surgeon who has a care for his or her own health is well advised to use a suction system of adequate capacity with the tip placed as close as possible to the impact point of the laser on the tissue. One such system is shown in Figure 6–1. This provides both variable flow rate and renewable inline filtration by activated charcoal to remove odor and particulates. It should be noted here that the typical operating room suction system is inadequate to cope with the smoke evolved by aggressive CO_2 laser vaporization of large tissue masses. It quickly becomes clogged with smoke condensates, and is rendered nonfunctional. The surgeon's rapport with the engineering staff and the operating room personnel are not enhanced by this result. The prevalent misconception in this case is that the smoke plume is not a matter for concern. Quite the contrary: it is a real hazard.

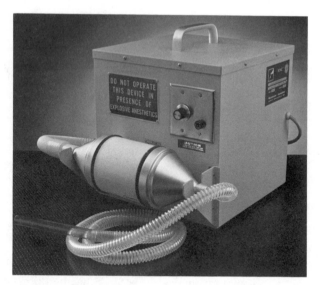

Figure 6–1. Smoke evacuator for use with CO_2 lasers in surgery. This unit offers variable flow, replaceable charcoal filter, and adaptors for different sizes of tubing. *(Courtesy of Stackhouse Associates, Manhattan Beach, California.)*

Intracorporeal Dissemination of Viable Cells

The CO_2 laser poses a vanishingly small risk of scattering viable cells into other parts of the patient's body, whether used for coagulation or vaporization. Because it seals small (0.5 mm or less) blood vessels and lymphatic ducts, it allows accurate surgery in a relatively bloodless field with a minimum of mechanical or manipulative contact with the tissue. In this respect it is superior to any other device available for the surgical treatment of malignancy, with the possible exception of the Nd:YAG laser when used to produce coagulatory necrosis. Though the Ar laser is not widely used to treat malignancies, essentially the same comments apply to it as well. It is the author's firm belief that the CO_2 laser, perhaps combined with the Nd:YAG, and used in conjunction with photoradiation (or photodynamic) therapy (PRT), will eventually become the premier modality for dealing with both primary and metastatic malignancies.

POSSIBLE HAZARDS OF WAVEGUIDE LASER TUBES WITH HIGH FREQUENCY EXCITATION

Since the advent of CO_2 lasers using sealed-off waveguide tubes in 1980, there have been rumors and allegations to the effect that the stray electric fields leaking from the power supplies and connecting cables of such lasers might be biologically harmful. Much confusion has arisen on this subject, which neither the Bureau of Radiological Health (BRH) of the U.S. Food and Drug Administration (FDA) nor the manufacturers of these lasers have done much to dispel. Each group has been reticent about making public comment on the allegations. However, the BRH has given its customary tacit approval to the makers of such lasers, who are selling them to hospitals and clinics in the United States and Canada. Actually, two federal agencies have jurisdiction over devices which can emit radio frequency (RF) electric fields: the BRH and the Federal Communications Commission (FCC). As the name implies, the BRH is concerned with situations in which radiation may affect health. The FCC is concerned with possible interference of such radiation with communications such as radio and television.

The FCC promulgates tables of the allowable radiated field strengths from various devices, such as physicians' paging receivers and transmitters, transmitters for garage door openers, cordless microphones, citizens'-band radios, and so on. Though these permitted levels of RF interference are functions of the frequency band in which they occur, the maximum permitted stray radiation from *any* device in the frequency ranges covered by these regulations is only 0.50 millivolt per meter (mV/m). The FCC specifies, and various manufacturers produce, field-strength meters (which are essentially small radio receivers) to measure such radiated interference. It can be readily calculated that the allowable radiated power density of a waveguide laser is four orders of magnitude below any irradiance which has ever been suggested to have any biologic effects. In view of the lack of experimental evidence to the contrary, it is the view of this author that the waveguide lasers now commercially available to the medical world (in the U.S. and Canada) are quite safe for long-term use in operating rooms, so long as each individual unit continues to meet the standards of both the BRH and the FCC regarding stray radiation.

IMPORTANT HAZARDS OF LASERS IN SURGERY AND THERAPY

Preliminary Observations

It is pertinent to observe that the safety record in the surgical and therapeutic uses of CO_2, Ar, and Nd:YAG lasers over the past 15 years shows an accident rate of about 0.5 percent (ratio of the number of accidents to the number of procedures done with lasers). This figure is difficult to determine accurately because not all of the accidents which occur are reported in the literature, few are reported in the public press, and the records of hospitals reporting accidents to governing agencies are privileged information. Though the present incidence of mishaps with medical lasers is certainly very low, it could be improved by better training and diligence on the part of the laser practitioners. The fatality rate has been much lower, and much more difficult to document, because surgeons and hospital administrators are understandably reluctant to discuss the problem for the record. The author knows anecdotally of four laser accidents which resulted in the death of the patient. To put this whole matter into proper perspective, it should be observed here that a carelessly wielded scalpel can cause more damage in a split second than a laser. If properly used, a laser is less hazardous than a knife, because it affords the surgeon better control and visualization of tissue destruction or removal, especially when a CO_2 laser is used with a binocular microscope. The average patient is probably at much greater risk from general anesthesia than from laser surgery. For the record, it should be stated here that *the malfunction of laser equipment is seldom a factor in traumatic laser accidents.* The overwhelming majority are caused by ignorance and/or negligence on the part of the laser operator.

Specific Hazards of Lasers

This section deals only with the following laser types: CO_2, Nd:YAG, Ar, dye, and helium-neon (He-Ne) lasers. The Ar laser, widely employed for the treatment of vascular diseases of the ocular fundus and less often for therapy of vascular skin lesions, has found no widely accepted uses in gynecology as yet. The gynecologic uses of the Nd:YAG are relatively few, e.g., coagulation of the uterine endometrium in cases of intractable menorrhagia. The dye laser has been increasingly used for photoradiation therapy, which has recently been employed for diagnostic as well as therapeutic purposes in treatment of malignancies of the female genitalia. These and other laser types, however, some of which are as yet not used medically, will find increasing applications not only in gynecology but in many other medical specialties. It is therefore only prudent for the reader of this text, who is presumably a gynecologist, to be familiar with the hazards of all the lasers now commonly employed in surgery and therapy.

The practitioner must bear in mind that *the destructive potential of any laser is directly proportional to its output of radiant power,* although different types of lasers may have different effects upon specific parts of the body at a given power level. In the following discussion, we shall define risk as the probability of an accident, multiplied by the severity of its sequelae. The significant hazards of laser surgery or therapy are listed in order of declining risk, and each is discussed in terms of cause, consequences, and means of prevention. Several of the specific hazards listed here are not likely to be encountered by the gynecologic laser surgeon. They are discussed here because a laser acquired by a hospital at the request of a gynecologist often gets used opportunistically by other specialists at the same institution, some or all of whom may not have had adequate training in the proper use of lasers. This is especially dangerous for otolaryngologists using the CO_2 and Nd:YAG lasers. Some of the listed hazards, although not presently related to gynecologic uses of lasers, may in the future become quite relevant as gynecologists put into practice some of the new laser techniques which are now still experimental.

Hazards of Laser-Ignited Combustion

Elastomeric endotracheal tubes used for providing the so-called positive end-expiratory pressure ventilation during surgery of all kinds under general anesthesia are often used during laser surgery in the same airway. These tubes have been the source of most of the morbidly serious and nearly all of the fatal accidents in laser surgery over the past decade. This danger is completely avoidable if the operator, during laser surgery in the intubated airway, uses only red silicone rubber or high silicon-elastomer tubes (Fig. 6–2) protected with reflective, adhesive-backed aluminum tape properly wrapped exteriorly (Fig. 6–3), and inflates the cuffs, covering them proximally with closely packed wet cottonoid patties of the neurosurgical variety (with retrieving strings attached). Alternatively, one of the newer high frequency positive pressure ventilatory techniques[7-10] using an all-metal cannula eliminates this hazard altogether. An unprotected elastomeric endotracheal tube however can be quickly punctured by the beam of either a CO_2 or a Nd:YAG laser at surgical power densities ($300\ W/cm^2$ or higher). This is espe-

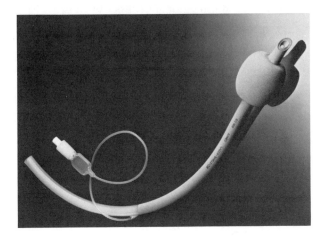

Figure 6-2. SURGITEK silicone endotracheal tubes. These tubes can withstand the beam of a CO_2 laser at surgical power densities for up to 30 seconds without protective aluminum wrapping. *(Courtesy of Medical Engineering Company, Racine, Wisconsin [division of Bristol-Meyers Co.].)*

cially true of polyvinylchloride (PVC) tubes, which should *never* be used during laser procedures in the airway; they are rapidly punctured by laser beams and burn fiercely in the presence of oxygen and/or nitrous oxide at concentrations of 35 percent or higher. During combustion, highly toxic gases are evolved, e.g., phosgene, which irritate the respiratory mucosa. The melted and burned PVC forms a sticky black coating on the tracheal and bronchial wall which is very difficult to remove during any postoperative emergency treatment. The red silicone or high

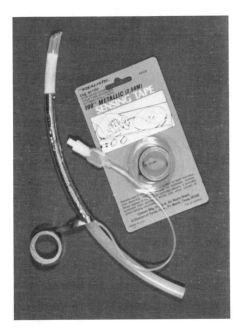

Figure 6-3. Silicone endotracheal tube with protective aluminum tape applied, starting at proximal side of the cuff and wrapping back to bifurcation of the inflating tube, using a 50 percent overlap of the turns. The aluminum tape shown is called "Sensing Tape," and is available from Radio Shack Corporation.

silicone elastomers resist puncture much longer than PVC, burn with less intense flames, and evolve no toxic combustion products. Once punctured, however, any of these tube types will burn like a blowtorch, with a flame which usually starts in the lumen but can quickly involve the exterior, and travels swiftly from the puncture site toward both the distal and proximal ends of the tube. Figure 6–4 (see Color Plate I*) shows a PVC endotracheal tube burning internally after deliberate ignition by a CO_2 laser while carrying a stream of pure O_2 internally. This most serious of all laser hazards in surgery has caused more than 35 severe burns of the respiratory tract in humans and at least 2 deaths to date. The tragedy is that these accidents are totally preventable. The gynecologist has a moral obligation to warn his colleagues in otolaryngology about this danger.

Ignition of Rectal Gas

Like a monopolar electrosurgical device (popularly called a "bovie"), a CO_2 or Nd:YAG laser can ignite gas expelled from the patient's rectum, if the methane content is high enough. The resulting explosive flare can cause severe burns of the patient's perianal area, buttocks, and thighs, as well as the surgeon's hands, arms, and face. This danger can be averted by presurgical evacuation of the patient's lower bowel, together with insertion of a wet cottonoid plug into the patient's anus. Though rectal gas is mostly air ingested with food, it sometimes contains enough methane to burn in room air. At least three such accidents have occurred to date.

Bronchoscopic Fires

In many medical centers today the flexible fiberoptic bronchoscope has largely replaced rigid bronchoscopes for diagnostic bronchoscopy, because the flexible scope allows viewing of the smaller branches of the tracheobronchial tree. Its flexibility also allows the beam of any laser which is transmissible through a quartz or glass optical fiber to be directed into these smaller bronchial passages which are not accessible by means of a rigid bronchoscope. For this reason, some of the less experienced laser bronchoscopists have used the Nd:YAG laser with flexible fiberoptic bronchoscopes to treat obstructive lesions of the airway below the larynx. Though diagnostic bronchoscopy can usually be done with only topical local anesthesia, bronchoscopic laser therapy often requires general anesthesia and positive end-expiratory pressure ventilation. Because the working lumen of the typical fiberoptic bronchoscope is not large enough to accommodate the laser fiber and still provide an adequate lumen for ventilation, the fiberoptic scope is inserted through the lumen of a rigid metal ventilating bronchoscope, or through a conventional endotracheal tube with inflated cuff, and ventilation is then provided in the usual manner during flexible bronchoscopy. This practice presents all the hazards of CO_2 laser surgery of the upper airway with an elastomeric endotracheal tube. Any incandescent particle produced by the Nd:YAG laser by irradiation of the tracheobronchial epithelium or of the endotracheal tube can quickly ignite both the endotracheal tube and the plastic covering of the fiberoptic bronchoscope in the oxygen-rich atmosphere. For this reason, it is inadvisable to use an elastomeric endotracheal tube as the cannula for insertion of the fiberoptic broncho-

---

*Color Plate I appears following p. 177.

scope. If the advantage of flexibility is deemed so compelling as to require the fiberoptic bronchoscope for laser therapy of the lower airway under general anesthesia, the fiberoptic scope should be introduced only via a conventional rigid stainless steel bronchoscope of adequate lumen. The plastic jacket of the fiberoptic scope can still be ignited by hot particles resulting from aggressive irradiation. This jacket will burn fiercely in gas mixtures having an O_2 or $O_2 + N_2O$ concentration of 35 percent or higher, producing a blowtorch-like flame which can seriously damage the whole lower airway right down to the alveoli. Furthermore, the small external diameter of the fiberoptic bronchoscope requires that its working lumen be too small to allow the passage of a suction cannula of sufficient capacity to cope with even moderate bleeding or to evacuate the smoke and vapor produced by the beam of the Nd:YAG laser. Though the Nd:YAG is an excellent hemostatic device, hemorrhage can be sudden and massive, flooding the target area before the operator can coagulate the bleeding vessel(s), and necessitating copious suction.

For these reasons, experienced Nd:YAG bronchoscopists like Dumon et al.[11] and Shapshay[12] use the fiberoptic scope for diagnosis and examination, and utilize only the conventional rigid metal ventilating bronchoscope in therapeutic laser bronchoscopy. With the impending advent of flexible fibers to transmit the beams of CO_2 lasers efficiently over lengths of 1 m or more within sheaths of small enough diameter to be used in flexible endoscopes, as described by Fuller and Beckman,[13] it can be expected that the CO_2 laser, already widely used for rigid bronchoscopy of the upper respiratory tract, will experience increased application in therapeutic and surgical bronchoscopy of the lower respiratory structures via flexible bronchoscopes. This will increase the risk of ignition of the plastic jackets of such scopes, and give further impetus to the trend back to rigid metal scopes for therapy and surgery with lasers in this region of the body.

Ignition of Surgical Drapes

The beam of either the CO_2 or the Nd:YAG laser will readily ignite dry combustibles in room air. Sterile drapes, cottonoid pads, surgical tape, rubber gloves, and scrub suits will burn when irradiated at surgical power densities (300 W/cm^2 and higher). The best preventive measure is to saturate with normal saline or sterile water all cloth or paper coverings near the surgical site. So long as liquid water is present, it will totally absorb the radiant energy of a CO_2 laser, carrying it away as latent heat of vaporization. The rays of the Nd:YAG laser will penetrate the water and be converted to heat in the protected material, which will be cooled by the evaporation of its absorbed water. The two lasers differ in the site of absorption of the radiant energy: rays at 10,600 nm are completely absorbed in the water, but those at 1064 nm (Nd:YAG) are transmitted through the water and absorbed in the drape material. In either case, the evaporation of water ablates the heat. *The surgeon must be careful to keep his gloved hands out of the beam,* which is *invisible* to the eye during its transit from the laser aperture to the laser target. Although virtually all infrared lasers now use a visible red beam from a He-Ne laser as an aiming designator, this also is invisible unless scattered by airborne smoke or reflected from a target surface. Plastic materials which will not absorb water should be removed from around the surgical site, or else covered by thick, wet cottonoids taped securely in place. Note also that any target surface can be protected from the beam of a CO_2 or Nd:YAG laser by covering it with *heavy gauge aluminum foil*, which must first be *minutely rumpled* to avoid specular (mirror-like) reflections, and then *taped in place*.

Vaporization of Surgical-Preparative and Diagnostic Liquids

These liquids, such as Betadine, Hibiclens, Lugol's and Schiller's stains, acetic acid, and toluidine blue, must be allowed to dry before the laser beam is fired at the surface(s) to which they have been applied. Despite their lack of flammability, such liquids strongly absorb the rays of a CO_2 laser (and the dark liquids absorb the rays of the Nd:YAG), and will be vaporized by the laser beam at surgical power densities. Their vapors are chemically active and can cause burns or irritation to the skin and eyes of the surgeon. *Alcohol, acetone, and hydrocarbon solvents must never be used near a laser beam because they are highly flammable.*

Ignition of Plastic Vaginal Specula

Some gynecologists regularly use disposable vaginal specula made of a plastic material. Though most of these will not sustain combustion in room air if momentarily ignited by the beam of a CO_2 laser *(the rays of the Nd:YAG are not strongly absorbed in most transparent plastics having no color)*, there is at least one brand which will burn readily in air after the source of ignition is removed. The author has learned anecdotally of an accident in which such a speculum was ignited by exposure to the beam of a CO_2 laser and burned rapidly before it could be extracted from the patient, causing severe vaginal burns. This hazard can be totally avoided by a trial exposure of every plastic speculum of unknown properties to the laser beam before vaginal insertion, and rejection of any specimen which sustains combustion in air. To be completely safe, one should avoid the use of plastic specula altogether by employing only stainless steel units when doing laser surgery or therapy through a vaginal speculum. If the gynecologist is concerned about possible reflection of the laser beam from the inner surfaces of the blades of the speculum (which, being concave, can refocus the beam on the vaginal wall), specially designed laser specula are available which will not reflect the impinging beam. Regarding reflections from solid surfaces, the reader must be aware of the following facts:

1. Every solid surface has irregularities when viewed under sufficient magnification.
2. The kind of reflection produced by a surface is determined by the ratio of the wavelength of the reflected light to the mean size of the irregularities.
3. When the mean irregularity (MI) is much larger than the wavelength (WL), reflections are diffuse; when the MI is comparable to the WL, reflections are diffracted and scattered; and when the MI is much smaller than the WL, the reflections are specular.
4. The color of an object (its spectrum of reflected visible light) is not a reliable indicator of its reflectance in the infrared portion of the spectrum.

Thus an object which appears black to the eye (like a cast iron skillet) will reflect strongly in the far infrared part of the spectrum at the wavelength of the CO_2 laser (10,600 nm). Reduction of reflectance for infrared radiation is accomplished either by coating the surface with a layer of a nonmetallic substance like aluminum oxide, which has both a rough surface and strong absorbance in the far infrared, or by roughening the surface of a metallic object by sandblasting or shot-peening. All metals have moderately high reflectance in the near infrared range and this increases to 90 percent or higher in the far infrared (from 3000 nm to 1 mm) portion of the spectrum. The most effective means of reducing the reflectance of metal surfaces at the CO_2 wavelength is roughening, which changes the reflection from specular to diffuse.

Accidental Trauma by Direct Action of Laser Beams

Perforation of Hollow Organs

As CO_2 and Nd:YAG lasers are used more frequently in endoscopic procedures (either flexible or rigid), this hazard will carry a progressively higher risk. The CO_2 laser, presently used only for rigid endoscopy, removes tissue more rapidly because the power density of its beam is totally absorbed in a very shallow (less than 0.1 mm) surface layer without lateral scattering, and it quickly bores a hole if stationary or cuts a groove if moving. The beam of the Nd:YAG laser, by contrast, is strongly scattered in soft tissue, so that the power density within the tissue is much lower than in the incident beam, thus making it much more difficult for the surgeon to vaporize the tissue. Nonetheless, because most surgical Nd:YAG lasers can deliver up to 100 W of CW radiant power to the tissue, they can cause vaporization. Like the CO_2 laser, *the Nd:YAG should be fired only in short, repetitive bursts when its beam is applied within the lumen of any hollow organ.* Furthermore, there is a latent danger peculiar to the Nd:YAG laser. Because of strong forward scattering in soft tissue, the point of maximum histologic power density is not at the irradiated surface, as with the CO_2 laser, but displaced forward along the beam axis into the tissue by as much as several millimeters. This phenomenon produces what has been described by Halldorsson and colleagues[14] as the "popcorn effect": an explosive rupture of the tissue as the temperature at the displaced point of maximum power density rises to the boiling level of 100°C. Because this point is surrounded by tissue and *concealed from the view of the surgeon,* the only forewarning is a progressive blanching, possibly followed by charring, of the irradiated surface before the explosion occurs. As the intratissue temperature rises through 60°C, the thermal coagulation of the proteins causes increased scattering and accentuates the popcorn effect. The popcorn effect usually occurs only after continuous irradiation of 10 to 20 seconds in duration. *It will happen even if the irradiated surface is flooded with liquid saline or high molecular weight dextran,* when the histologic power density is high enough to cause vaporization of cellular water. Figure 6–5 shows schematically the effects of Nd:YAG laser radiation in soft tissue.

Obviously such explosive destruction of tissue is undesirable. Not only can it scatter viable malignant cells from a tumor, but it can also cause rupture of the wall of a hollow organ during an endoscopic procedure. *Perforation of the wall of the esophagus or trachea can quickly expose one or more of the great blood vessels to damage by the laser beam (CO_2 or Nd:YAG) and the very imminent possibility of a sudden, fatal hemorrhage.* This has happened to at least two

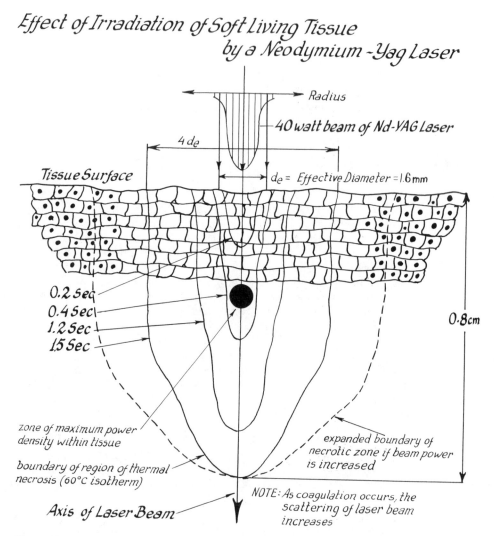

Figure 6–5. Schematic illustration of effects of Nd:YAG irradiation in soft living tissue, showing extent of isothermal surfaces as functions of time after onset. *(Adapted from Halldorsson et al.[14])*

human patients. In this regard, the CO_2 laser is capable of much faster puncture than the Nd:YAG. The full extent of tissue destruction, however, is always visible to the user of a CO_2 laser, thus allowing much more precise control. To quote the old teaching maximum, "what you see is what you get" with the CO_2 laser. The Nd:YAG, on the other hand, gives its operator only a poor visual indication of tissue damage, but counterbalances this deficit by producing lower histologic power density for a given beam diameter and power. When the rapid boring of the CO_2 is compared to the popcorn effect of the Nd:YAG, giving due weight to the difference in visualization of damage, these two laser types pose about equal risks of fistulization. With either type, *cautious intermittent irradiation during endoscopy is highly advisable.*

Rigid laparoscopy is now done routinely with the CO_2 laser, particularly for the removal of ectopic endometriosis in the pelvic peritoneal cavity. Though this is a safe procedure in skilled hands, there is a possible risk of perforating one or more of the viscera. At best, single puncture laparoscopy gives the surgeon a two-dimensional view with distorted perspective. The dual puncture technique offers some improvement in depth perception. With the advent of suitable flexible fibers for the CO_2 laser beam, there will be increasing use of this laser in flexible laparoscopy, making more of the peritoneal cavity accessible without laparotomy. The Nd:YAG laser will quite probably be utilized for laparoscopic procedures as more surgeons discover the advantages of near infrared radiation, particularly in the management of metastatic abdominal malignancies. With both of these lasers, *the risk of accidental visceral puncture is high. Laparoscopic laser irradiation should be done cautiously and intermittently, with adequate suction to remove vapor,* so that the surgeon has a clear visual field at all times.

Abdominal procedures with lasers, through a laparotomy, now routinely done for lysis of adhesions, fimbrioplasty, fallopian reconstruction, etc. pose a much lower risk of visceral perforation by the laser beam. The surgeon, however, must remember to *provide adequate backstopping* for the laser beam, either by cottonoids soaked in normal saline or by mechanical implements designed for this purpose. *Glass backstops should not be used.* They crack and shatter after repeated impacts of the laser beam (CO_2), scattering almost invisible fragments which are nearly impossible to find and remove.

Injury to Neural Tissue
Extreme caution and lasing in short bursts are advisable when removing lesions on or near important nerves. The CO_2 is the laser of choice for neurosurgical excision or vaporization. The Nd:YAG is useful in coagulation of highly vascular lesions such as aneurisms and hemangiomas, and in coagulation of large meningiomas prior to vaporization by CO_2 laser or removal by ultrasonic aspiration.

Injury to Eyes
The handbooks on general laser safety[15,16] usually regard this as the most serious hazard of lasers to humans. In the setting of a scientific laboratory, an industrial plant, or a military operation, this is quite true. In the operating room or laser clinic, however, a very different set of conditions prevails. Statistically, the incidence of eye injuries by lasers (excluding the obvious category of deliberate or accidental injuries in the ophthalmic applications of lasers) is very low in surgery and therapy. The physiologic and emotional consequences of eye injuries to the victim are quite severe, and this hazard would rank higher on our list were it not for its low incidence. The low rate of laser accidents involving eyes in medical applications is probably the result of a high level of awareness of the hazard on the part of physicians and nurses.

Damage to eyes by laser beams is not the same for all wavelengths. Both the location of the damage, i.e., cornea, lens, or fundus and maximum safe radiant exposure are functions of wavelength. In general, the radiant energy of visible lasers passes harmlessly through the cornea, aqueous, lens, and vitreous of the eye to the retina and choroid, where it is converted to heat, except for a very small amount which produces the electrochemical reactions which generate visual sensations in the rods and cones. The argon laser, with wavelengths of 488 and 514 nm (blue and green, respectively), takes advantage of this fact to produce coagulation of the pigmented and vascular structures of the fundus. The rays of near-infrared lasers, like those of the Nd:YAG at 1064 nm, though not visibly perceptible by the eye, are primarily absorbed by the fundus also. There is, however, some small absorption of near-infrared rays by the cornea, lens, capsule, and vitreous; this absorption becomes significantly enhanced if the cornea, lens, or capsule is cataractous. Such absorption is not essential to the process by which the new (since 1977) class of ultra-short-pulsed Nd:YAG lasers cause precise focal perforations of the posterior capsule in patients who have previously had their cataractous natural lenses replaced by plastic implants and later develop opacities of the posterior remnant of the capsule. These lasers cause very localized destruction of molecular, cytologic, and histologic architecture by virtue of the intense electric fields (10^8 V/m and higher) associated with their rays in the vicinity of the focal point of the beam. The small f-number of the focusing lens, together with the exceedingly short duration of the pulses of laser energy (a few picoseconds to many nanoseconds, depending upon the pulsing method) produce focal power densities of 1×10^{10} W/cm^2 and higher. The enormous electric fields of these rays literally strip the outer-shell electrons off the atoms in the tissue and form a plasma consisting of about equal concentrations of free electrons and positive ions at temperatures of 15,000°C or higher. The diameter of the damaged region is usually a small fraction of a millimeter. Shock-wave and thermal effects are usually insignificant because of the small energy per pulse (a few millijoules).

At the far-infrared wavelength (10,600 nm) of the CO_2 laser, all of the radiant energy is converted to heat at the surface of the cornea or the sclera. Though not yet available as radiation from medical lasers, far-ultraviolet rays (100 to 315 nm) are strongly absorbed at the outer scleral or corneal surface; near-ultraviolet rays (315 to 400 nm) are primarily absorbed by the lens. Far-ultraviolet rays from excimer lasers have been proposed as cutting energy for such corneal surgery as radial keratotomy to correct visual defects like myopia resulting from inadequate refraction of the cornea and lens. The radiant energy at these wavelengths is totally absorbed in a very shallow depth of tissue and scattering is insignificant. Thus far-ultraviolet lasers, if suitably developed and if approved by the U.S. FDA, may become competitive with CO_2 lasers in certain precise surgical applications.

The safest practice is to require everyone in a laser operating room or treatment area to wear protective eyeshields when the laser is in use. The spectral transmission characteristics of these eyeshields must be chosen according to the wavelength(s) to be screened out. For the invisible rays of the CO_2 laser, ordinary corrective glasses or industrial safety goggles or face shields will provide adequate *temporary* protection, while allowing high transmission of the visible spectrum for eyesight. It must be remembered that, *at surgical power densities (300 to 500,000 W/cm^2), the focused beam of a CO$_2$ laser will eventually puncture glass or plastic* of the thickness used in ordinary eyeglasses and safety shields. The impact of the beam upon the surface of the eyeshield will produce a *visible warning* in the form of cracking, crazing, flame, or smoke which alerts the wearer to get his or her head out of the beam. Safety goggles or face shields which can be worn over corrective glasses are preferable, because they provide shielding at the sides and over the eyebrows. The surgeon need not wear any eyeshield against the beam of a CO_2 laser when looking through a binocular surgical microscope, because the several thicknesses of internal optical glass give adequate protection at this wavelength. This is not true, however, for the rays of visible and near infrared lasers. When visible lasers are used, e.g., the argon laser, with ophthalmoscopes or endoscopes, these scopes must be provided with automatic shutters which cut off transmission of the light to the operator's eyes while the laser beam is on, or with slip-on viewing lenses which transmit the visible spectrum except for the strongly attenuated region around the wavelength(s) of the laser.

Eyeshields for visible lasers must attenuate the incident radiation to a level which is safe for direct viewing of the laser beam over a time interval at least as long as that which the eyeshield itself can endure without damage. If we arbitrarily take this time as 10 seconds, then we can calculate the maximum permissible eye exposure for direct (intrabeam) viewing of the laser beam, as well as the attenuation factor needed in the eyeshield, for any given power density in the direct laser beam. In 1976, the American National Standards Institute (ANSI) promulgated a set of maximum permissible exposures for intrabeam viewing of lasers, and these have been adopted by government and industry as standards for protection of eyes against laser radiation. These ANSI Standards, Z 136.1 of 1976, state that the maximum permissible exposure (mpe) of the human eye to the direct beam of a laser whose wavelength lies in the range 400 to 700 nm is 1.0×10^{-3} W/cm^2, for a 10-second exposure. Taking the highest power density available from a medical laser in this spectral range, namely 20 W averaged over a Gaussian focal spot of 0.1 mm effective diameter, or 200,000 W/cm^2, we see that a protective eyeshield must attenuate this direct beam by a factor of 200,000,000. Because of the large numerical values of attenuation required for eye protection, it is customary to specify attenuation in terms of *optical density,* (OD) where

$$OD \equiv \log_{10} (\text{attenuation}). \tag{6-2}$$

Hence the optical density of a safe eyeshield for 10-second exposure to any Ar laser must be 8.3 at the wavelengths of 488 and 514 nm. The dye laser, usually operated between 600 and 700 nm in photoradiation therapy, produces much lower power densities than Ar. Because the laser operator must be able to see the surgical site and its surroundings while wearing the eyeshield, the spectral variation of OD in the eyeshield must be such that it is low (less than 1.0) over as much of the visible spectrum as possible, and high only around the wavelength(s) that must be screened out.

For the spectral range 1060 to 1400 nanometers, and a 10-second exposure, the ANSI Standards show that the mpe is 5.0×10^{-3} W/cm^2. The maximum power available from the present Nd:YAG lasers used in medical applications is 150 W. Averaged over a Gaussian beam of focal effective diameter of 1.0 mm, this gives a power density of 15,000 W/cm^2. To reduce this to 5 mW/cm^2 requires an attenuation of 3,000,000. The equivalent optical density is 6.5. The eyeshield must allow good transmission of visible light for viewing the surgical site.

Good eyeshields can usually be obtained from the manufacturers of the lasers against which protection is sought. Alternatively, the surgeon or hospital safety officer can procure them directly from a maker of such devices, e.g., Glendale Optical Company. Some notes of caution are in order here. Most of the eyeshields for visible and near infrared lasers have distinct color when viewed by reflected or transmitted light. *It is not easy, however, for the prospective user of an unidentified eyeshield to judge its spectral transmittance or optical density merely by looking through it. The laser practitioner should never rely on an unknown eyeshield while using a laser simply because that shield looks like one which is known to be effective. In fact, it is highly advisable to test every eyeshield before it is worn for the first time,* even if it has been newly obtained from a reputable manufacturer. The engineering department of the hospital will often have a multirange radiant power meter available; this can be used to make a quick test of a new eyeshield by placing the shield across the defocused beam of the laser and measuring the power transmitted, on the appropriate meter range. The incident power of the unattenuated beam can be measured either by the power meter on the laser console or by the multirange external meter (on the appropriate scale) with the eyeshield removed from the beam. The power meter must have at least seven decade ranges from 100 W down to 10^{-5} W, because the optical densities required for adequate protection of eyes are in the order of seven. Such a meter, Model 460, is made by EG&G Electro-Optics of Salem, Mass. It has seven decade ranges, measures maximum power levels up to 1000 W, and has a choice of five specific wavelengths in the range of 200 to 1100 nm. It is not necessary to test plastic or glass eyeshields for CO_2 laser beams in this fashion, because any plastic, glass, or quartz in a thickness of 1 mm or more will have an optical density of 20 or higher at 10,600 nm.

If subjected to power densities in the range of 300 to 20,000 W/cm^2, eyeshields for visible and near infrared lasers may be damaged (crazing, cracking, or melting). Before putting on a previously used eyeshield, the prospective wearer should examine it for signs of such damage, and discard it if they are present.

However, wearing eyeshields is not enough, by itself, to guarantee safety for the eyes of surgical personnel. The laser surgeon must train the surgical assistants to disarm (inactivate) the laser routinely when it is not being actively used to irradiate the patient. The surgeon must then ask an assistant to rearm the laser for firing the next time it is needed. This simple procedure will avoid accidental lasing of any unintended target if the surgeon should accidentally depress the foot switch while the laser aperture (emission port) is pointed in any direction but at the intended target. The articulated arm and handpiece or the surgical microscope used with a CO_2 laser will often be swung aside while the surgeon uses suction or mechanical instruments, thus creating a danger of accidentally lasing one of the surgical assistants. This danger is even greater with the slender, ultra flexible optical fiber used to deliver the beam of an Ar or Nd:YAG laser: when not restrained by the operator's hand, it can whip around randomly like a live snake. Fortunately, the divergence of a focused CO_2 laser beam beyond the focal point of the handpiece or the microscope, or the conical expansion of the beam of an Ar or Nd:YAG laser away from the free end of the delivering fiber, reduces the power density in inverse proportion to the square of the distance. For practical purposes, the power density falls to noninjurious levels for 10-second direct viewing at a distance of 15 m from the emission port of the laser applicator (micromanipulator, handpiece, or fiber), for any medical laser now in common use. This fact, however, should not be used as an excuse for failing to wear eyeshields or to disarm an idle laser.

An exceptionally dangerous condition exists when a CO_2 laser is energized while its articulated arm is not terminated at its distal end by a handpiece or a micromanipulator, or some device containing a focusing lens. The beam emerging from the unterminated distal end of the articulated arm is highly collimated and has a diameter typically in the order of 1 cm. At a power of 100 W, such a beam will have an average power density of 110 W and a central power density of 255 W/cm^2, if it is Gaussian. Because of its collimation, this beam will have negligible divergence in distances of 100 m or more. Even a power level of 30 W under these conditions will produce dangerous power densities at great distances.

Contrary to popular opinion, *the He-Ne laser beam used as an aiming designator is not safe for direct viewing.* Typically, these lasers deliver 2 to 5 mW of radiant power. At the He-Ne wavelength of 633 nm, virtually all of the light striking an eye is absorbed by the retina and choroid. The human eye can safely endure a 10-second exposure to a power density of only 1 mW/cm^2 at this wavelength. However, an aiming beam of 2.0 mW focused to a spot of 1.0 mm has a central power density of 0.51 W/cm^2, or 510 times the safe level! Although postfocal divergence will reduce this power density with distance, the diameter of the He-Ne beam entering the final focusing lens of the laser system may be considerably smaller than that of a CO_2 or Nd:YAG laser; this means that its f-number will be much larger than that of the primary beam and its divergence angle much smaller. Furthermore, *eyeshields for CO_2 or Nd:YAG lasers do not filter out the He-Ne wavelength;* if they did, the operator could not see the aiming beam as it reflects from the target. *The laser operator should scrupulously avoid looking directly into the aiming beam.*

The BRH requires that every laser sold in the United States bear certain warning labels. Each opening or port through which laser radiation can emerge during normal operation must be labeled with the legend LASER APERTURE. There is, then, no excuse for anyone in the laser operating room or treatment area to look directly into a laser aperture without knowing that it is an exit port for the laser beam. *Any laser aperture should be treated with the same respect accorded to the muzzle of a loaded gun.*

Finally, *warning signs should be conspicuously placed on each access door to a laser operating room or treatment area,* prohibiting the entry of unauthorized persons and requiring those who do enter to put on the appropriate eyeshields. The laser personnel and safety officers must always be mindful of the old proverb, "Familiarity breeds contempt." This is true of those who work around lasers for long periods with no mishaps. Carelessness gradually replaces caution, sometimes with tragic results. Those in charge of lasers in the hospital or clinic must be vigilant to prevent this from happening.

Injury to Other Body Parts

For laser room personnel, avoidance of this hazard depends upon strict adherence to a procedural rule requiring that the laser be disarmed when not being used to irradiate the patient. Since all medical lasers have a standby position of the power control switch, this is easy to do. Fortunately, laser injuries to the skin cause immediate, intense pain which triggers reflexive withdrawal of the irradiated part from the laser beam, provided that it is not anesthetized. Moreover, superficial laser injuries heal quickly, often without scars.

The laser patient, however, will usually be anesthetized, at least locally, and therefore unprotected by neuromuscular reflexes. *If the patient is under general anesthesia, his or her eyes should be covered by thick, wet cottonoid pads of 4-inch × 4-inch size taped securely in place over eyelids previous taped shut* after subblepheral application of a bland ocular ointment. If conscious, a patient should wear the same protective eyeshield as the medical personnel. Those portions of the patient's anatomy surrounding the surgical site should be covered only by sterile drapes or pads soaked in sterile water or normal saline. *Epidermal areas may be covered, alternatively, with rumpled, heavy gauge aluminum foil taped in place.* This diffusely reflects the laser beam. There remains the hazard of specular reflection from the polished surface of a metal instrument. Usually such surfaces will be convex, with short radii of curvature, thus producing rapidly divergent reflections which greatly reduce the power density over short distances from the instrument. In most cases, such reflections will not cause serious trauma to nearby organic structures, but the surgeon must be constantly alert to avoid prolonged reflective exposures. This hazard can be greatly diminished by having all surgical hand instruments sandblasted or shot-peened to produce a rough satin finish. Blackening by chemical treatment (e.g., anodizing) is effective in the visible and near infrared portions of the spectrum, but not at the CO_2 wavelength of 10,600 nm, unless a thick layer of oxide is deposited by the process.

Inappropriate or Unskilled Use of Lasers

This is usually the result of inexperience or lack of basic training on the part of the laser practitioner. Four common mistakes are possible:

1. Using the wrong laser for the purpose, e.g., Nd:YAG to vaporize or CO_2 to coagulate
2. Using the wrong power density for the procedure
3. Applying the laser beam to the tissue for too long or too short a time
4. Failing to remove or destroy all the diseased tissue because the depth and margins of the irradiation are inadequate.

The sequelae of these mistakes can be serious, and include recurrence of viral or malignant lesions, postoperative pain, and scarring, and preoperative hemorrhage. To use lasers effectively in surgery and therapy, it is necessary to understand the biophysics of laser light in living tissue. A discussion of some specific problems follows.

Laser Treatment of an Unidentified Lesion
Sound medical judgment should dictate that a laser not be used to vaporize or coagulate a lesion which is not fully accessible or of unknown extent, cytology, or histology. Biopsies must be taken *before* lasing. If the lesion cannot be fully destroyed by laser alone, then excise, amputate, or combine these with prior debulking by laser. Do not rely on the mistaken belief that a laser can magically cure disease without irradiating all of it so as to vaporize, excise, or thermally necrotize the entire morbid mass.

Excess Thermal Necrosis

In using a CO_2 laser, the operating rule to remember is simple: *Apply the highest power density at which your achieved coordination of eyes, mind, and hands will allow you to vaporize or cut tissue without greater destruction than you intend.* This technique minimizes the time of tissue exposure to the laser beam, and thus the unwanted thermal necrosis of adjacent healthy tissue. Normally the CO_2 laser will not be the instrument of choice to obtain hemostasis in vessels larger than 0.5 mm. However, presurgical injection of a suitable vasoconstrictor, e.g., vasopressin, in appropriate dosage directly into the tissue at and near the surgical site, or mechanical compression of a major feeding artery, will significantly enhance the hemostatic effect of the CO_2 laser at power densities up to 10,000 W/cm^2. If major bleeding occurs during surgery with the CO_2 laser and a Nd:YAG is not available, the proper hemostatic technique is to reduce the power density (by defocusing and/or lowering the power) until visible vaporization stops, and then "paint" the laser beam randomly and slowly over the hemorrhagic area until bleeding stops. This may take as long as a minute. Liquid blood overlying or overflowing the area must first be removed by suction and/or absorbent tamponade, before lasing at low power density will be effective. If the bleeding cannot be stopped this way within about 60 seconds or less, then other methods must be employed. *Prolonged lasing at low power density causes extensive thermal necrosis by hemispherical conduction of heat* away from the beam impact site to the surrounding tissue.

In using a Nd:YAG laser the objective is, or should be, coagulation per se. Because of the relatively deep axial penetration and strong omnidirectional scattering at 1064 nm, Nd:YAG radiation can quickly coagulate tissue volumes up to several cubic centimeters, either for hemostasis or for deliberate necrosis. It is inherently a much more effective tool for mass coagulation than either a CO_2 laser or an electrosurgical device, because it produces more voluminous heating than the CO_2 laser and better volumetric definition with more uniform histologic temperature than the electrocautery. The unpredictable density and spatial distribution of the high frequency electrosurgical current produce nonuniform coagulation, and tissue damage at fairly remote points by electric resistance heating.

Halldorsson and Langerholc[17] have demonstrated that, at depths up to 2 mm into a bladder wall irradiated in vitro by a Nd:YAG laser delivering 40 W in a 3-mm beam, the temperature elevations are about 2.5 times as high as those achievable by a CO_2 laser at the same time after onset of irradiation. In this comparison, the incident power density of the Nd:YAG beam was 489 W/cm^2, where that of the CO_2 was only 6 W/cm^2 (the characteristic power density of thermal conduction at a surface temperature of 100°C). Raising the incident power density of the CO_2 laser beam would only cause rapid vaporization of the bladder surface without further elevation of its temperature, upon which the rate of thermal conduction to the interior is solely dependent. The situation would not be markedly different in vivo, except that the characteristic power density of thermal conduction would be somewhat higher (perhaps about 10 W/cm^2) because of the increased water content of living tissue. Furthermore, in vivo, at depths of a centimeter or more, the difference in temperature elevations achievable by the Nd:YAG and CO_2 would be still greater. For deep coagulation, the CO_2 laser is no match for the Nd:YAG under any conditions.

At depths beyond its absorption distance (0.1 mm produces 99.95 percent absorption in water), the beam of a CO_2 laser can heat tissue only by thermal conduction into the mass, since its radiant energy is all converted to heat within this very shallow layer below the irradiated surface. The Nd:YAG easily wins the coagulation contest with the CO_2 because its much *deeper radiant penetration* and strong scattering produce far *higher power density of radiation in the bulk of the tissue,* where it is instantly converted to heat, so that *every point becomes a source of thermal energy.* By contrast, the process of thermal conduction, the only physical mechanism by which a CO_2 laser can heat any material beyond its absorption depth, requires a *decrease of temperature* with distance away from the tiny volume impacted by the beam.

Delayed Thermal Necrosis

It must be remembered that the death of tissue heated to a necrotizing temperature below 100°C is not instantaneous. Cells on the periphery of a coagulated tissue mass may undergo relatively slow physiologic death, which can take hours or even days after the irradiation. *If tissue has been too aggressively irradiated by the Nd:YAG surgeon or therapist, the ultimate volume of destruction can be much greater than intended.* Therefore a Nd:YAG laser should be applied cautiously and in repetitive bursts no longer than about 1 second each, whenever the output power is more than 30 W or so. If this precaution is not observed during endoscopy of, say, the trachea or esophagus, the surgeon may be confronted some time later with pneumothorax or pneumomediastinum resulting from tumor necrosis which is not structurally compensated by scar formation. Though this is not so great a hazard with the Nd:YAG laser as with the technique of photoradiation therapy (PRT), it cannot be ignored.

Fistulization by Photoradiation Therapy

Photoradiation therapy is finding some applications in the airway, digestive tract, female genital tract, and body surfaces for the conservative treatment of malignancies. Its use may very probably soon be extended to adjuvant therapy in general surgery. In cases where extensive infiltration by a tumor has occurred in the wall of a hollow viscus, tumor necrosis can result in a fistula. The morbid sequelae can readily be imagined by the reader, and need not be recited here. Once again, as with other forms of laser therapy, *cautious, intelligent application of this technique is mandatory.* Furthermore, the entire surface of the hematoporphyrin derivative (HpD)-injected patient's body is highly susceptible to photonic necrosis for up to 100 hours by sunlight or bright indoor illumination.

PREVENTION OF LASER ACCIDENTS

The laser modality has much to offer the gynecologist and other specialists in terms of precise, effective, conservative treatment of several maladies. Like any other modality, it has its own unique advantages, limitations, and dangers. Injuries and fatalities caused by medical lasers are occurring as this is written. *At any given rate of incidence, the total number of mishaps will continue to rise.*

Sooner or later, in a litigious society like ours, lawsuits will result and the sensation hungry news media will publicize them. The federal government, which has heretofore shown admirable restraint regarding medical lasers, may be impelled to place onerous restrictions on the use and further development of this highly promising means of surgery and therapy.

Regulation of Medical Lasers

The Role of the Hospital

The administration of the hospital is the key agency in setting and enforcing standards for the safe use of lasers in surgery and therapy. Ideally, these functions should be the province of the governing board of some professional organization chartered for this purpose. However, no such organization now exists, although some of the established medical specialties now recognize the laser as a valid modality. These specialties have scarcely promulgated even guidelines, let alone standards, for the safe and effective use of lasers, or for the accreditation of laser practitioners. Therefore, at present, the only effective means of ensuring the proper use of lasers in medical applications is the control that every hospital already exerts over its medical and surgical staffs.

The majority of laser injuries in hospitals and clinics have occurred because a neophyte operator of a laser did not receive adequate prior training in its proper use, or disregarded the advice of those who did. The hospital administration can reduce the incidence of laser accidents to the statistically inevitable minimum by simply requiring that every laser aspirant on the staff must take one or more continuing medical education (CME) accredited courses in laser surgery-therapy, followed by an individual preceptorship under an experienced laser practitioner, before being allowed to use a laser in treating a patient. These training programs are now so numerous and moderately priced that there is no excuse for failing to require them for accreditation in laser practice.

The hospital should appoint one member of its institutional review board or committee to serve as the laser control officer, with responsibility for the establishing of accreditation standards for laser practice in all specialties, and the authority to promulgate and enforce rules for the proper use and maintenance of all lasers at that institution. As part of this process, one simple element can greatly reduce the hospital's risk of litigation by disgruntled patients: the adoption of a standard form of informed patient consent, to be signed by both the patient and the laser practitioner prior to laser treatment. This is mandatory in the case of the Nd:YAG laser, and highly advisable for all other types whether required or not by governmental regulations. A suggested model format which the author has recommended to various institutions for which he has served as a laser consultant, is shown in Figure 6–6. Figure 6–7 shows a model format of practitioner's affidavit of competence to perform laser surgery or therapy. Though this latter form may be resented by the untrained or inexperienced practitioner, it will be of considerable value to the hospital or clinic in its own defense if a malpractice suit is brought following a laser accident or a laser procedure of which the results were unsatisfactory.

INFORMED CONSENT TO LASER TREATMENT

I, _____(name of patient)_____ , have read the written material given to me, describing the uses of lasers in therapy and surgery, and I have heard the spoken description of the _____(type of laser)_____ laser and its beneficial uses in therapy and surgery given to me by _____(names of physicians, surgeons, or paramedical persons)_____ on _____(date)_____ . I certify that I understand all of this information, and that I hereby agree to have the following surgical or therapeutical procedure(s) performed upon me: _____

_____

_____

by _____(name(s) of surgeon(s) and other participating persons)_____ , using an FDA-approved laser, among other devices, in such a manner and to such extent as the aforenamed person(s) may decide is indicated, on the basis of his, her, or their training and experience in _____(medical specialty)_____ and in laser therapy and/or surgery. I have been told by the aforenamed informants that no warranty can be made by them to me regarding the medical, surgical, or cosmetic quality of the results of this procedure, except that they will perform the procedure(s) described above in a manner consistent with the accepted standards of United States medical and surgical practice generally, and of _____(medical specialty)_____ in particular. My signature below attests to the truth of the statements made herein.

SIGNED: _____ (patient)

WITNESS: _____(other than patient or physician)_____

PHYSICIAN IN CHARGE: _____

DATE: _____

Figure 6–6. Suggested format for obtaining informed consent of the patient to laser surgery or therapy.

Governmental Controls

Both the federal government of the United States and the governments of many of the individual states have imposed regulations on the use of lasers in therapy and surgery. In a general way, these regulations bear more heavily on those who manufacture and sell lasers than upon those who use them. These regulations, if they refer to licensed medical or surgical professionals at all, generally presume that the individual's license to practice is prima facie evidence of competence to use lasers in the course of treating patients, wherever the use of lasers is deemed safe, proper, and effective in the opinion of the medical profession generally, the practitioner's specialty in particular, on the cognizant authorities at the institution where the individual practices. The sheer number and diversity of state laws and regulations make a discussion of them here impractical and impertinent to the topic of laser safety in surgery and therapy.

PHYSICIAN'S AFFIDAVIT
OF COMPETENCE TO PERFORM
LASER THERAPY OR SURGERY

I, _____(name of physician)_____ , hereby certify that I have received formal training and instruction qualifying me for CME credits in laser therapy and/or surgery
in _____(medical specialty)_____ , and that I have been approved by the cognizant
authorities of this institution, _____(name and address of hospital or clinic)_____

_____

as a qualified practitioner of laser therapy and/or surgery in my specialty at this
institution.

SIGNED: _____(signature of physician)_____

DATE: _____

Figure 6-7. Suggested format for surgeon's affidavit of competence to perform laser surgery or
therapy.

The federal government, through the agency of the FDA, in the Department of
Health and Human Services, imposes restrictions on the manufacture, sale, and
use of lasers for medical purposes. Specifically, the Bureau of Radiological Health
(BRH)* and the Bureau of Medical Devices (BMD) of the FDA have jurisdiction
over medical lasers. These regulatory powers, as they refer to lasers, may sometime
be placed entirely in the hands of the BRH, but at the moment both bureaus have
authority, fortunately not conflicting, over medical lasers. The rules of the BRH
deal almost exclusively with those who make, sell, and service medical lasers as
business activities. They are published in the Code of Federal Regulations, 21
CFR 1040. This and other information relevant to lasers is available by writing to
the Bureau of Radiological Health, Division of Compliance, U.S. Dept. of Health
and Human Services, Rockville, Maryland 20850.

These regulations became effective for all laser products manufactured for use
in the United States after August 1, 1976. Essentially, 21 CFR 1040 does the
following:

1. It sorts all lasers into classes according to accessible emission limits, i.e.,
   the total radiant power or energy which can fall upon a target external to
   the laser, as functions of wavelength and the duration of radiant emission.
   These are Classes I, II, III, and IV. (Virtually all lasers used for surgery
   and therapy are in Class IV, most dangerous.)

---

*After this chapter had been completed the BRH and the BMD were combined into the National
Center for Devices and Radiological Health (NCDRH).

2. It requires that manufacturers place certain labels on each laser to show its class, output characteristics, warnings to operators, and the aperture(s) through which radiation can emerge (Fig. 6–8).
3. It sets limits on the collateral radiation emissible by a laser during normal operation, e.g., x-rays which may be emitted by high voltage components, and light emitted by pumping lamps.
4. It establishes tests which must be made by the manufacturer to show that the laser product complies with the regulations.
5. It sets performance requirements for lasers, e.g., protective housings, safety interlocks, emission indicators, beam attenuators (shutters), and location of controls.
6. It imposes requirements on the manufacturer to keep certain records and make certain periodic reports to the BRH.

In addition to the general requirements for all lasers set forth in 21 CFR 1040, §1040.11 thereof sets forth certain special requirements for medical laser products.

These requirements are extremely detailed, and there is little value in reciting them here. They are well summarized and explained by Sliney and Wohlbarsht[16] in their excellent handbook on laser safety, to which the interested reader can refer. Only the laser safety officer of the hospital is likely to derive much practical benefit from a study of these regulations. Suffice it here to say that the only lasers having any biomedical application which are not in Class II (hazardous), Class III (hazardous-dangerous), or Class IV (most dangerous) are the low powered (under 1.0 mW) lasers now being used rather extensively in treating racehorses for pain and tendonitis. These are usually solid state diode lasers producing wavelengths in the range of 800 to 950 nm.

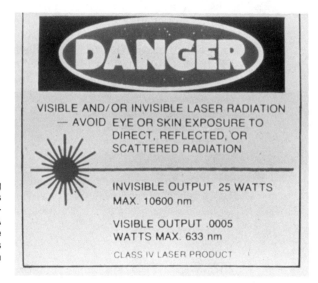

Figure 6–8. Typical warning label for a CO_2 surgical laser, as required by the Bureau of Radiological Health of the U.S. FDA Not shown, but also required, are labels designating the apertures through which laser radiation can emerge.

The Bureau of Medical Devices (BMD) of the FDA has operational jurisdiction over all medical hardware from tongue depressors to computerized tomographic scanners. The BMD places all such devices into one of three categories:

Class I   Simple devices of long usage, historically, which are well understood and not used for life support, e.g., fever thermometers

Class II   More complex devices, but proved by long usage and well understood; not for life support; must meet prescribed standards of performance, e.g., electrosurgical devices

Class III   More complex devices, used for life support and/or still under clinical investigation. These devices must be used under specific protocols approved by the institutional review committee of the hospital and under *Investigational Device Exemptions* (IDEs) approved by the BMD, e.g., Nd:YAG lasers and ultrasonic phacoemulsifiers

For virtually all known applications (and, by "grandfather" extension, to nearly any conceivable future application), the CO_2 laser is in BMD Class II, as is the Ar laser. The Nd:YAG laser, however, is at this writing still in BMD Class III for all applications presently being studied. This fact should not deter the gynecologist or other specialist from undertaking a study program of surgery or therapy with the Nd:YAG laser, because the manufacturers of these devices have already collaborated with various physicians and hospitals to prepare approved protocols and secure IDEs for those applications now being studied. These IDEs can readily be extended to include new investigators, by getting an approved protocol from a manufacturer and submitting it to the BMD with a formal request to be added to the list of investigators authorized to use the Nd:YAG laser under the existing IDE. Because of the wide clinical experience now accumulated in the several recognized uses of the Nd:YAG, obtaining permission from the BMD for studying new applications is a relatively routine procedure, in which the laser manufacturer may often provide assistance at no charge to the physician.

INTERACTION OF LASER LIGHT WITH LIVING TISSUE

This is an exceedingly complex subject, which has been discussed in great detail in many books and articles. For the interested reader who wishes to pursue the subject in greater depth than our basic presentation here, a good starting point is the book edited by Hillenkamp, Pratesi, and Sacchi.[18] The following presentation is intended to give the reader a qualitative understanding of what happens when a laser beam strikes biologic tissue. The emphasis is practical, and theory is presented only as an aid to comprehension of basic principles.

The coherence, collimation, and monochromaticity of laser light make it possible to focus laser beams down to very small spots, having minimum diameters of a few wavelengths, in which the power density can exceed a million watts per square centimeter. This ability to achieve tiny focal spots or large beam diameters at will, together with the resultant variation in power density, is probably the most important single advantage of the laser in surgery and therapy. Of secondary importance is the spectral purity of laser light. Although few, if any, photobiologic phenomena require light of such narrow spectral linewidth, the ability to put all the radiant power of the source into one or a few wavelengths is of great advantage in treatment of those diseases for which optical radiation is useful.

The effects of radiation from medical lasers on living tissue fall into three basic categories:

1. *Heating.* This is the absorption of radiant energy by the molecules of the tissue, with conversion into heat and increase of temperature.
2. *Stimulation or moderation of chemical reactions.* This is the conversion of radiant energy into stored chemical energy, in stable compounds, or its conversion into thermal energy which causes breakage of complex molecular structures, or its excitation of photosensitizers which chemically interact with living tissue. These effects occur at low power densities.
3. *Mechanical disruption of histologic structure.* This is the result of pressure waves or of bulk movement of tissue caused by rapid vaporization of intra- and extracellular water or other cytologic materials heated by absorbed radiation.

When a laser beam strikes the surface of a tissue mass, there is a reflection of some fraction of the incident power. Of the remaining radiant power, which penetrates the tissue, some will be converted to other forms of power, such as heat flow, or to radiation at different wavelengths, e.g., fluorescence, or chemical energy storage, e.g., photosynthesis in green plants. Some of the penetrating radiation may be transmitted through, or scattered out of, thin tissue sections. Once inside the tissue, the incident rays of the laser beam will, in general, no longer retain their original collimation, because of scattering from particles and molecules in the tissue. Each scattered ray will itself be scattered repeatedly, and along each trajectory between scattering centers there will be absorption of the radiant power by the constituents of the tissue. The great majority of this absorbed energy is converted to heat, which flows from the conversion sites to other parts of the tissue by thermal conduction and/or convection, e.g., in the vasculature. This thermal power may be converted into mechanical energy flow in the form of pressure waves (acoustic transients), or kinetic energy flow in the form of mass movements of tissue and vapor.

If we therefore trace a path parallel to the axis of the incident laser beam, and measure the power density at points along this straight line, we find that it has a maximum value, p, just outside the tissue surface. Just inside the tissue surface the ongoing power density, p_o, is lower than p because some of it, p_r, is reflected at the surface. As we go deeper into the tissue along this straight line, the internal (histologic) power density, p_i, diminishes steadily because of the combined effects of scattering and absorption. These facts are quantitatively summarized in the simple expression of Bouguer's law (often attributed to Beer or Lambert):

$$p_i = (p - p_r)\, \epsilon^{-Az}, \tag{6-3}$$

where p_i is the power density on the beam axis inside the tissue, (power)/(area); p is the power density on the beam axis just outside the tissue; p_r is the power density reflected from the surface on the beam axis; ϵ is the base of the natural logarithms, = 2.71828 (numeric); A is the attenuation coefficient, (length)$^{-1}$; and z is distance below the tissue surface measured along the axis of the beam. The attenuation coefficient is the sum of two parts:

$$A = \alpha + \beta, \qquad (6\text{-}4)$$

where α = the absorption coefficient, and β = the scattering coefficient.

For the complex structures of living tissues, which contain a bewildering variety of chemical constituents, particulate inclusions, and physical arrangements of these, Bouguer's law is only an approximation to what actually happens as a beam of light traverses an organism. It tells us that absorption and scattering of light in tissue is color dependent, because the coefficients α and β are functions of wavelength for the elements and structures which constitute the tissue.

Scattering

Scattering in tissue is an exceedingly complex phenomenon, depending upon the size of the scattering elements relative to the wavelength of the radiation, their density, and their spatial organization. There are two basic kinds: Rayleigh scattering and Mie scattering. Rayleigh scattering occurs when the scattering elements (which can be molecules, particulates, or whole cells) are much smaller in size than the wavelength of the scattered light. For a given material medium, the Rayleigh coefficient β is inversely proportional to the fourth power of the wavelength, and the intensity of the scattered light does not vary drastically with the angle of the scattered ray off the axis of the laser beam. At an angle of 90 degrees, i.e., perpendicular to the beam, the scattered intensity is one-half as strong as that in the forward or backward direction along the beam axis. Rayleigh scattering is the predominant kind in all pure solids, liquids, and gases as well as in true solutions, for wavelengths in the ultraviolet, visible, and near infrared portions of the spectrum, because in these the scattering elements are atoms and molecules. Mie scattering occurs when the scattering elements are comparable in size or larger than the wavelength of the scattered light. It is characterized by a strong dependence of the scattered intensity on the direction of the scattered ray relative to the beam axis, being most intense for small angles off the direction of the forward beam and very weak for other directions, especially parallel and opposite to the direction of propagation. The Mie coefficient declines with increasing wavelength, but at a much smaller rate than the Rayleigh coefficient. For particles much larger than the wavelength, the light is no longer scattered, but undergoes reflection and refraction.

There are some common examples of these phenomena which are familiar to all of us. The sky appears blue on a clear day because the white light of the sun is Rayleigh scattered by air molecules, most strongly at the blue end of the visible spectrum. Clouds, however, with fine water droplets cause Mie scattering; because the variation of scattered intensity is much less wavelength dependent, they appear white or grey.

To obtain some estimate of the relative importance of Rayleigh and Mie scattering in the medical uses of lasers, it is instructive to consider the range of sizes for the scattering elements in living tissues: atoms, molecules, and particulate inclusions, such as organelles within cells. Very approximately, these are as follows:

Inorganic Molecules:	0.01–1.0 nm
Organic Molecules:	1.0–1000 nm
Organelles:	1000–100,000 nm
Cells:	100,000–1,000,000 nm

From this tabulation we can see that water, cytosol, and plasma cause Rayleigh scattering for all medical lasers (400 nm $\leq \lambda \leq$ 10,600 nm). Large organic molecules, such as proteins, polypeptides, and polysaccharides, will cause Mie scattering for visible and near infrared lasers, but Rayleigh scattering for far infrared (CO_2). Small organelles cause Mie scattering for visible and near infrared lasers and Rayleigh scattering for far infrared. Large organelles and cells cause reflection and refraction for all medical lasers. Because of the inverse dependence of Rayleigh scattering on the fourth power of wavelength, the rays of the CO_2 laser are negligibly scattered in living organisms. The rays of visible lasers and near infrared are significantly scattered by the Mie effects, which predominate in biologic tissue and liquids. By comparison, the magnitude of the Rayleigh effects is small. Because of the extreme complexity of even one living cell, calculation of scattering coefficients from measurements made on pure substances is a futile exercise. As yet, little or no work has been done in the empiric determination of β-values for various kinds of animal tissue in vitro or in vivo, but this would be a worthwhile undertaking.

Absorption

Absorption of optical radiation by the molecules found in living tissue is strongly wavelength dependent. It is predominantly in the ultraviolet range 200 nm $\leq \lambda \leq$ 315 nm. For the range from 315 to 400 nm, only a small number of biomolecules show even a moderate absorption. In the visible and near infrared, 400 $\leq \lambda \leq$ 1400 nm, virtually no biologic molecules exhibit any absorption unless absorbing chromophores are naturally or artificially attached to them. Artificial chromophores can be dyes topically applied or parenterally introduced. Photosensitizers, such as psoralens or hematoporphryins, can be intravenously injected to cause optical absorption in this range of wavelengths. In the far infrared, where 1400 $\leq \lambda \leq$ 20,000 nm, all biomolecules have strong absorption because of vibrational energy bands.

Hence it can be said that human cells and tissues in their natural state are virtually transparent to laser radiation from Ar, He-Ne, dye, and Nd:YAG, except for erythrocytes and melanocytes, which contain two of the most important natural chromophores, hemoglobin and melanin, respectively. Absorption curves for these substances are shown in Figure 6–9. The curves for oxyhemoglobin and deoxyhemoglobin show the maximum difference in absorption at about 670 nm. Oxygen saturation in vivo can be found by measuring the relative absorption of blood in vivo at this wavelength (or the relative reflection). Rather than the pronounced peaks and valleys which characterize the absorption spectrum of hemoglobin, there is a smooth decline of absorbance for melanin as wavelength

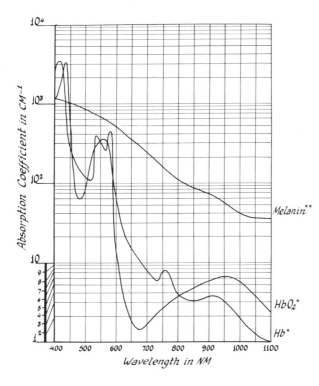

Figure 6–9. Absorption coefficient as a function of wavelength for oxyhemoglobin (HbO₂), deoxyhemoglobin (Hb), and melanin. HbO₂ and Hb are in a physiologic solution of 150 mg/liter in aqueous solution. The melanin curve shown corresponds to the concentration found in very dark skin; for fair caucasian skin, multiply the values shown by 10^{-1}. Key: *concentration = 150 mg/L; **in black skin. (Adapted from Hillenkamp.[19])

increases. At wavelengths where the absorption of hemoglobin is stronger than that of melanin, i.e., 400 to 430 nm, laser light could be used to destroy superficial vasculature, e.g., hemangiomas or telangiectasias, without serious damage to overlying or underlying skin. Conversely, at wavelengths where melanin is more strongly absorbent than hemoglobin, pigmented lesions like nevi can be selectively treated. This occurs at 488 nm (Ar) and 694 nm (ruby), and generally throughout the range from 450 to 700 nm.

Coefficients for Medical Lasers

Several investigators[12,18–20] have published values for α and/or β at the 1064-nm wavelength of the Nd:YAG in substances such as water, clear albumin, melanin, hemoglobin, and bladder wall tissue. The numerical values are not precise, but give us an idea of approximate magnitudes (all values are in cm^{-1}):

	Melanin[a]	HbO₂	Hb	Water	Albumin	Stomach or Bladder
α	3.5	3.3	0.8	0.18	0.15	0.11
β						5–10

[a]Physiol. Conc. = 150 g/l

It is probably safe to assume that the scattering coefficient of Nd:YAG rays in cells containing melanin and hemoglobin is not dramatically different from that of cells from the bladder wall. The significance of these numbers is that the absorption of Nd:YAG rays by the two major chromophores in animal tissue is the same (and within an order of magnitude of that of deoxyhemoglobin), while the absorption of nonpigmented tissue (the in vitro bladder lacked blood) is about the same as that of pure water or a clear serum. Furthermore, the scattering coefficient of unpigmented tissue is about equal to the absorption coefficient of the major coloring agents in living tissue. In addition, Halldorsson and Langerholc[14] have noted that the denaturation of protein at temperatures above 57°C causes greatly increased scattering, as evident from their experiments with clear albumin irradiated by the Nd:YAG laser.

The upshot of all this is that the Nd:YAG laser is almost ideally suited to voluminous heating of organic tissues and fluids irrespective of their natural coloration. For clear liquids, like water, blood plasma, and cytoplasm, and in unpigmented cells, the absorption coefficient is almost constant at about 1 to 2 percent of the scattering coefficient, a nearly optimum ratio for filling a large volume of tissue with radiation and converting it to heat within that volume. For pigmented cells containing either melanin or oxyhemoglobin, the absorption coefficient of Nd:YAG rays is about equal to the scattering, thus reducing the heated volume for a given beam diameter and power from what it would be in colorless tissue, but still allowing relatively deep penetration into blood for superior hemostasis in comparison to Ar and CO_2 lasers. For deoxygenated blood, the Nd:YAG produces a heated tissue volume which is larger than that for arterial blood but less than that for colorless tissue. Finally, one very important characteristic of Nd:YAG radiation is its strong forward scattering in tissue, probably due to a predominance of Mie effects over Rayleigh, which displaces the point of maximum histologic power density forward into the tissue on the beam axis. Although this effect was discussed under Perforation of Hollow Organs in this chapter (the popcorn effect) as a hazard, it is also a distinct advantage when used intelligently, because it produces higher histologic temperatures in depth than could be achieved by a hypothetical laser having the same coefficients of absorption and scattering but having predominantly Rayleigh scattering, where backscatter is as strong as forward scattering.

By contrast, the light of the Ar laser is not strongly absorbed or scattered by clear liquids and colorless tissue. Though there is a dearth of published information about the absorption and scattering coefficients at 514 nm in unpigmented tissue, the approximate values appear to be $\alpha = 0.01$ cm^{-1} and $\beta = 0.08$ cm^{-1}. It is evident that the scattering of Ar laser light in biologic liquids is due to Mie effects caused by large organic molecules, because a theoretic calculation of the Rayleigh scattering coefficient of pure water at 514 nm gives a value of 1×10^{-7} cm^{-1}. The rays of the Ar laser, because of the small magnitude of α and β, penetrate deeply into tissue and clear biologic liquids, with insignificant scattering. This means that the illuminated volume of tissue is essentially the effective beam area at the tissue surface multiplied by the thickness of the tissue, where major pigments are absent. The measured transmission of the structures of the human eye shows that this is so: about 83 percent of the light entering the cornea of a normal eye is transmitted to the retina at a wavelength of 514 nm.

A very different situation exists when Ar laser light irradiates hemoglobin or melanin, or any pigment whose spectral reflectance, i.e., color, is low at the blue side and high at the red side of the visible range. The absorption coefficient of hemoglobin at 514 nm is about 112 cm^{-1}, for either the oxygenated or reduced form. Hence the ratio of absorption to scattering for the rays of argon lasers in blood is $\alpha/\beta = 1400$. The corresponding depth for 99.9 percent absorption is only 0.62 mm. In melanin, the absorption coefficient for Ar light is about 1000 cm^{-1} and the corresponding absorption depth is 0.069 mm. The ratio of α to β is 12,500. The net effect of all this is to make the Ar laser quite useful in the coagulation of blood in small vessels or shallow vascular lesions, and in vaporization of strongly pigmented tissue which is yellow, orange, or red in color. For coagulation of large volumes of tissue however, it is ineffective no matter what the color. This explains why the Ar laser has failed in attempts to control massive gastrointestinal bleeding, but has been successful in treating nevi, angiectatic skin lesions, and proliferative vascularization of the ocular fundus.

The CO_2 laser is unexcelled for precise cutting or vaporization of tissue, irrespective of color or the histologic structure of the tissue. The absorption coefficient of water at the CO_2 wavelength of 10,600 nm is 770 cm^{-1} as measured by Bayly.[21] For biologic liquids like cytosol, plasma, and cerebrospinal fluid, the values of α are not dramatically different than that for pure water. In fact, for the whole gamut of substances from which human and animal bodies are composed, the value of absorption coefficient at 10,600 nm is of the order of 1000 cm^{-1}. Hence more than 99.9 percent of the power of a CO_2 laser beam is absorbed (converted into heat) in a depth of 0.1 mm beyond the first surface of incidence. *Scattering of CO_2 laser rays is completely negligible in all absorbing materials,* which is to say virtually all substances except most metals, a few intermetallic compounds, and some metal halides. The significance of these facts for the CO_2 laser is that it is ideally suited to precise tissue destruction with minimum transfer of heat to adjacent regions. It is poorly suited, however, to the task of voluminous heating for purposes of hemostasis, hyperthermia, or thermonecrosis.

All of the foregoing discussion can be summarized concisely in the following observations:

1. Lasers whose absorption depth is 0.1 mm or less for all tissue colors and whose ratio α/β is greater than 10,000 are superb photonic scalpels but poor coagulators. These are all far-infrared.

2. Lasers whose absorption depth is between 1 and 100 cm for the gamut of biologic materials and whose ratio α/β is between 0.01 and 1.0 are excellent photocoagulators but poor scalpels. Wavelengths fulfilling these criteria are all in the near-infrared.

3. Lasers which do not fulfill the foregoing criteria generally may still be useful for irradiation of particular biologic materials or tissues to produce specific effects. Examples are the dye laser tuned to 577 nm to coagulate blood in proliferative ectatic vasculature with minimal damage to surrounding skin, and the same laser tuned to 630 nm for activation of hematoporphyrin in cells of malignant tumors, where absorption by the tumor tissue itself would seriously attenuate light at the shorter wavelengths at which the hpd shows stronger absorption.

In the first two observations, it is tacitly assumed that the laser has a high enough power output and/or small enough beam diameter to produce histologic power densities adequate for the purpose.

Reflection

In general, when light strikes an interface between two media which differ in chemical composition or physical structure, some of the incident power density will be reflected back into the medium of origin. When a beam of light from a laser impinges on the surface of living tissue, the relative intensity of this reflection is wavelength dependent. Unfortunately, numerical values of reflectance for various types of animal tissue are scarce. The skin has probably been the subject of more reflectance measurements than any other body tissue, and these values give some general idea of the way in which reflectance varies with wavelength. Tabulated below are some approximate values of skin reflectance (ratio of p_r to p):

Laser	λ nm	Dark Skin (%)	Fair Skin (%)
	300	4	4
	400	10	32
Ar	514	12	43
Dye	700	33	65
Nd:YAG	1064	43	52
CO_2	10,600	6	6

For ultraviolet rays, which produce sunburn or tanning, the reflectance is low and the absorbance is high. Reflectance, as would be expected for creatures who survive and function in an environment filled with visible light, is moderate to high through the visible range. It falls to a level minimum value at about 4000 nm and is constant out to more than 50,000 nm. The reflectance values for dark skin are approximately those of tissue containing melanin anywhere in the body, while those for fair skin are probably representative for nonpigmented tissue, i.e., not containing melanin or hemoglobin. These numbers show that visible and near infrared lasers lose a large fraction of their incident power density by reflection at the surface of incidence. While this reflection is not generally hazardous to the attending personnel in a laser treatment area, because the reflection is diffuse, it does significantly reduce the power density which penetrates the tissue.

Only the CO_2 laser is relatively unaffected by reflection, another reason why it is the most suitable laser for cutting and vaporizing tissue. Not only reflection at the first surface must be considered, but reflections from organelles within cells are equally important. The radiation of the CO_2 laser is insensitive to target color, so these internal reflections have little effect upon its action in tissue. For the visible and near infrared lasers, however, notably the Nd:YAG, internal reflections play a major role in the scattering of light within cells and tissues. So-called Mie scattering is actually a composite of true scattering, refraction, and diffuse reflection.

Thermal Effects

As the direct and scattered rays of a laser traverse living tissue, they are progressively absorbed and converted into heat, which is random vibrational energy of the molecules. At every absorption center, the conversion of radiant energy to heat is essentially instantaneous, so that tissue being irradiated behaves as if it had a distributed group of point sources of heat. From each of these point sources of heat, there will be conduction of the thermal energy to all other points whose local temperatures are lower than that of the source point. For homogeneous and isotropic substances, the phenomenon of heat conduction has been extensively studied in both the steady and transient states. A transient state can be said to exist when the rate of thermal energy input to a substance is unequal to the rate at which it can be removed either by conduction away from the source, or by mass movements of the material in the form of solid, liquid, or vapor. In general, transient states will exist when the time duration of energy input to the material is much shorter than the time required for that material to remove the same amount of energy from the input site, as well as after the sudden cessation of energy input. During transient states, temperatures are changing; in steady states, temperatures are constant.

In tissue which is absorbing radiation, the temperature at every point where this radiation is being converted to heat will rise with time until heat is removed at a rate equal to that at which it is generated. We can phrase this concisely by saying that the tissue temperature will rise as long as the absorbed power density exceeds the removed power density. When the absorbed power density is enormously greater than the removed, the temperature of the tissue will rise rapidly to the point where cytosol and extracellular water boil, and the resulting steam will become superheated. The pressure can rise to several hundred atmospheres, causing a blast which propagates a shock wave before it in all directions outward from the irradiated volume. This is an uncontrollable effect which is never deliberately induced in present day surgery or therapy with lasers. However, a controlled rise of temperature to or below the boiling point of water is the objective in all laser surgery and in much laser therapy (except for laser-induced analgesia and photoradiation therapy). For surgery with the CO_2 laser, the temperature must reach $100°C$ within microseconds to milliseconds, so that rapid vaporization of cellular water occurs in an equilibrium state such that the absorbed radiant power is always equal to the rate at which energy is carried away by steam. Water is an excellent medium for this process, because it has a constant temperature of vaporization if constant pressure (atmospheric in this case) is maintained. For coagulative therapy, as with the Ar and/or the Nd:YAG laser, the histologic temperature must reach a value in excess of $60°C$ but lower than $100°C$ within a time-lapse of 0.01 to 10 seconds. Thermal equilibrium is not reached in these cases unless the heating culminates in vaporization, which is not advisable with these lasers, but the skilled practitioner controls the peak temperature by applying the radiation in short bursts of suitable magnitude and duration.

Equilibrium Conditions

Characteristic Power Density of Thermal Conduction

When the CO_2 laser destroys soft tissue it does so by rapidly boiling cytosol to form steam at atmospheric pressure or slightly higher and at a temperature of about 100°C. Because its absorption coefficient in water is very high, and its scattering coefficient is negligible, the impact volume of the tissue is essentially equal to the effective area of the beam multiplied by the absorption depth. This volume is usually very small: an effective diameter of 1.0 mm produces an impact volume of $0.1 \text{ mm} \times \pi/4 \times (1.0 \text{ mm})^2 = 0.0785 \text{ mm}^3$. The temperature within the impact volume quickly reaches the boiling point and remains constant unless the pressure of the steam rises above atmospheric, which it does not do unless either the power density is very high (megawatts/cm^2) or the irradiated volume is within a cul-de-sac from which the steam cannot readily escape. If the beam is stationary, the result is the boring of a hole whose diameter is about equal to the effective diameter of the beam (see reference 23 for a detailed discussion of the meaning and computation of effective diameter), and whose depth increases steadily with time as long as the irradiation continues. The shape of the crater in any cross-sectional plane passing through the beam axis will be an approximate geometric replica of the profile of power density for the beam in that plane. The wall of this crater, except near its rim, is an isothermal surface at about 100°C because it is the interface at which the laser rays are boiling the cellular water. This situation is illustrated in Figure 6–10, which shows schematically the crater made by a CO_2 laser beam in soft tissue.

Because the crater wall is at constant temperature, the conduction of heat away from the wall to the depths of the surrounding tissue is determined only by the change of temperature with time and distance between the wall and the tissue remote (more than 5 mm) from the crater, where circulation of lymph and blood carries away the heat so as to maintain a constant tissue temperature of 37°C. Immediately after the onset of boiling within the crater, the temperature of the surrounding tissue is still at 37°C, but rises with time because the outflowing thermal power is absorbed by this tissue mass at a rate of about 4 watt seconds (joules) per gram for every degree Celsius of temperature increase. Within a few seconds at most, the temperature of each point along every line perpendicular to the crater wall will reach a quasi-equilibrium temperature lying between 100°C and 37°C. At a distance of 5 mm or more, depending upon the nature of the tissue, the temperature will remain at normal body level. During this process, of course, the crater will be growing larger as irradiation continues, but its dimensions will not grow dramatically, because a 100 W CO_2 laser can vaporize only about 0.04 cm^3 of soft tissue in one second. The temperature in the tissue immediately surrounding the crater will decrease with distance in an exponential manner along every line normal to the crater wall. The slope of this exponential curve will always be greatest at the crater wall and fall toward zero where the temperature holds at 37°C. The thermal power density at any point along one of the lines of heat flow can be calculated from Fourier's equation of heat conduction:

$$p_t = -c_t \frac{dT}{dx} \text{, (power)/(area),} \tag{6–5}$$

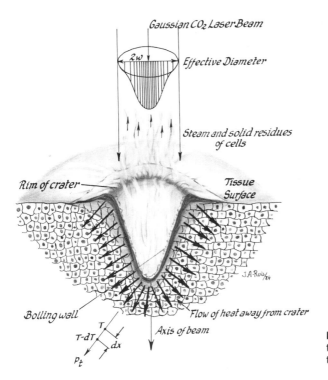

Gaussian CO₂ Laser Beam

Effective Diameter

Steam and solid residues of cells

Rim of crater

Tissue Surface

Boiling wall

Flow of heat away from crater

Axis of beam

J.A.Ruiz/84

Figure 6–10. Schematic illustration of crater formation in soft tissue by a CO_2 laser.

where c_t is the thermal conductivity of the tissue (water), (power)/(length × temp. diff.); dT/dx is the temperature gradient along path x, (temperature change)/(length).

From Equation 6–5 it can be seen that the thermal power density is greatest at the wall of the crater and declines with distance into the surrounding depths of tissue, because the temperature gradient falls. (The minus sign merely signifies that the temperature decreases with increasing distance.) This decrease of thermally conducted power density with distance must occur, because the lines of heat flow diverge away from the crater and so the total power conducted away is flowing through an ever-increasing cross-section of tissue.

Clearly, if the situation of thermal equilibrium just described is to be maintained, the incident power density from the beam of the CO_2 laser must be at least equal to that which is thermally conducted away from the wall of the crater. This equilibrium value of p_t at the boiling surface of the crater is called the characteristic power density of thermal conduction. A little thought will show that this is the maximum value of power density which can be removed by a particular kind of tissue in a state of thermal equilibrium with a concentrated source of heat like a CO_2 laser beam at one point. In the transient state which exists just after the onset of irradiation, the tissue can thermally absorb much higher power densities than it can conduct away in the steady state, but only until the temperature at each point has reached an equilibrium value.

Obviously the soft tissue in a human body is neither homogeneous nor isotropic. Heat is removed from the crater wall not only by conduction through the cytoplasm trapped within individual cells, but also by convection of blood and lymph in the local vessels. The thermal conductivity of this heterogeneous medium is not the same everywhere. These departures from ideality notwithstanding, we can obtain from Equation 6–5 a good approximation to the characteristic power density of thermal conduction for soft tissue. The average thermal conductivity for water, which constitutes 70 to 90 percent of soft tissue, is $c_t = 6.92 \times 10^{-3}$ W/cm°C between 37 and 100°C. Measurements made by Mihashi et al[22] with small thermocouples implanted in a living canine tongue at various distances from the impact crater of a CO_2 laser show that the temperature gradient at the boiling wall is somewhere between -1000 and -2000°C/cm. If we take -1500°C per cm as a typical value, then Equation 6–5 gives

$$p_{ct} = 10.4 \text{ W/cm}^2. \tag{6–6}$$

The significance of this quantity is that *the temperature of the tissue cannot be brought to the boiling point and tissue water evaporated by a CO_2 laser (or any other type, for that matter) unless the applied power density in the beam is greater than this critical value.*

We can define p_{ct} for other tissue, e.g., bone, as the power density thermally conducted away from a crater wall when the major constituent of that tissue has reached its vaporization temperature. Because bone has a much higher thermal conductivity than water, and its minerals evaporate at incandescent temperatures, p_{ct} for bone is much higher. Its value has not been measured, but it is probably in the order of 100 W/cm². The surgeon who wishes to perform osteotomy with the CO_2 laser and avoid extensive thermal necrosis of adjacent bone should use applied power densities well above 10,000 W/cm². Super pulsing (see the next section) is highly advisable in this procedure.

If the objective of laser irradiation is merely hyperthermia, the power density within the tissue must not exceed p_{ct}; otherwise, rapid rise of temperature and boiling of cytosol will occur. Note, however, that scattering will reduce the histologic power density to levels well below that of the incident beam for near infrared lasers, especially the Nd:YAG. For this reason, the Nd:YAG can operate at relatively high power densities in the incident beam without causing vaporization.

Practical Information for CO_2 Laser Surgery

As is illustrated in Figure 6–10, the shape of the defect created by a CO_2 laser is essentially the same as the profile of power density in the incident beam. This is true whether the beam is stationary or moving. The difference between the two cases is merely that the depth of the defect (crater if stationary, or groove if moving) is inversely proportional to the linear speed at which the beam sweeps across the tissue. This is not true for visible and near infrared lasers, which are poorly suited anyway to creation of defects, unless the tissue is previously stained with an appropriate dye or is naturally pigmented.

In Figure 6–10, the wavy lines emanating from the crater indicate vapor, which emerges upward with a velocity in the order of 3 m/s. This jet of steam carries with it the dehydrated organelles of the ruptured cells. As they pass through the direct beam of the laser, these are heated to incandescence and burn (oxidize) in the ambient air, giving rise to a thick plume of malodorous smoke, whose hazards have been discussed in the first part of this chapter. The uninformed observer, seeing this smoke, often concludes erroneously that burning is the mechanism by which the CO_2 laser destroys living tissue. This is not true, as can readily be demonstrated by blanketing the target area with a nonoxidizing gas like CO_2, He, or Ar: the smoke disappears, but vaporization of tissue continues.

To vaporize the aqueous liquids (cytosol, lymph, and plasma) in soft tissue, the laser beam must deliver 2522 watt seconds (joules) of energy to each cubic centimeter (gram) of tissue, starting from normal body temperature of 37°C. The power density of the incident beam must, of course, be well above 10 W/cm^2 at all points within the effective diameter. The depth of the resulting crater at every point in any cross-sectional plane passing through the beam axis (this plane must be perpendicular to the sweep direction of a moving beam) is proportional to the power density at that point. Around the outer fringe of the beam, however, where the power density at some radius becomes too low for vaporization (less than p_{ct}), the rays of the laser will only coagulate and char the tissue. This effect produces a raised rim around the crater, resembling that of a volcano, consisting of dead (cooked) tissue, whose radial extent and axial depth depend upon the power density profile of the beam, the peak power density of this profile, and the total time of irradiation. At low power densities, relatively long irradiation times are needed to vaporize a given mass of tissue. Consequently, the profile of temperature versus distance from the crater approaches the limiting value for thermal equilibrium, in which each point of surrounding tissue reaches the maximum possible temperature and the lateral extent of temperature rise above 37°C increases to 5 mm or so. The curves of Figure 6–11, which are derived from the data of Mihashi et al.,[22] show that the tissue temperature at any point along a line of heat flow comes close to its equilibrium value after about 1 second of irradiation at surgical power den-

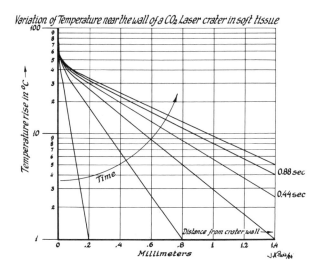

Variation of Temperature near the wall of a CO_2 Laser crater in soft tissue

Temperature rise in °C →

Distance from crater wall →

0.88 sec

0.44 sec

Time

Millimeters

Figure 6–11. Temperature rise as a function of distance from the wall of a crater, and time after onset of irradiation by a CO_2 surgical laser in soft tissue. *(Adapted from Mihashi et al.[22])*

sities, i.e., greater than 300 W/cm^2, and that the limiting curve of temperature versus distance goes out to 5 mm or so before falling back almost to normal body temperature. Longer irradiation will not significantly raise the temperature at any point away from the crater unless the beam is moved so that the crater wall lies closer to the point. The lateral extent of tissue temperatures at or above 60°C at thermal equilibrium is only about 0.5 mm as long as the water content is 75 percent or higher and the neighboring vasculature and lymphatics are functional. In highly vascular tissue, the lateral dimension of this necrotic zone may be less.

The foregoing facts lead us to a significant conclusion: the maximum depth to which a CO_2 laser can achieve coagulation, e.g., for hemostasis, is only about 0.5 mm for a stationary beam or one moving in a straight line. This is also the maximum diameter of a vessel which can be transected by a CO_2 laser beam and achieve automatic hemostasis. By randomly sweeping the beam at about 10 W/cm^2 over a surface area of a few square centimeters, a surgeon can produce an apparent heat source large enough so that the lines of heat flow into the tissue remain parallel to each other and perpendicular to the uncratered surface over a bleeding vessel. This maintains a higher thermal power density in the tissue below the surface, and may extend the depth of coagulation to a few millimeters. A much more effective technique employing this same scheme is to place a flat, satin-finished, metal tampon plate about 1.5 cm square on the surface of the tissue and irradiate the back (proximal) side so as to produce a uniform heat source over the unknown bleeder. The tampon, of course, can be irradiated at higher power density than 10 W/cm^2 to raise its temperature quickly.

Because of its small impact volume and the body's natural mechanisms for removal of heat, the CO_2 laser is very forgiving of the surgeon's errors regarding thermal trauma to adjacent tissue. Its use however can be optimized by applying the beam to the tissue in a series of short bursts whose duration is between 1.0 and 100 μsec, with a maximum repetition rate of about 5 percent of the reciprocal of the burst duration. This is equivalent to saying that the repetition period is 20 times the burst duration. The profile of intensity versus time for each burst should be as nearly rectangular as possible, though in commercial systems the bursts usually have steep leading edges and long exponential tails. Several makers of CO_2 lasers now offer such systems, with adjustable burst duration and repetition rate. This technique is known by the somewhat unfortunate name of super pulsing, which is reminiscent of the long discredited Q-switching used in early Nd-glass and ruby lasers, which were so rightly castigated by Ketcham and his coworkers[2,3] in the late sixties. The modern systems used in CO_2 lasers, however, utilize electronic pulsing of the power supply for the laser tube; this does not produce such short pulses nor high peak power. Super pulsing is most useful for fine incisions (as in fallopian resection prior to reanastomosis) or ablation of small lesions near critical structures. It is of little value for vaporization of large tissue masses, such as meningiomas in the skull, which can be safely ablated in a CW mode. It has the disadvantage for large lesions of reducing the average power, unless the peak power is suitably raised to compensate.

Thermal trauma to the tissue surrounding the crater made by a CO_2 laser in soft tissue is not just a matter of temperature; time is also a factor, as indicated by the cell-survival curve of Figure 6–12. This curve is actually a band having a

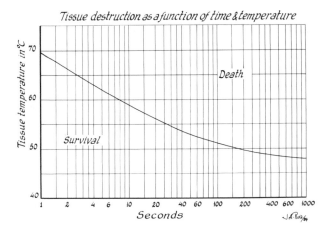

Figure 6-12. Curve of cell death or survival as functions of time and temperature elevation.

vertical width of $\pm 3°C$ or so. From it we can quickly see that cells can readily survive temperatures of 50°C for 10 seconds, but will die at this temperature in 5 minutes. Furthermore, because of histologic synergism, death of a few cells at the time of surgery can result in morbidity later. *The skilled surgeon will apply the CO_2 laser beam to the tissue for the shortest time needed to achieve the intended result.* The morbid sequelae of inept use of the CO_2 laser include postoperative scarring, pain, and hemorrhage, which can usually be avoided by intelligent use of this unique device.

Quantitative Relationships in CO_2 Laser Surgery

Though the surgeon will seldom calculate in advance the depth of an incision or the time required to ablate a given mass of tissue, it is instructive to have some approximate formulas which show the effect of each parameter on the result. Each of the following is based upon the assumption that the applied power density in the laser beam is at least ten times the characteristic power density of thermal conduction, that the tissue is at least 80 percent water, and that the beam strikes the tissue perpendicular to its surface. The power density profile of the beam is assumed to be Gaussian.

Power Density of the Beam

This is the most important operating parameter of a CO_2 surgical laser. The surgeon should have an approximate idea of the magnitude of the power density in his laser beam at all times. *The exact magnitude is not critical; range is important.* It must be remembered that few, if any, of the CO_2 lasers commercially available for surgery produce a truly Gaussian (TEM_{00}) beam. The Gaussian mode is highly desirable in fine cutting or boring of holes, but mode shape (power density profile) is not of prime importance when the beam is swept repeatedly over the tissue to evaporate a large mass, so long as the sweep is performed in at least two *rasters* (patterns of closely spaced parallel lines) perpendicular to one another.

Average Power Density over the Effective Diameter

To a good approximation, this parameter is given by

$$p_{aw} = \frac{100 \times (\text{total beam power in watts})}{(\text{effective beam diameter in millimeters})^2},$$ **(6–7)**

where p_{aw} is expressed in W/cm^2. The exact formula would have the factor 110 in the numerator rather than 100. Given the usual deviations from Gaussian mode and the difficulty of measuring effective diameter, however, this approximate formula is good enough.

Effective Diameter

For practical purposes, this is the diameter of a coaxial circle normal to the beam axis through which 86 percent of the total beam power is flowing. It is measurable to a reasonable approximation by exposing a clean wooden tongue depressor to the focal point of the laser beam for 0.1 second at a power of 10 W, and then measuring the diameter of the charred spot with a millimeter rule under a microscope at about 25× magnification.

Central Power Density in the Beam

For a true Gaussian profile, the power density of the beam is highest at the center (on the axis):

$$p_c = 2.32\ p_{aw}.$$ **(6–8)**

Appropriate Range of Power Density

Destruction of tissue without thermal trauma is incompatible with attainment of maximum hemostasis. Hemostasis therefore declines as power density increases and tissue exposure time decreases. The hemostasis referred to here is that which is automatically achieved as the laser beam transects tissue in one sweep; it is not obtained when the beam cuts vessels whose diameter is larger than about 0.5 mm. The following tabulation is intended only as a guide, not as an absolute prescription; it gives average power densities:

Tissue Effect	Range of Power Density in W/cm^2
Coagulation only	10
Coagulation with superficial vaporization	10–100
Vaporization with little coagulation	100–1000
Cutting	1000–10,000
Ultra rapid incision	10,000–500,000

Note that it requires 45 W through an effective diameter of 0.1 mm to produce 500,000 W/cm^2. This is attainable in several surgical lasers currently available.

Magnitude of the Defect Created by a CO_2 Laser Beam

Although there have been a few empiric measurements of crater diameter, depth, and volume for both stationary and moving beams of CO_2 lasers, it is hard to find consistency in the results reported by various authors. The following formulas, which are given without derivation, are based upon the assumption of a Gaussian beam evaporating *gelatin* (which is 95 to 98 percent water in a collagen matrix) at a power density of at least 300 W/cm^2 (average). The reader will recognize that gelatin is not representative of living soft tissue in any respect except its thermal constants of specific heat, conductivity, and density. A comprehensive, meticulous experimental study is needed to establish formulas for estimating the size of laser-created defects in various types of human tissue. The following relationships, however, show which factors are important and their relative effects. They take account of reflection.

Depth of Crater Produced by a Stationary CO_2 Laser Beam
The central depth is

$$z_c = \frac{0.96^* \times (P_0 \text{ in watts}) \times (t \text{ in seconds})}{(d_e \text{ in mm})^2} \text{ mm,} \qquad \textbf{(6-9)}$$

where P_0 is the total power in the beam; t is the total time of exposure; and d_e is the effective diameter (usually denoted by 2w).

Depth of Groove Produced by a Moving CO_2 Laser Beam
The central depth is

$$z_c = \frac{0.060^* \times (P_0 \text{ in watts})}{(v \text{ in cm/sec}) \times (d_e \text{ in mm})} \text{ mm,} \qquad \textbf{(6-10)}$$

where P_0 is the total power in the beam; v is the linear speed of the beam; and d_e is the effective diameter of the beam.

Mass of Tissue Vaporized by a CO_2 Laser Beam
The total mass vaporized is independent of the sweep speed of the beam. It is given by

$$M = \frac{k_f \times (P_0 \text{ in watts}) \times (t \text{ in seconds})}{2522^*} \text{ g,} \qquad \textbf{(6-11)}$$

where k_f is a numerical factor depending upon d_e, the power density profile, and the total beam power. If the power density of the beam is above 100 W/cm^2 everywhere within a coaxial circle of diameter 1.5 d_e, the value of k_f is 0.95. If the power density everywhere is 10 W/cm^2 or less, k_f is zero.

---

*The numerical constants are not dimensionless.

PRACTICAL INFORMATION FOR ND:YAG LASER SURGERY

Except when it is combined with a CO_2 laser for microsurgery, the beam of the Nd:YAG laser is usually delivered through a flexible optical fiber of about 0.5 to 1.0 mm in core diameter. Depending upon the details of the lens system used to focus the beam into the proximal end of this fiber, the divergence angle of the beam emerging from the fiber can be as great as 5 degrees or so. This makes computation of the average power density at the tissue difficult, because the distance between the fiber tip and the tissue is not easy to judge when the beam is applied via an endoscope. Even if the incident power density at the tissue surface were known, the scattering of the laser beam by the tissue makes it virtually impossible to compute the power density within the tissue. Figure 6–5 shows in schematic form the effects of scattering upon the redistribution of power density of the beam of a Nd:YAG laser in soft tissue. This figure is based upon the results of Halldorsson and Langerholc.[14] It illustrates the approximate size and location of the isothermal surfaces to be expected when soft tissue is irradiated for time durations up to 15 seconds at 40 W and an average incident power density of $1560 \ W/cm^2$.

The most significant facts in this situation are the forward displacement of the zone of maximum histologic power density and the high ratio of the diameter and depth of the coagulation volume to the diameter of the incident beam. The danger posed by this is the popcorn effect, which has been discussed in the first part of this chapter. Also important is the increase of scattering as the tissue proteins are denatured. This is quite probably due to the increased density of free amino acids released by the fracturing of large protein molecules by thermal vibration resulting from elevated temperature.

Because of the extreme structural complexity of large organic molecules, there are large numbers of energy states and interstate transitions, whose energy values are low. Near and far infrared photons can be absorbed by these giant molecules, setting them into various modes of vibration. Because the bonding energies of long chain molecules are relatively low, they can be fractured by long wave radiation of low power density. Conversely, it also appears that near infrared radiation at low intensity can stimulate long chain formation. The results of Castro et al.[24,25] in experiments done at Harbor General Hospital in Torrance, California in 1982 indicate that both synthesis and degeneration of collagen molecules can be stimulated by irradiation with the Nd:YAG laser at low intensities. This is a highly promising field of study which could lead to a host of new applications for near infrared lasers in therapy and bioengineering.

Meanwhile, the uses of the Nd:YAG in therapy and quasi-surgery are growing. These are largely endoscopic applications intended to necrose and shrink tumors obstructing respiratory, alimentary, and urinary passages of the body. With elapse of time, there will undoubtedly be a growing use of the Nd:YAG as an ancillary to outright surgery with the CO_2, for hemostasis in highly vascular organs like the liver and kidney, which may even outpace its present hemostatic advantages in gastrointestinal bleeding.

The thermonecrotic effects of the Nd:YAG in tumor therapy are quite different from the vaporization of lesions by a CO_2 laser. Nd:YAG irradiation literally cooks tumor tissue, making it friable and amenable to removal by suction. Postnecrotic manipulation of dead tumor tissue presents none of the disseminatory hazards of sharp dissection which cause metastasis of malignant tumors during the manipulation of tumor masses in bloody fields resulting from scalpel surgery. Present indications are that the Nd:YAG will play an increasingly important role in the treatment of primary and metastatic malignancies now considered inoperable.

REFERENCES

1. Mirhoseini M, Muckerheide M, Cayton MM: Transventricular revascularization by laser. Lasers in Surg Med 2:187–198, 1982
2. Ketcham AS, Minton JP: Laser radiation as a clinical tool in cancer therapy. Fed Proc Suppl 14 24(1):S-159, 1965
3. Ketcham AS, Hoye RC, Riggle GC: A surgeon's appraisal of the laser. Surg Clin North Am 47(5):1249, 1967
4. Osterhuis JW: Tumor Surgery with the CO_2 Laser: Studies with the Cloudman S-91 Mouse Melanoma. Groningen, Netherlands, Veenstra-Visser, 1977
5. Bellina JH, Stjernholm RL, Kurpel JE: Analysis of plume emissions after papovavirus irradiation with the carbon dioxide laser. J Repro Med 27(5):268–270, 1982
6. Mihashi S, Ueda S, Hirano M, et al: Some problems about condensates induced by CO_2 laser irradiation. In Atsumi K (ed): Transactions, 4th Congress of the International Society for Laser Surgery. Tokyo, Intergroup Corp, 1981, pp 2-25–2-27
7. Kirby RR: High-frequency positive-pressure ventilation (HFPPV): What role in ventilatory insufficiency? Anesthiology 52:109–110, 1980
8. Borg U, Eriksson I, Sjostrand U: High-frequency positive-pressure ventilation (HFPPV): A review based upon its use during bronchoscopy and for laryngoscopy and microlaryngeal surgery under general anesthesia. Anesth Analg 59(8):594–603, 1980
9. Eriksson I, Sjostrand U: Effects of high-frequency positive-pressure ventilation (HFPPV) and general anesthesia on intrapulmonary gas distribution in patients undergoing diagnostic bronchoscopy. Anesth Analg 59(8):585–593, 1980
10. Babinski M, Smith RB, Klain M: High-frequency jet ventilation for laryngoscopy. Anesthesiology 52:177–180, 1980
11. Dumon JF, Meric B, Garbe L, et al: YAG laser resection of tracheobronchial lesions (600 treatments). In Atsumi K (ed): New Frontiers in Laser Medicine and Surgery. Amsterdam, Netherlands, Casparie, 1983, pp 271–279
12. Shapshay SM: Lasers in Bronchology. Otolaryn Clin North Am (in press)
13. Fuller TA, Beckman H: Carbon dioxide laser fiberoptics in endoscopy. In Atsumi K (ed): New Frontiers in Laser Medicine and Surgery. Amsterdam, Netherlands, Casparie, 1983, pp 76–80
14. Halldorsson T, Langerholc J, Senatori L, Funk H: Thermal action of laser irradiation in biological material monitored by egg-white coagulation. Appl Opt 20(5):822–825, 1981
15. Mallow M, Chabot L: Laser Safety Handbook. New York, Van Nostrand Reinhold, 1978
16. Sliney D, Wohlbarsht M: Safety with Lasers and Other Optical Sources. New York, London, Plenum Press, 1980
17. Halldorsson T, Langerholc J: Thermodynamic analysis of laser irradiation of biological tissue. Appl Opt 17(24):3948–3958, 1978
18. Hillenkamp F, Pratesi R, Sacchi CA (eds): Lasers in Biology and Medicine, New York, London, Plenum Press, 1980
19. Hillenkamp F: Interaction between laser radiation and biological systems. In Hillenkamp F, Pratesi R, Sacchi CA (eds): Lasers in Biology and Medicine. New York, London, Plenum Press, 1980, pp 37–68

20. Halldorsson T, Rother W, Langerholc J, Frank F: Theoretical and experimental investigations prove Nd:YAG laser treatment to be safe. Lasers Surg Med 1(3):253–262, 1981
21. Bayly JG, Kartha VB, Stevens WH: The absorption spectra of liquid phase H_2O, HDO, and D_2O from 0.7 μm to 10 μm. Infrared Phys 3:211, 1963
22. Mihashi S, Jako GJ, Incze J, et al: Laser surgery in otolaryngology: Interaction of CO_2 laser and soft tissue. Ann NY Acad Sci 267:263–294, 1976
23. Fisher JC: The power density of a surgical laser beam: Its meaning and measurement. Lasers Surg Med 2(4):301–315, 1983
24. Castro D: Effects of laser on DNA synthesis and collagen production in human skin fibroblast cultures. Paper presented at 3rd annual meeting of the American Society for Laser Medicine & Surgery, New Orleans, Jan 1983. Audio cassette No. 26
25. Castro D: Wound healing: Biological effects of collagen metabolism in pig skin treated with Nd:YAG laser in comparison to thermal burn. Paper presented at the 3rd annual meeting of the American Society for Laser Medicine & Surgery, New Orleans, Jan 1983. Audio cassette No. 41

7

The Histology of CIN, VIN, and VAIN

Barbara Winkler
Ralph M. Richart

INTRODUCTION

Despite the availability of cytologic screening and improved diagnostic and therapeutic techniques, squamous cell carcinoma of the cervix remains among the five leading causes of cancer deaths in women in the United States, and, in countries in which cytologic screening is not routinely available, cervical carcinoma remains the leading cause of female cancer deaths. The 1984 cancer statistics for the United States project over 45,000 new cases of cervical carcinoma in situ and 16,000 new cases of invasive cervical carcinoma annually and estimate that 7000 deaths will occur from cervical carcinoma.[1] The incidence of preinvasive and invasive squamous cell carcinoma of the lower female genital tract including the vulva, vagina, and cervix has steadily been increasing in young women, highlighting the fact that genital squamous neoplasia continues to be a disease of major public health concern in the United States.[2]

Most of the recent advances in the control of invasive carcinoma of the female genital tract have been made in the identification and treatment of squamous cancer in its preinvasive, or intraepithelial, stage.[3] The concept of squamous intraepithelial neoplasia is predicated on the observation that there is a continuum of histologic changes that precede invasive squamous cell carcinoma, and, as a corollary, that when these histologic changes are reproducibly identified and diagnosed and their corresponding macroscopic lesions treated appropriately, the development of invasive cancer can be prevented.[4] The use of the diagnostic term "intraepithelial neoplasia" implies that there is a precursor lesion, i.e., a lesion which, if left untreated, has a statistically significant—albeit individually unknown—risk of developing into invasive carcinoma at some time in the future. Old definitions separating squamous epithelial dysplasia and carcinoma in situ implied an arbitrary distinction between the biology of the different grades of intraepithelial lesions which is not supported by scientific evidence. Instead, the scientific evidence corroborates the concept of a lesional spectrum or continuum which is similar biologically at all grades and is distinguished only by minor quantitative differences.[5] The basic schematic for intraepithelial neoplasia is an adaptable and dynamic system by which diagnostic classifications and terminology and their corresponding clinical applications may be updated based on current investigation and therapeutic advances. The morphologic definitions and the pathologic classifications of neoplastic alterations of the genital squamous epithelium are currently being reworked because of the rapidly accumulating clinicopathologic studies of the relationship between human papillomavirus (HPV) infection, HPV-induced epithelial abnormalities, and intraepithelial neoplasia. Studies of these HPV-induced, condylomatous lesions have demonstrated that they share many of the histologic and biologic features of intraepithelial neoplasia, and their identification has dramatically altered the diagnostic approach to lesions of the genital squamous epithelium.

CERVICAL INTRAEPITHELIAL NEOPLASIA

Most of the information on which the intraepithelial neoplasia concept is based is derived from studies of cervical intraepithelial neoplasia (CIN), and its clinicopathologic correlates serve as the foundation for our understanding of squamous precursor lesions in other sites. CIN is a disease of young women with a mean age for carcinoma in situ of approximately 35 years, preceding by 15 years the mean age for invasive carcinoma.[6] The annual reported incidence of CIN is two to four times the annual incidence of invasive cervical carcinoma, and the age-specific incidence curve for CIN appears to be moving to the left, as both the incidence and prevalence of CIN are rising steadily, particularly in teenagers and women under 30.[2,7] CIN appears to arise solely within the transformation zone and, on the basis of glucose-6-phosphate dehydrogenase studies, appears generally to be unifocal. Within the transformation zone CIN expands by mechanical, confluent growth to replace the adjacent epithelium and may spread into the endocervical canal or even the endometrial cavity. It does not involve the native portio epithelium.[2,8–10]

The epidemiology and pathogenesis of CIN and invasive cervical cancer have been studied extensively, and the defined risk factors are summarized in Table 7–1. The data suggest that there is a causal relationship between sexual activity, particularly young age at first intercourse and multiple sexual partners, and CIN. CIN has all the characteristics of a sexually-transmitted disease. The evidence points to an oncogen which acts preferentially on the immature transformation zone and is spread by venereal transmission.[11]

Two venereally-transmitted viruses, the human papillomavirus (HPV) and the herpes simplex virus (HSV), have received serious attention as possible etiologic agents in intraepithelial neoplasia and squamous carcinoma of the female genital tract. The HPVs are a heterogeneous group of DNA viruses which cause proliferation of the squamous epithelium in a variety of body sites, including the skin and mucosal surfaces such as the oral cavity, larynx and tracheobronchial tree, esophagus, bladder, anus, and genitalia of both sexes. They have most commonly been identified as the causative agents of the common skin wart (verruca vulgaris) and the genital wart (condyloma acuminatum).[12] The papillomaviruses are remarkably species-specific and site-specific, producing morphologically distinct

TABLE 7–1. EPIDEMIOLOGIC RISK FACTORS FOR CIN

Sexual Activity
  Independent Variables
    Early sexual activity
    Multiple sexual partners
  Dependent Variables
    Multiple pregnancies
    "High-risk" male sexual partner
    Early age first pregnancy
    Early age first marriage
    Unstable marital history
    Low socioeconomic status
Sexually-Transmitted Diseases (especially HPV and HSV)
Immunosuppression

lesions in different body sites, depending on the virus type involved.[13] HPVs transform cells in vitro and are known to be oncogenic in experimental and animal systems.[12,14–16]

Some 28 types of HPV are now recognized (Table 7–2), and it is apparent that their clinical expressions are distinctive.[17] Malignant transformation by particular types of HPV has been documented in the skin lesions of patients affected by epidermodysplasia verruciformis, and there is now substantial circumstantial evidence to link HPV to both benign and malignant squamous cancers of the mucosal surfaces as well.[18–20]

The incidence of HPV infection of the lower genital tract has increased as much as sixfold in the last decade alone, and it is now reported that cytologic evidence of HPV infection is detectable in as many as 3 percent of women under the age of 30, implying that there are a large number of infected individuals and an enormous pool for the propagation of the infection.[20,21] HPV infections in both men and women are rapidly increasing in incidence and prevalence with between 60 and 85 percent of the sexual partners of HPV-infected individuals developing genital condylomata in an incubation period averaging 2 to 3 months.[22]

In the male, intraurethral and flat condylomata of the penile shaft may serve as a "hidden" source of HPV infection and may be documented by careful examination in 60 to 80 percent of the male partners of women with lower genital tract neoplasia.[23–25] This documentation of previously unsuspected penile condylomata fits well into the epidemiologic characterization of the "high-risk" male (Table 7–3) and further substantiates the role of sexually-transmitted disease in the genesis of CIN.[26–33] In homosexual males, the incidence of anal and perianal condylomata is especially high and is associated with a 25 to 50 times increased risk of developing anal squamous cell carcinoma, a rare clinical entity before the HPV epidemic.[34–36]

The epidemiologic evidence for an association between HPV infection of the cervix and CIN is manifold. Since Meisels et al. first described flat condylomata of the cervix in 1977, it has become apparent that many cases previously diagnosed as mild dysplasia, or CIN 1, are actually manifestations of HPV infection, and some authors have reclassified up to 70 percent of low grade CINs as such.[20,37,38]

TABLE 7–2. HUMAN PAPILLOMAVIRUSES

Type	Usual Clinical Presentation
1	Plantar and Palmar warts (verruca plantares)
2	Common warts (verruca vulgaris)
3	Juvenile flat wart (verruca plana)
4	Plantar and common warts
5	EDV[a]
6	Genital warts (condyloma acuminatum) Laryngeal papilloma GTN[b]
7	Butcher wart
8,9	EDV
10	Juvenile flat wart (verruca plana) EDV
11	Genital warts (condyloma acuminatum) Laryngeal papilloma GTN
12	EDV
13	Focal epithelial hyperplasia of oral cavity
14,15	EDV
16	GTN, Bowenoid papulosis
17	EDV
18	GTN, Bowenoid papulosis
19–25	EDV
26–28	Immunosuppressed host

[a]EDV, epidermodysplasia verruciformis.
[b]GTN, genital tract neoplasia (males and females).
(Adapted from Broker T, Cold Spring Harbor Laboratories, Cold Spring Harbor, NY. Personal communication.)

In addition, in histologic analyses, 25 to 50 percent of high grade CIN lesions have coexisting or intermixed condylomatous features.[20,37,38] It is clear that HPV infection of the cervix is several times more prevalent than true CIN and that the presence of HPV may alter both the acquisition and time course of CIN. Crum et al., Meisels et al., and others have documented that patients with concomitant HPV infection and CIN are younger than patients with CIN alone and that their lesions

TABLE 7–3. INCREASED RISK OF CERVICAL CARCINOMA IN PARTNERS OF "HIGH RISK" MALE: EPIDEMIOLOGIC CHARACTERIZATION

History of genital carcinoma (especially penile carcinoma)
History of cervical carcinoma in first wife
Low socioeconomic status
Sexually-transmitted disease (especially penile condyloma)

are acquired and progress at a faster rate.[20,39,40]

Other infectious agents, particularly herpes simplex virus, and other etiologic factors including nutritional influences and environmental, iatrogenic or chemical carcinogens (Table 7–4) have been implicated in the genesis of CIN.[41–50] These observations need not be dismissed because of the enfolding story on HPV as they might act as cofactors. Herpes simplex virus (HSV) has received a great deal of attention in relation to the etiology of CIN with studies linking HSV to CIN and cervical cancer epidemiologically and biologically. These studies have been summarized in detail by Nahmias et al. and Fenoglio et al.[51,52] Our understanding of oncogenesis is now based on the interaction of initiators and promotors, and it is probable that most cancers result from a series of multiple etiologic events with neoplastic transformation as an endpoint.[53,54]

Several recent investigations have suggested that HSV and HPV may interact in producing human genital carcinoma. Zur Hausen hypothesized that the two viruses act synergistically with HSV as a mutagenic stimulus on already proliferating cells infected by HPV (Fig 7-1).[55] Furthermore, it is notable that HSV has been localized in genital condylomata by in situ hybridization and that HPV DNA, usually present as an unintegrated plasmid in infected cells, is found to be integrated into the host cell DNA when the cells have previously been infected with HSV.[52,56,57] The immune system obviously plays a role in this multifactorial process, and there is a well-documented epidemiologic association between immunosuppression and both condylomata and neoplasia of the lower female genital tract. Carcinoma of the cervix comprises 8 percent of de novo cancers in organ homograft recipients, among whom there is a 14-fold increase in the incidence of intraepithelial neoplasia when compared with immunocompetent controls. Condylomata of the female genitalia have also been reported to be increased in incidence in the immunosuppressed host with a greater propensity to multifocality, large size, and resistance to therapy. The development of neoplastic changes and invasive carcinoma is reported to occur with greater frequency in the condylomata of immunosuppressed individuals. It has been proposed that the relationship

TABLE 7–4. PROPOSED AGENTS IN A MULTIFACTORIAL ETIOLOGY OF CIN

Infectious
   Human papillomavirus
   Herpes simplex virus

Nutritional
   Folic acid deficiency
   Vitamin A deficiency
   Vitamin C deficiency

Chemical
   Cigarette smoking
   Chemical carcinogens
   Chemotherapy (e.g., alkylating agents, methotrexate)
   Steroid hormones
   Immunosuppressive therapy

Irradiation

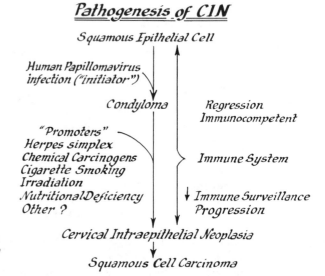

Figure 7–1. The important risk factors for CIN. *(Adapted from Zur Hausen H.[55])*

between immunosuppression and squamous neoplasia may occur as the combined effects of decreased immune surveillance, increased susceptibility to oncogenic viruses, and/or the direct cytostatic or cytotoxic effects of therapeutic agents such as azathioprine and corticosteroids.[58–60]

The epidemiology and pathogenesis of CIN are areas of active research interest, and extensive reviews continue to be available.

From the standpoint of the surgical pathologist and of the clinician, however, the major topics are differential diagnosis and clinicopathologic correlation. This is of particular importance today because the recent recognition of HPV-induced epithelial abnormalities has forced a revision of the histologic definitions by which intraepithelial neoplasia is diagnosed.

The cytologic and histologic hallmark of HPV infection is the koilocyte, an enlarged, superficial, squamous epithelial cell with vacuolated, clear cytoplasm, forming a perinuclear halo and a wrinkled hyperchromatic nucleus (Fig. 7–2). The koilocyte, first described by Koss in 1956, has only in recent years been recognized as a cytopathic effect of HPV infection.[61] Other features of HPV infection include epithelial hyperplasia with varying degrees of widening of the intermediate squamous epithelial layer (papillomatosis), elongation of the rete pegs (acanthosis), basal hyperplasia, abnormal keratinization with hyperkeratosis, dyskeratosis, bi- or multinucleation, and giant cell formation. Varying degrees of cytologic atypia and pleomorphism may also be present in HPV-induced condylomatous lesions, but, in general, the basal polarity, organization, and maturation remain intact, although there may be somewhat disordered growth in the intermediate and superficial layers characterized primarily by the ballooning koilocytes (Fig. 7–3).

The macroscopic and histologic manifestations of HPV infection are diverse. Macroscopically, HPV (condylomatous) lesions present in a variety of ways. The classic and easily recognized condyloma acuminatum is an exophytic, papillary

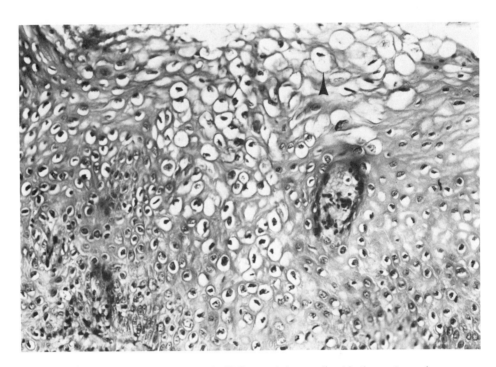

Figure 7–2. Flat condyloma of the cervix. Koilocytosis is prominent in the center and upper portions of this field. The koilocyte *(arrow)* is an enlarged cell with clear cytoplasm and a pyknotic nucleus.

tumor, often with prominent hyperkeratosis, papillomatosis, and acanthosis (Fig. 7–4). These occur most commonly on the vulva, perineal, and perianal skin, although they may also be present as smaller lesions on the mucous membrane of the introitus, vagina, and cervix. Less florid condylomata may be seen as circumscribed, hyperplastic lesions with surface epithelial spikes produced by projections of fibrovascular papillae uplifting the squamous epithelial surface. The flat condyloma described by Meisels et al. presents as a slightly raised, circumscribed lesion with an undulating surface and has been of particular interest.[62] The flat condylomata may occur on the vulva, vagina, or cervix and may easily be confused macroscopically, colposcopically, and histologically with intraepithelial neoplasia (Fig. 7–3). These flat condylomata occur most commonly on the cervix and are now recognized as forming the bulk of what was previously defined as mild dysplasia or CIN 1.

HPV infection is commonly multifocal, and, when florid condylomata of the vulva are identified, vaginal and/or cervical lesions may be observed in greater than 70 percent of patients.[20,62,63] The natural history of HPV infection is one of remission in 40 to 80 percent of patients and unpredictable recurrence or reinfection. Persistent lesions occur in 50 to 70 percent of patients, and progression occurs in about 10 percent of patients in 2 to 3 years.[20,62,64]

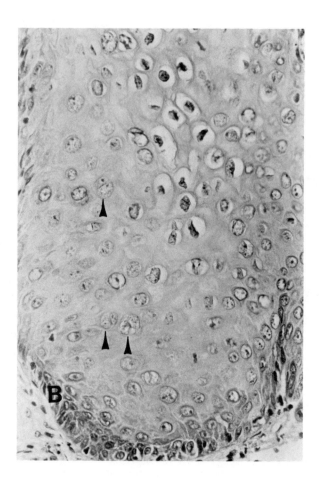

Figure 7–3. Condyloma acuminatum. There is only mild proliferation of the basal layer (B) which maintains its usual polarity and organization. Bi- and multinucleated cells *(arrows)* are frequent. Koilocytes are seen in the mid- and upper portion of the field. *(Courtesy of Dr. Christopher P. Crum, New York. N.Y.)*

In the cervix, the distribution of flat condylomata differs from that of CIN in that condylomata may be multiple and may often occur on the portio epithelium. HPV may also infect the immature squamous epithelium of the transformation zone and present as atypical immature squamous metaplasia with a full thickness population of metaplastic epithelial cells with orderly basal polarity, mild basal hyperplasia, mild pleomorphism, and only focal or minimal koilocytosis. Atypical immature metaplasia is identified in approximately one-third of patients with cervical condylomata, may have an endophytic growth pattern, and can be distinguished from CIN by its uniform nuclear chromatin, preserved polarity, and lack of abnormal mitotic figures (Fig. 7–5).[65]

The classic lesions of intraepithelial neoplasia have a progressive loss of epithelial maturation, absent glycogenization, and cellular disorientation accompanied by a loss of polarity and a crowded growth pattern with nuclear atypia, pleomorphism, and an increased nuclear-to-cytoplasmic ratio (Fig. 7–6). Although the entire epithelium is populated by atypical cells, the grading of intraepithelial neoplasia is classically based on the proportion of the epithelium occupied by neo-

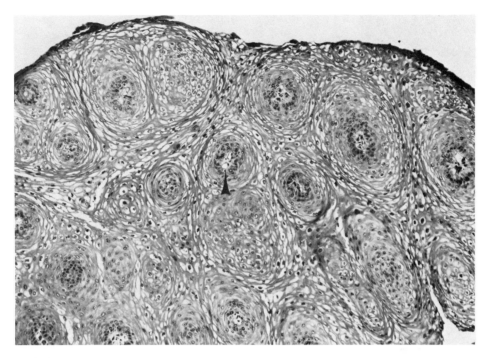

Figure 7–4. Condyloma acuminatum. Cross-sections of acanthotic pegs are prominent, surrounding fibrovascular cores *(arrow).*

plastic basal-type cells: Grade 1, lower third; Grade 2, lower third to two-thirds; and Grade 3, two-thirds to full thickness (Figs. 7–7 through 7–9). The progression rates, transit times, lesional size, and endocervical distribution vary directly with increasing severity of the grade of the CIN. The transit times of varying grades of CIN have been reported by Barron and Richart who estimated the progression in severity from one grade to the next to be 3 to 6 years in CIN 1, 2 years in CIN 2, and 1 year in CIN 3. In their study, however, they noted that only 50 percent of patients with low grade CIN lesions progressed to CIN 3 and that spontaneous regression of CIN 1 and 2 occasionally occurred. Retrospectively, the absence of progression in some patients and the spontaneous regression in others is accounted for by the reclassification of at least some of these lesions as flat condylomata. It is estimated, however, that at least 70 percent of CIN 3 (carcinoma in situ) will progress to invasive cancer in a 10-year period.[4,5,66,67]

Since cervical condylomata have such a high rate of spontaneous regression and low rate of progression, a central issue in recent years has been defining reproducible criteria for differentiating condyloma from CIN. This may be especially difficult because, as has been noted previously, condyloma may frequently coexist with CIN, and there are lesions which so incorporate the features of both HPV infection and CIN as to make differential diagnosis virtually impossible using conventional cytologic criteria. In addition, with the increased awareness of flat con-

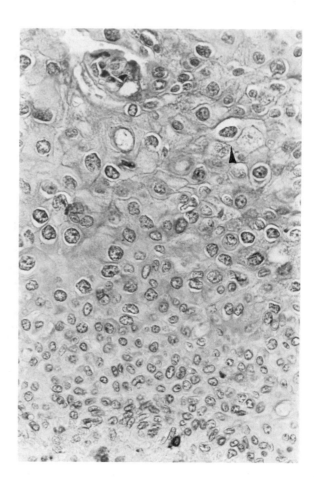

Figure 7–5. Atypical immature metaplasia, metaplastic epithelium with cytologic atypia, and rare koilocytes *(arrow)*. Koilocytes are uncommon and frequently poorly formed but are diagnostic. *(Courtesy of Dr. Christopher P. Crum, New York, N.Y.)*

dyloma of the cervix, there has been increased diagnostic use of the terms condyloma and koilocytosis with mounting concern that underdiagnosis of CIN may occur and that some patients will escape adequate treatment and surveillance.[68] This is especially important in view of the high incidence of HPV and the estimated 600,000 to 1,000,000 individuals infected.[21]

The diagnostic features of condyloma (principally koilocytosis) and CIN (principally pleomorphism) superficially appear to be easily discernible. However, Meisels et al. have described a subgroup of cervical condylomata to which they have given the designation "atypical condylomata" which have significantly more atypia than do the usual condylomata and which have a substantially greater risk of progression to CIN.[20,69] Other investigators have also noted such "transition lesions" bewteen cervical condyloma and CIN, and it has now been accepted that such transition lesions and, indeed, cervical condylomata themselves be incorporated into the defined spectrum of precursor lesions to cervical cancer. This schematic is summarized in Figure 7–10.

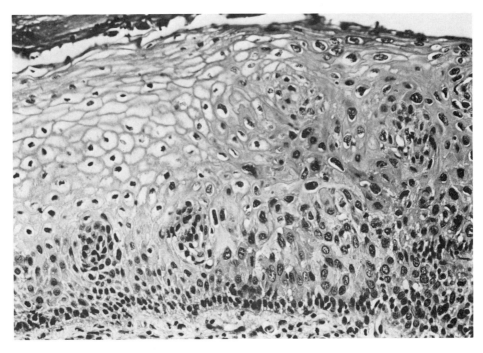

Figure 7–6. Junction between flat condyloma and normal cervical epithelium. Contrast the normal epithelium on the left with the condyloma on the right. The transition from normal to condyloma is usually abrupt as is seen here. The lesion has poor maturation and glycogenization. The epithelium is crowded and disorganized. Numerous hyperchromatic and pleomorphic nuclei are present, but abnormal mitotic figures (AMFs) are absent.

A number of investigative techniques have been used to define parameters by which HPV-induced flat condyloma may be differentiated from CIN including immunohistochemistry, nuclear DNA content analysis, and molecular hybridization. Immunoperoxidase staining with a broadly cross-reactive antibody to HPV localizes the viral protein capsid antigen to nuclei of superficial koilocytes (Fig. 7–11). Positive staining, however, depends upon the number of viral particles present and requires whole, fully assembled viral particles, terminal differentiation, and squamous maturation for HPV antigenic expression. HPV antigens may be detected by immunohistochemistry in 50 to 80 percent of the cases of typical flat and acuminate condyloma, and their presence correlates well with the demonstration of intranuclear HPV particles as seen by electron microscopy in these lesions (Fig. 7–12). The frequency of positive staining varies inversely with increasing degrees of epithelial atypia and maturational abnormality. The lack of sensitivity, even in obvious condyloma, and the occasional positive staining in definitely neoplastic, albeit koilocytotic, cervical lesions, diminishes the usefulness of HPV immunoperoxidase as a routine diagnostic tool.[65,70–74]

Other laboratory techniques for viral identification in tissue section such as in situ hybridization have, as yet, been unsuccessful for HPV because of their small

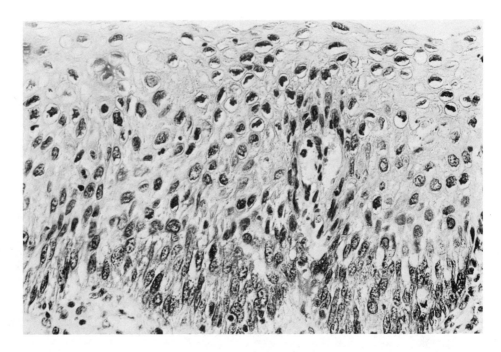

Figure 7-7. CIN grade 1 (mild dysplasia in the classic nomenclature). The lower third of the epithelium is occupied by overlapping basal-type cells with coarse, granular nuclear chromatin. There is maturation and some glycogenization of the upper two thirds of the epithelium. The superficial cells are atypical with enlarged hyperchromatic nuclei and clear vacuolated (koilocytotic) cytoplasm.

size, low copy number, and patchy distribution, even in overt acuminate condyloma. Identification of viral transcription products, RNA, and proteins, is in progress, but they have not yet been characterized.

Because of recent technical advances in antibody production, immunohistochemistry, and molecular hybridization, a number of new markers for squamous epithelia have become available and have been valuable in understanding normal and abnormal epithelial differentiation. Biochemical markers for squamous differentiation, including keratins and the envelope protein involucrin, demonstrate the presence of terminal maturation in the benign condylomata even though their protein distribution is altered. Involucrin expression and the production of the high molecular weight keratins indicative of normal squamous maturation are absent in contrasting high grade neoplastic lesions but may or may not be present in histologically defined low or midgrade CIN. Involucrin, necessary for cross-linkage of intermediate and superficial squamous cells, may be detected rapidly by immunohistochemistry, and, although currently being investigated, the preliminary data suggest that it may be useful in differential diagnosis, particularly when combined with other laboratory methods.[75-78] The study of prekeratin and keratin distribution in these lesions as an adjunct to histologic evaluation is hampered by the labor intensive techniques required, and substantive results are pending. New

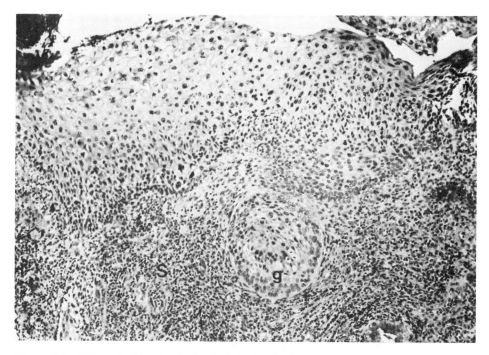

Figure 7–8. CIN grade 2 (moderate dysplasia in the classic nomenclature). Basaloid cells occupy approximately one half to two thirds of this epithelial lesion. Gland involvement (g) is seen. The stroma (S) contains a dense infiltrate of chronic inflammatory cells.

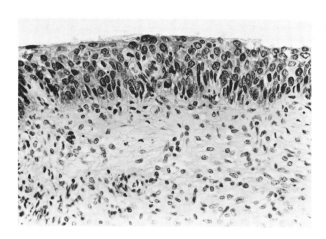

Figure 7–9. CIN grade 3 (severe dysplasia/carcinoma in situ in the classic nomenclature). The epithelium is made up of basal-type neoplastic cells. The nuclei are highly atypical, and AMFs are present.

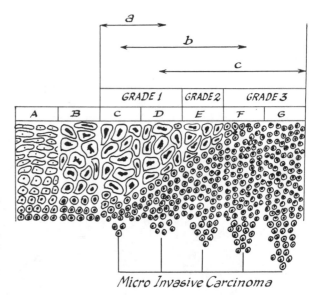

Figure 7–10. Precursors of cervical squamous cell carcinoma: a, Atypical condyloma; b, CIN with koilocytosis; c, CIN; A, Normal; B, Condyloma; C, Very mild dysplasia; D, Mild dysplasia; E, Moderate dysplasia; F, Severe dysplasia; G, In situ carcinoma.

Micro Invasive Carcinoma

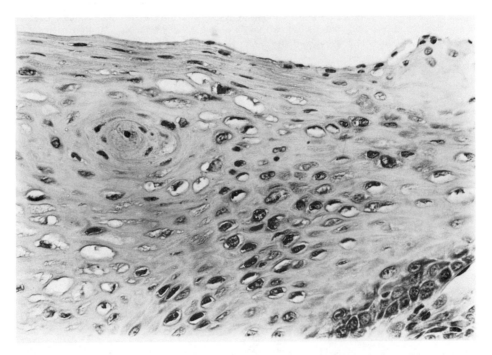

Figure 7–11. Localization of HPV antigens by immunoperoxidase. Positive staining is indicated by the presence of a dark intranuclear precipitate. Numerous positive cells are seen in this field.

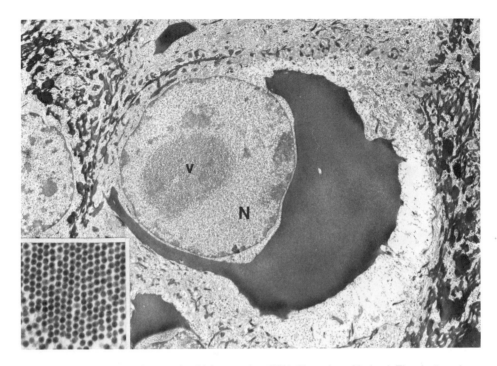

Figure 7–12. Electron micrograph with intranuclear HPV. (N, nucleus, V, virus). The electron dense material seen on the right of the nucleus is aggregated cytoplasmic keratin, indicating dyskeratosis in this cell. Further on the right there are thick bundles of tonofilaments, also a feature of HPV infection. *(Insert—lower left):* High power of intranuclear HPV particles. The viral shape is an icosadeltahedron. Magnifications × 5000. Insert: × 60,000. *(Courtesy of Dr. Rabia Mir, New York, N.Y.).*

antigenic expression by neoplastic cells may also be useful in the classification of these cervical lesions, but these data are as yet unavailable.[79–82] Epithelial membrane antigen may be localized by immunohistochemistry to neoplastic cervical epithelium, although it is absent in normal squamous tissue, serving normally as a surface marker for transitional and glandular epithelium. Its distribution and diagnostic usefulness are currently being studied.[83]

One of the most useful techniques in the evaluation of epithelial neoplasia has been nuclear DNA content analysis by Feulgen microspectrophotometry. As a result of such studies, it has been found that the ploidy level as determined from the distributional histogram of the nuclear DNA content serves as a fairly accurate predictor of biologic behavior, particularly in nonendocrine dependent tumors and is a useful tool in differentiating benign, condylomatous lesions from CIN. The typical condylomata are composed of a polyploid cell population, whereas all grades of "true" intraepithelial neoplasia are characterized by an aneuploid cell population.[84–89] The value of the ploidy level as a predictor of biologic behavior in cervical lesions is exemplified in a prospective study by Fu et al. in which it was found that 100 percent of lesions which progressed to invasive cancer were aneuploid by Feulgen DNA microspectrophotometry as were 95 percent of the lesions which persisted. Diploid or polyploid lesions, on the other hand, regressed in 91 percent of patients and persisted in only 9 percent.[84] It is well recognized that changes in nuclear DNA content are accompanied by cytologic atypia with aneuploidy producing the most severe cytologic alterations diagnosed morphologically as anisonucleosis, hyperchromasia, chromatin clumping, and irregularity in the nuclear membrane. Polyploidy also produces cytologic atypia, characterized primarily by anisonucleosis, but it is usually of a milder degree.

In lesions in which high degrees of polyploidy overlap between low degrees of aneuploidy, cytologic differentiation between the two may be difficult or impossible. The most reliable histologic criterion for detecting aneuploidy is the presence of morphologically abnormal mitotic figures (AMFs). This correlation has been corroborated in a number of studies in which the presence of AMFs was linked to finding an aneuploid cell population, even in lesions with the extensive koilocytosis associated with HPV infection (Fig 7–13).

It is well known that HPV infection induces cellular changes, including cytoskeletal abnormalities, spindle abnormalities, cell fusion, and multinucleation, and it is plausible that a polyploid cell population may provide the background for the mitotic derangements that lead to abnormal chromosome numbers (aneuploidy) and CIN. The change from polyploidy to aneuploidy would be accompanied by an increase in atypia and in the frequency and morphologic irregularity of the mitoses and a corresponding decrease in koilocytosis (Fig. 7–14). There have

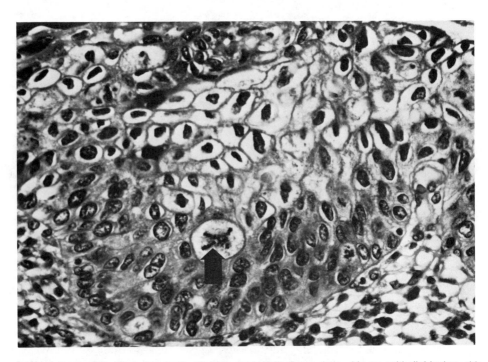

Figure 7–13. CIN with koilocytosis. Quadripolar mitotic figure *(arrow)* in an epithelial lesion with extensive superficial koilocytosis. These koilocytotic cells, however, have cytologic evidence of neoplasia, most importantly, increased nuclear-to-cytoplasmic ratio, and hyperchromatism.

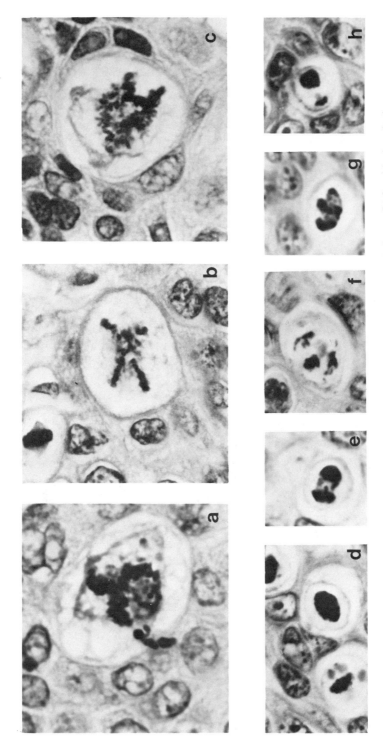

Figure 7–14. Morphologic diversity of abnormal mitotic figures. **(a)** Tripolar mitotic figure. **(b)** Quadripolar mitotic figure. **(c)** V-shaped mitotic figure. **(d)** Clumped, densely aggregated chromosomes. **(e)** Metaphase with clumped, densely aggregated chromosomes. **(f, g)** Three-group metaphase. **(h)** Two-group metaphase.

147

been several studies of so-called transition lesions. In one, rare abnormal mitotic figures were found in basically polyploid condylomatous cervical lesions which stained positively for HPV by immunoperoxidase. In the other, 14 percent of aneuploid lesions stained positively for HPV.[87-89]

Recent studies by molecular hybridization suggest that different HPV types may infect the genitalia and that these different viral types may have differing oncogenic potentials. This observation is similar to the observations of differing rates of malignant transformation by different HPV types in the skin lesions of patients with epidermodysplasia verruciformis. Several authors have studied the more common genital HPVs and have noted that HPV types 6 and 11 are generally associated with the usual, "nonatypical" flat and acuminate condylomata, whereas HPV types 16 and 18 are associated with the atypical condylomata, transition lesions, CIN, and invasive squamous cell carcinoma.[91-98] Other HPV types, including HPV types 2, 3, and 10, have also been identified in both benign and malignant genital lesions but less commonly than HPV types 6, 11, 16, and 18. The HPV constituents of condylomata and HPV-containing CIN are highly complex and, within the lesions in a single patient or within a single lesion, may present heterogeneous genomic patterns, suggesting that infection by multiple subtypes and possible recombinants or mutations may take place, consistent with the morphologic diversity of these lesions.[98]

Gissman and Zur Hausen have found HPV type 6 in 60 percent and HPV type 11 in 30 percent of acuminate condylomata, whereas HPV type 16 or 18 is detect-

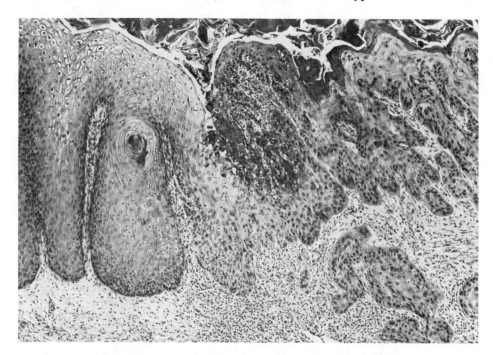

Figure 7-15. Squamous cell carcinoma with adjacent and overlying cervical condyloma. The epithelial lesion to the left is characteristic of an endophytic condyloma with minimal atypia. Immediately adjacent to it *(right)* is an invasive squamous cell carcinoma.

able in less than 10 percent. Their findings of HPV types 16 and 18 in over 75 percent of invasive cervical carcinomas as well as in substantial numbers of in situ squamous lesions in genital and extragenital sites suggest that these particular viral types have a high risk of malignant conversion (Fig. 7–15). The concept of HPV types 16 and 18 as viral types with carcinogenic potential is substantiated by the finding that HPV types 16 and 18 are integrated into the host cell DNA, whereas HPV types 6 and 11, with a low risk of malignant conversion, are found as free, unintegrated plasmids.[94,99] In correlating HPV type with histology, Crum et al. have further corroborated the hypothesis of HPV type 16 as a marker of neoplasia and have found that the subgroup of koilocytotic cervical lesions defined as an aneuploid precursor by the presence of abnormal mitotic figures is also defined by the presence of HPV type 16.[97]

The major limitations of nuclear DNA analysis and HPV typing by molecular hybridization is that, despite their sensitivity as predictors of biologic behavior, these techniques are too time consuming and expensive to be of routine use diagnostically. Instead, an assessment of the presence and type of AMFs can be applied at the level of conventional diagnostic pathology and, as they correlate well with nuclear DNA content and with HPV type and natural history (Table 7–5), they can be used to distinguish between the low-risk, polyploid HPV types 6 and 11 infections and the high-risk aneuploid HPV types 16 and 18 lesions.

TABLE 7–5. SUMMARY OF CONTRASTING HISTOLOGIC FEATURES OF CERVICAL CONDYLOMA AND CIN[a]

Major Criterion	Condyloma[b]	CIN
Clinical		
Age	20–30	Late 20–30
Age incidence	Decreasing	Decreasing
Cervical portio	+	−
T-zone	+	+
Multifocal	+	−
Regression	+/−	−
Progression	Low risk	High risk
Histologic		
Koilocytosis	+	+/−
AMFs	−	+
Basal polarity	+	−
Chromatin clumping	−	+
Anisonucleosis	+	+
Multinucleation	+	+
Biologic		
DNA content	Polyploid	Aneuploid
IMPO[c] (HPV)	+	−
HPV-type	6/11	16/18
IMPO (involucrin)	+	−
Clonality	Polyclonal/monoclonal	Monoclonal

[a]This table outlines the opposite ends of the spectrum. Obviously, transitional lesions would share some features of both as outlined in the text.
[b]Includes flat condyloma and atypical squamous metaplasia (atypical immature metaplasia).
[c]Immunoperoxidase staining.

The present data suggest a lesional spectrum with benign condyloma at one end, possibly representing a "preprecursor" lesion and established CIN at the other end with a significant risk of developing into invasive carcinoma. Between these two poles, fall the transition lesions which, sharing histologic features of both HPV infection and CIN, have been designated in the literature as atypical condyloma or CIN with koilocytosis or condylomatous features. Whatever their pathogenesis and their relationship to HPV, because these transition lesions significantly overlap clinically, biologically, and histologically and because their prospective risk is, at present, undefined, we believe they should be managed as CIN lesions with appropriate clinical surveillance until their natural history can better be delineated.

VULVOVAGINAL NEOPLASIA

The natural histories of vulvar intraepithelial neoplasia (VIN) and vaginal intraepithelial neoplasia (VAIN) are distinct from that of CIN, and, although histologic comparisons between CIN, VIN, and VAIN are valid, biologic and clinical comparisons cannot completely be validated because investigative approaches to VIN and VAIN have yielded contrasting results as summarized in Table 7-6.

The epidemiology of vulvar intraepithelial neoplasia and vaginal intraepithelial neoplasia have not been well studied because of the difficulty in accumulating sufficiently large numbers of cases for statistical analysis. Although the exact inci-

TABLE 7–6. CONTRASTING FEATURES OF THE NATURAL HISTORY AND PATHOLOGY OF CIN VERSUS VIN/VAIN

Major Criterion	CIN	VIN/VAIN
Clinical		
Age	Late 20–30	>30
Age at incidence	Decreasing	Decreasing
Multifocal	—	+
Regression	—	+/−
Recurrence posttherapy	Small	Frequent
Progression	High risk	Unknown risk, ? < 10%
Squamous cell carcinoma	Common	Rare
	Mean age = 50	Mean age = 60–70
	Incidence ↓ with ↑ age	Incidence ↑ with ↑ age
HPV-associated	+	+
Histologic		
Koilocytosis	+/−	+/−
AMFs	+	+
Biologic		
DNA content	Aneuploid	Aneuploid
Clonality	Monoclonal	Polyclonal
HPV-type	16/18	16/18
	? others	? others

dence of VIN and VAIN is not known, several studies suggest that the overall incidence of both VIN and VAIN is increasing and that the average age of women with these lesions is decreasing.[100–104] This may be due to an actual increased incidence of VIN and VAIN or may simply reflect increased surveillance and detection. At present, VIN and VAIN are uncommon when compared to CIN, and, although invasive cervical cancer is a common disease, both vulvar and vaginal squamous carcinoma are relatively rare with a limited clinical impact. Squamous cell carcinoma of the vagina and vulva, in contrast to cervical carcinoma, are diseases of the elderly with peak age incidences in the sixth and seventh decades respectively. The incidence increases with increasing age.[101,104]

The epidemiologic risk factors for vulvovaginal neoplasia and squamous cell carcinoma are controversial and poorly documented. The most apparent risk factor for both VIN and VAIN is concomitant or antecedent CIN. Twenty-five to 30 percent of cases of VIN are associated over time with CIN, and 80 percent of women with VAIN have been found to have been treated previously for CIN or squamous cell carcinoma of the cervix.[101,104,105] This association between vulvovaginal intraepithelial neoplasia and CIN has led to the idea of a "lower genital tract neoplasia syndrome" (LGTNS) which associates these asynchronous, multifocal intraepithelial neoplasms with a shared embryologic and pathogenetic origin.[106–110]

Immunosuppression is also a risk factor for VIN and VAIN, both of which occur with increased frequency and a greater tendency to multifocality in the immunosuppressed host.[60,110,111] As with CIN, HPV infection has been associated epidemiologically and statistically with vulvar and vaginal neoplasia.[112] In many cases of VIN and VAIN, direct continuity between condylomatous and neoplastic epithelium may be observed. VIN is associated with antecedent or concomitant HPV infection in 20 to 60 percent of cases. HPV-associated VIN and VAIN occurs in younger patients, and HPV has been implicated in the decreasing age incidence of VIN and VAIN because of the frequent association between condyloma and vulvovaginal carcinoma, particularly in the uncommon cases of young women in whom invasive cancer has been observed.[101,112] HPV-specific structural proteins have been identified histochemically in the nuclei of some neoplastic lesions. Further documentation has been provided by the isolation of HPV DNA by molecular hybridization in intraepithelial neoplasms of the vulva and vagina as well as in verrucous carcinomas and the usual squamous cell carcinomas of these sites.[91,94,96,99]

VIN and VAIN are diseases characterized by multifocality and polyclonality. Their natural history, including transit times and risk of progression, has not been well defined, although the apparent risk of these lesions progressing to invasion is considerably less than that of CIN.[101,113–117] VIN generally presents as slightly raised, single or multiple plaque-like lesions which may occur anywhere on the vulvar surface involving both the keratinized skin and mucous membranes. VIN may extend into the pilosebaceous units of the skin whose usual depth is approximately 2 mm (Fig. 7–16). Many VIN lesions are hyperpigmented, resulting from both melanin deposition in basal keratinocytes and from melanin uptake in dermal macrophages. VAIN also presents as single or multiple irregular plaques, most commonly occurring in the anterior or posterior walls of the upper third of the vagina. VIN often occurs in association with condylomata and the lower genital

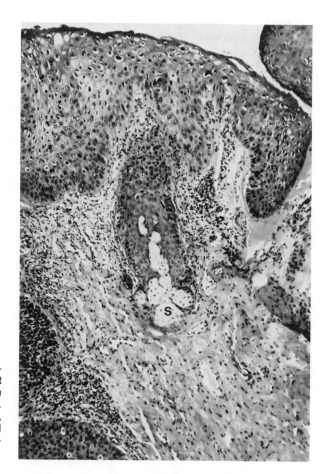

Figure 7–16. VIN 2 with extension into a pilosebaceous unit (S). The epithelial changes seen in VIN are similar to those in CIN. Note the superficial koilocytosis, nuclear hyperchromatism, and pleomorphism, as well as numerous abnormal mitotic figures.

tract neoplasia syndrome with the greatest risk of progression occurring in the elderly and the immunosuppressed. Less than 10 percent of VIN lesions appear to progress to invasive carcinoma, but in over 50 percent of cases of invasive vulvar carcinoma there is an adjacent VIN lesion present, implying that at least some VIN lesions have a malignant potential, although their biology cannot be predicted on an individual basis.[118,119]

Because of its multifocal, polyclonal nature, VIN frequently recurs following treatment, but it may regress spontaneously without treatment.

Spontaneous regression of VAIN is also well documented. However, the DNA content of VIN and VAIN does not appear to be as accurate a predictor of biologic behavior as has been observed in the cervix, and, even though the presence of aneuploidy in VIN correlates well with the degree of histologically observed abnormalities, several authors have reported the regression of aneuploid vulvar and vaginal lesions without therapy.[100,101,107,109,112,120–122]

The use of the diagnostic term VIN encompasses several synonymous systems of nomenclature as outlined in Table 7–7.[123] Grading and histologic identification

TABLE 7–7. SYNONYMS FOR VIN

Hyperplastic vulvar dystrophy with atypia	
Mild	VIN 1
Moderate	VIN 2
Severe	VIN 3
Mixed vulvar dystrophy with atypia	
Mild	VIN 1
Moderate	VIN 2
Severe	VIN 3
Carcinoma in situ	VIN 3
Bowen's disease	VIN 3
Erythroplasia of Queyrat	VIN 3
Carcinoma simplex	VIN 3

of VIN and VAIN parallels that of CIN (Fig. 7–10). Differential diagnosis from vulvovaginal condyloma is based on the presence of atypia, pleomorphism, loss of basal polarity, and the finding of AMFs as described in CIN, although clinicopathologic correlations are less clear with VIN and VAIN because of the substantially lower risk of progression.

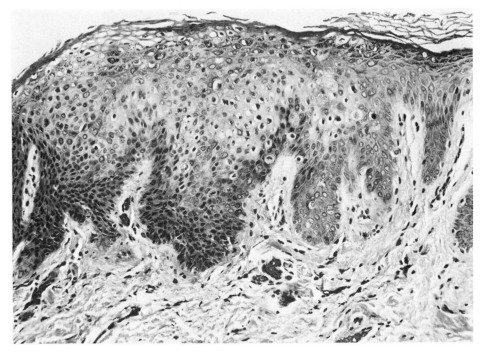

Figure 7–17. Bowenoid papulosis. The histology is indistinguishable from VIN and must be defined clinically. Hyperkeratosis and hypergranulosis are seen in the superficial epithelium on the right. Scattered koilocytes are present, best seen in the surface on the left. Despite their histologic appearance, the lesions of Bowenoid papulosis may regress spontaneously.

In some cases, as with CIN, the differential diagnosis of atypical vulvovaginal lesions with koilocytosis may be exceedingly difficult. This is particularly true in the case of vulvar Bowenoid papulosis, the biology and natural history of which is of particular interest with regard to the relationship between HPV infection and neoplastic alterations of the squamous epithelia. Bowenoid papulosis, although histologically indistinguisable from typical VIN, is distinctive clinically in that it consists of multiple, glistening, hyperpigmented papules, may occur in children, and commonly regresses spontaneously within 6 months to 1 year (Fig. 7–17). Bowenoid papulosis is being reported with increasing frequency in males as well as females. Its diagnostic recognition is dependent on the finding of the papular gross lesions and must be distinguished from VIN. The association of Bowenoid papulosis with concomitant or subsequent CIN has been described. The high rate of spontaneous regression in Bowenoid papulosis is of exceptional interest because these lesions have been found to be aneuploid by DNA microspectrophotometry and to contain not only HPV types 6 and 11 but also HPV types 16 and 18, the apparent markers of irreversible neoplasia in the cervix.

Further clinicopathologic studies are required to document the epidemiology and natural history of VIN and VAIN and Bowenoid papulosis and to investigate further the factors responsible for the apparent disassociation in vulvovaginal neoplasia between biologic behavior, ploidy levels, HPV types, and histology, which correlate so well in the natural history of intraepithelial neoplasia in the nearby cervix.

ACKNOWLEDGMENT

The authors would like to acknowledge the technical assistance of Ms. Barbara Lezynski and Mr. William Oxberry in the preparation of photographs for this manuscript.

REFERENCES

1. Silverberg E: Cancer Statistics, 1983. CA 33:9, 1983
2. Berkowitz RS, Ehrmann RL, Lavizzo-Mourey R, Knapp RC: Invasive cervical carcinoma in young women. Gynecol Oncol 8:311, 1979
3. Richart RM: The patient with an abnormal Pap smear: Screening techniques and management. N Engl J Med 302:332, 1980
4. Richart RM: Cervical intraepithelial neoplasia: A review. Pathol Annu 8:301–328, 1973
5. Ferenczy A: Cervical intraepithelial neoplasia. In Blaustein A (ed): Pathology of the Female Genital Tract, 2nd ed. New York, Springer-Verlag, 1982
6. Cramer DW, Cutler SS: Incidence and histopathology of malignancies of the female genital organs in the United States. Am J Obstet Gynecol 118:443, 1974
7. Sadeghi SB, Hsieh EW, Gunn SW: Prevalence of cervical intraepithelial neoplasia in sexually-active teenagers and young adults. Am J Obstet Gynecol 148:726, 1984
8. Smith JW, Townsend DE, Sparks RS: Genetic variants of glucose-6-phosphate dehydrogenase in the study of carcinoma of the cervix. Cancer 28:529, 1971
9. Richart RM, Lerch V: Time-lapse cinematographic observations of normal human

cervical epithelium, dysplasia, and carcinoma-in-situ. J Natl Cancer Inst 37:317, 1966

10. Ferenczy A, Richart RM, Okagaki T: Endometrial involvement by cervical carcinoma-in-situ. Am J Obstet Gynecol 110:590, 1971
11. Fenoglio CM, Ferenczy A: Etiologic factors in cervical neoplasia. Semin Oncol 9:349, 1982
12. Zur Hausen H: Human papillomaviruses and their possible role in squamous cell carcinomas. Curr Top Microbiol Immunol 78:1, 1977
13. Gross G, Pfister H, Hagedorn M, Gissman L: Correlation between human papillomavirus (HPV) type and histology of warts. J Invest Dermatol 78:160, 1982
14. Olson C, Gordon DE, Robl MG, Lee KP: Oncogenicity of bovine papillomavirus. Arch Environ Health 19:827, 1969
15. Garrett WFH, Murphy J, O'Neil BW, Larid HM: Virus-induced papillomas of the alimentary tract of cattle. Int J Cancer 22:323, 1978
16. Lancaster WD, Olson C: Animal papillomaviruses. Microbiol Rev 46:191, 1982
17. Howley PM: The human papillomaviruses. Arch Pathol Lab Med 106:429, 1982
18. Orth G, Favre M, Breitburg F, et al: Epidermodysplasia verruciformis: A model for the role of papillomaviruses in human cancer. In Essex M, Todaro G, Zur Hausen H (eds): Viruses in Naturally Occurring Cancer. Cold Spring Harbor, NY, Cold Spring Harbor Laboratory Press, 1980, Vol A, p 259
19. Zur Hausen H, de Villiers EM, Gissman L: Papillomaviruses and human genital cancer. Gynecol Oncol 12:124, 1981
20. Meisels A, Morin C, Casas-Cordero M: Human papillomavirus infection of the uterine cervix. Int J Gynecol Pathol 1:75, 1982
21. Centers for Disease Control: Morbidity, Mortality Weekly Report 32:306, 1983
22. Oriel JD: Natural history of genital warts. Br J Vener Dis 47:1, 1971
23. Benedictis TJ, Marmar JL, Praiss DE: Intraurethral condylomata acuminata management and review of the literature. J Urol 118:767, 1977
24. Ray B: Condyloma acuminatum of the scrotum. J Urol 117:739, 1977
25. Levine RU, Crum CP, Herman E, et al: Cervical papillomavirus infection and intraepithelial neoplasia: A study of male sexual partners. Obstet Gynecol 64:16, 1984
26. Rotkin ID: A comparison review of key epidemiological studies in cervical cancer related to current searches for transmissible agents. Cancer Res 33:1353–1367, 1973
27. Kessler II: Venereal factors in human cervical cancer: Evidence from marital clusters. Cancer 39:1912–1919, 1977
28. Martinez I: Relationship of squamous cell carcinoma of the cervix uteri to squamous cell carcinoma of the penis. Cancer 24:777–780, 1969
29. Graham S, Priore R, Graham M, et al: Genital cancer in wives of penile cancer patients. Cancer 44:1870–1874, 1979
30. Cartwright RA, Sinson JD: Carcinoma of penis and cervix. Lancet 1:97, 1980
31. Maggregor JE, Innes G: Carcinoma of penis and cervix. Lancet 1:1246–1247, 1980
32. Smith PG, Kinlen LJ, White GC, et al: Mortality of wives of men dying with cancer of the penis. Br J Cancer 41:422–428, 1980
33. Stein DS: Transmissible venereal neoplasia. Am J Obstet Gynecol 137:864, 1980
34. Daling JR, Weiss ND, Klopfenstein LL, et al: Correlates of homosexual behavior and the incidence of anal cancer. JAMA 247:1988, 1982
35. Lee SH, McGregor DH, Kuziez MN: Malignant transformation of perianal condyloma acuminatum: A case report with review of the literature. Dis Colon Rectum 24:462, 1981
36. William DC: Venereally-transmitted anal warts: Medical aspects. Human Sexuality 11:77, 1977
37. Purola E, Savia E: Cytology of gynecologic condyloma acuminatum. Acta Cytol 21:26, 1977

38. Surjanen KJ, Heinonen UM, Kauraniemi T: Cytologic evidence of the association of condylomatous lesions with dysplastic and neoplastic changes in the uterine cervix. Acta Cytol 25:17, 1981
39. Boon ME, Fox CH: Simultaneous condyloma acuminatum and dysplasia of the uterine cervix. Acta Cytol 25:393, 1981
40. Crum CP, Egawa K, Barron B, et al: Human papillomavirus infection (condyloma) of the cervix and cervical intraepithelial neoplasia: A histological and statistical analysis. Gynecol Oncol 15:88, 1983
41. Clarke EA, Morgan RW, Newman AM: Smoking as a risk factor in cancer of the cervix: Additional evidence from a case control study. Am J Epidemiol 115:59, 1982
42. Romney SL, Palan PR, Dattagupta C, et al: Retinoids and the prevention of cervical dysplasias. Am J Obstet Gynecol 141:890, 1981
43. Wassertheil-Smoller S, Romney SL, Wylie-Rosset J, et al: Dietary vitamin C and uterine cervical dysplasia. Am J Epidemiol 114:714–724, 1981
44. WHO Scientific Group: Neoplasia of the uterine cervix. In WHO Scientific Group: Steroid Contraception and the Risk of Neoplasia. (Technical Report Series 619). World Health Organization, Geneva, Switzerland, 1978, pp 26–33
45. Melamed MR, Flehinger BJ: Early incidence rates of precancerous lesions in women using oral contraceptives. Gynecol Oncol 1:290–298, 1973
46. Swan SH, Brown WL: Oral contraceptive use, sexual activity, and cervical carcinoma. Am J Obstet Gyencol 139:52–57, 1981
47. Robboy SJ, Truslow GY, Anton J, Richart RM: Role of hormones, including diethylstilbestrol in the pathogenesis of cervical and vaginal intraepithelial neoplasia. Gynecol Oncol 12:S98, 1981
48. VanNiekerk WA: Cervical cells in megaloblastic anemia of puerperium. Lancet 1:1277, 1962
49. Whitehead N, Reyner F, Lindenbaum J: Megaloblastic changes in the cervical epithelium: Association with oral contraceptive therapy and reversal with folic acid. JAMA 226:1421–1424, 1973
50. Butterworth CE, Hatch KD, Gore H, et al: Improvement in cervical dysplasia associated with folic acid therapy in users of oral contraceptives. Am J Clin Nutr 35:73–82, 1982
51. Nahmias AJ, Roizman B: Infection with herpes simplex viruses 1 and 2. N Engl J Med 289:667, 719, 781, 1983
52. Fenoglio CM, Galloway DA, Crum CP, et al: Herpes simplex virus and cervical neoplasia. In Fenoglio CM, Wolff M (eds): Progress in Surgical Pathology, Vol 4. New York, Masson, 1981 pp 45–82
53. Barron BA, Cahill MC, Richart RM: A statistical model of the natural history of cervical neoplastic disease: The duration of carcinoma-in-situ. Gynecol Oncol 6:196–205, 1978
54. Barron BA, Richart RM: A statistical model of the natural history of cervical carcinoma based on a prospective study of 557 cases. J Natl Cancer Inst 41:1343, 1968
55. Zur Hausen H: Human genital cancer: Synergism between two virus infection or synergism between a virus infection and initiating events? Lancet 2:1370, 1982
56. Burnett TS, Gallimore PH: Personal communication 1982, Cold Spring Harbor, NY
57. La Porta RF, Taichma LB: Human papilloma viral DNA replicates as a stable episome in cultured epidermal keratinocytes. Proc Natl Acad Sci USA 79:3393, 1979
58. Shorkri-Tobibzadeh S, Koss LG, Molnar J, Romney S: Association of human papillomavirus with neoplastic processes in the genital tract of four women with impaired immunity. Gynecol Oncol 12:S129, 1981
59. Lutzner MA: Immunopathology of papillomavirus-induced warts and skin cancers in immunodepressed and immunosuppressed patients. Semin Immunopathol 5:53, 1982

60. Winkler B, Norris JH, Fenoglio CM: The female genital tract. In Ridell RH (ed): Pathology of Drug-Induced and Toxic Diseases. New York, Churchill Livingstone, 1982

61. Koss LG, Durfee GR: Unusual patterns of squamous epithelium of the uterine cervix: Cytologic and pathologic study of koilocytotic atypia. Ann NY Acad Sci USA 63:1235, 1956

62. Meisels A, Fortin R, Roy M: Condylomatous lesions of the cervix, II. Cytologic, colposcopic, and histopathologic study. Acta Cytol 21:379, 1977

63. Roy M, Meisels A, Fortier M, et al: Vaginal condylomata: A human papillomavirus infection. Clin Obstet Gynecol 24:261, 1981

64. Bellina JH: The use of the carbon dioxide laser in the management of condyloma acuminatum with eight-year follow-up. Am J Obstet Gynecol 147:375, 1983

65. Crum CP, Egawa K, Fu YS, et al: Atypical immature metaplasia (AIM): A subset of human papillomavirus infection of the cervix. Cancer 51:2214, 1983

66. Richart RM, Barron BA: A follow-up study of patients with cervical dysplasia. Am J Obstet Gynecol 105:386, 1969

67. Barron BA, Richart RM: A statistical model of the natural history of cervical carcinoma, II. Estimates of the transition time from dysplasia to carcinoma-in-situ. J Natl Cancer Inst 45:1025, 1970

68. Kaufman R, Koss LG, Kurman RJ, et al: Caution in interpreting papillomavirus-associated lesions (Letter). Obstet Gynecol 62:269, 1983

69. Meisels A, Roy M, Fortier M, et al: Human papillomavirus (HPV) infections of the cervix: The atypical condyloma. Acta Cytol 25:7, 1981

70. Kurman RM, Shah KH, Lancaster WD, Jenson AB: Immunoperoxidase localization of papillomavirus antigens in cervical dysplasia and vulvar condylomas. Am J Obstet Gynecol 140:931–935, 1981

71. Ferenczy A, Braun L, Shah KV: Human papillomavirus (HPV) in condylomatous lesions of cervix. Am J Surg Pathol 5:661–670, 1981

72. Syrjanen KJ, Pyrhonen S: Immunoperoxidase demonstration of human papilloma virus (HPV) in dysplastic lesions of the uterine cervix. Arch Gynecol 233:53–61, 1982

73. Kurman RJ, Jenson AB, Lancaster WD: Papillomavirus infection of the cervix, II. Relationship to intraepithelial neoplasia based on the presence of specific viral structural proteins. Am J Surg Pathol 7:39–52, 1983

74. Gupta JW, Gupta PK, Shah KV, Kelly DP: Distribution of human papillomavirus antigen in cervicovaginal smears and cervical tissues. Int J Gynecol Pathol 2:160–170, 1983

75. Said JW, Nash G, Sassoon AF, et al: Involucrin in lung tumors: A specific marker for squamous differentiation. Lab Invest 49:563–568, 1983

76. Warhol MJ, Antoniolo DA, Pinkus GS, et al: Immunoperoxidase staining for involucrin: A potential diagnostic aid in cervicovaginal pathology. Human Pathol 13:1095, 1982

77. Antoniolo DA, Fu YS, Warhol M, et al: Multifactorial approach to the detection of cervical squamous cell dysplasia. Lab Invest 48:4A, 1983

78. Warhol MJ, Pinkus GS, Rice RH, et al: Papillomavirus infection of the cervix, III. Relationship of the presence of viral structural proteins to the expression of involucrin. Int J Gynecol Pathol 3:71, 1984

79. Fuchs E, Green H: Changes in keratin gene expression during terminal differentiation of the keratinocyte. Cell 19:1033–1042, 1980

80. Croissant O, Bonneaud G, Orth G: Detection of the vegetative viral DNA replication in papillomavirus-induced tumors by in-situ molecular hybridization. Cr Acad Sci Paris 274:614, 1972

81. Mole R, Levy R, Czernobilsky B, et al: Cytokeratins of normal epithelia and some neoplasms of the female genital tract. Lab Invest 49:599, 1983

82. Löning TH, Kühler CH, Caselitz J, Stegner HE: Keratin and tissue polypeptide antigen profiles of the cervical mucosa. Int J Gynecol Pathol 2:105–112, 1983
83. Bamford PN, Ormerod MG, Sloane JP, Warburton MJ: An immunohistochemical study of the distribution of epithelial antigens in the uterine cervix. Obstet Gynecol 61:603, 1983
84. Fu YS, Reagan JW, Richart RM: Definitions of precursors. Gynecol Oncol 12:S220–5231, 1981
85. Shevchuk MM, Richart RM: DNA content of condyloma acuminatum. Cancer 49:489, 1982
86. Fu YS, Reagan JW, Richart RM: Precursors of cervical cancer. Cancer Surv 2:359, 1983
87. Fu YS, Braun L, Shah KV, et al: Histologic, nuclear DNA, and human papillomavirus studies of cervical condyloma. Cancer 52:1705–1711, 1983
88. Fujii, T, Crum CP, Winkler B, et al: Human papillomavirus infection and cervical intraepithelial neoplasia: Histopathology and DNA content. Obstet Gynecol 63:99, 1984
89. Winkler B, Crum CP, Fujii T, et al: Koilocytotic lesions of the cervix: The relationship of mitotic abnormalities to the presence of papillomavirus antigens and nuclear DNA content. Cancer 53:1081, 1984
90. Gissman L, Zur Hausen H: Partial characterization of viral DNA from human genital warts (condylomata acuminata). Int J Cancer 25: 605, 1980
91. Gissman L, DeVilliers EM, Zur Hausen H: Analysis of human genital warts (condylomata acuminata) and other genital tumors for human papillomavirus Type 6 DNA. Int J Cancer 29:143, 1982
92. Kurman RL, Sanz LE, Jenson AB, et al: Papillomavirus infection of the cervix, I. Correlation of histology with viral structural antigens and DNA sequences. Int J Gynecol Pathol 1:17–28, 1982
93. Durst M, Gissman L, Ikenberg H, Zur Hausen H: A papillomavirus DNA from a cervical carcinoma and its prevalence in cancer biopsy samples from different geographic regions. Proc Natl Acad Sci USA 80:3812, 1983
94. Gissman L, Wolnik L, Ikenberg H, et al: Human papillomavirus types 6 and 11 DNA sequences in genital and laryngeal papillomas and in some cervical cancers. Proc Natl Acad Sci USA 80:560, 1983
95. McCance DJ, Walker PG, Dyson JL, et al: Presence of human papillomavirus DNA sequences in cervical intraepithelial neoplasia. Br Med J 287:784, 1983
96. Okagaki T, Twiggs LB, Zachow KR, et al: Identification of human papillomavirus DNA in cervical and vaginal intraepithelial neoplasia with molecularly cloned virus-specific probes. Int J Gynecol Pathol 2:153–159, 1983
97. Crum CP, Ikenberg H, Richart RM, Gissman L: Human papillomavirus type 16 and early cervical neoplasia. N Engl J Med 310:880, 1984
98. Schneider PS, Krumholz BA, Topp WC, et al: Molecular heterogeneity of female genital wart (condylomata acuminata) papillomaviruses. Int J Gynecol Pathol 2:329, 1984
99. Zur Hausen H, Giessman L, Boshart M, et al: Presence of human papilloma virus in genital tumors. J Invest Dermatol 83:26^s–28^s, 1984
100. DiSaia PJ, Creasman WT, Rich WM: An alternate approach to early cancer of the vulva. Am J Obstet Gynecol 133:825, 1979
101. Friedrich EG, Wilkinson EJ: The vulva. In Blaustein A (ed) Pathology of the Female Genital Tract, 2nd ed. New York, Springer-Verlag, 1982
102. Green TH, Jr: Carcinoma of the vulva: A reassessment. Obstet Gynecol 52:462, 1978
103. Hilliard GD, Massey FM, O'Toole RV: Vulvar neoplasia in the young. Am J Obstet Gynecol 135:185, 1979

104. Blaustein A, Sedlis A: Diseases of the vagina. In Blaustein A (ed) Pathology of the Female Genital Tract, 2nd ed. New York, Springer-Verlag, 1982, pp 59–98

105. Zacur H, Genadry R, Woodruff JD: The patient at risk for development of vulvar cancer. Gynecol Oncol 9:199–208, 1980

106. Lopez de la Osa Garces L (ed): Etiology and pathogeny of carcinoma of the vulva. In Aspects and Treatment of Vulvar Cancer. Basel, S Karger, 1972, pp 4–15

107. Friedrich EG, Wilkinson EJ, Fu YS: Carcinoma-in-situ of the vulva: A continuing challenge. Am J Obstet Gynecol 136:830, 1980

108. Hansen LH, Collins CG: Multicentric squamous cell carcinomas of the lower female genital tract. Am J Obstet Gynecol 98:982, 1967

109. Wilkinson EJ, Friedrich EG, Fu YS: Multicentric nature of vulvar carcinoma-in-situ. Obstet Gynecol 58:69, 1981

110. Woodruff JD, Davis JH, Jones HW, et al: Correlated investigative techniques of multiple anaplasias in the lower genital canal. Obstet Gynecol 33:609, 1969

111. Simpkins PB, Chir B, Hill MGR: Intraepithelial vaginal neoplasia following immunosuppressive therapy treated with topical 5-Fu. Obstet Gynecol 46:360, 1975

112. Crum CP, Braun, LA, Shah KV, et al: Vulvar intraepithelial neoplasia: Correlation of nuclear DNA content and the presence of a human papillomavirus (HPV) structural antigen. Cancer 48:468–71, 1982

113. Jones I, Buntine D: Progression of vulval carcinoma-in-situ. Aust NZ J Obstet Gynaecol 18:274, 1978

114. Kaufman RH, Gardner HL: Intraepithelial neoplasia of the vulva. Clin Obstet Gynecol 8:1035, 1965

115. Buscema J, Woodruff JD, Parmley TH, Genadry R: Carcinoma-in-situ of the vulva. Obstet Gynecol 55:225, 1980

116. Gallup DG, Morley G: Carcinoma-in-situ of the vagina. Obstet Gynecol 46:339, 1975

117. Woodruff JD: Carcinoma-in-situ of the vagina. Clin Obstet Gynecol 24:485–501, 1981

118. Buscema J, Stein J, Woodruff JD: The significance of the histological alterations adjacent to invasive vulvar carcinoma. Am J Obstet Gynecol 137:902–909, 1980

119. Buscema J, Woodruff JD: Progressive histobiologic alterations in the development of vulvar cancer. Am J Obstet Gynecol 138:146–150, 1980

120. Rutledge F, Sinclair M: Treatment of intraepithelial carcinoma of the vulva by skin excision and graft. Am J Obstet Gynecol 102:806, 1968

121. Skinner MS, Sternberg WH, Ichinose H, Collins J: Spontaneous regression of Bowenoid atypia of the vulva. Obstet Gynecol 42:40, 1973

122. Fu YS, Reagan JW, Townsend DE, et al: Nuclear DNA study of vulvar intraepithelial and invasive squamous neoplasm. Obstet Gynecol 57:643, 1981

123. International Society of the Study of Vulvar Disease: New nomenclature for vulvar disease: Report of the Committee on Terminology. Obstet Gynecol 47:122–124, 1977

8

Colposcopy

Louis Burke

INTRODUCTION

The basic requirement for any expertise in laser surgery of the cervix, vagina, and vulva is a good basic knowledge of colposcopy. Without this knowledge, not only will improper application of the laser method be applied to the pathology, but more importantly, irreparable harm will be done to the patient. It is imperative that the laser surgeon have a working expertise in colposcopy. This chapter endeavors to review and update this expertise.

Colposcopy is the magnification of stratified squamous epithelium of the cervix, vagina, and the vulva, by means of a strong light and a low-powered binocular microscope of 4 to 40 times magnification (Fig. 8–1). The colposcopic image is determined by the nature of the surface epithelium and the vascular arrangement within the connective tissue stroma. The epithelial cell numbers, morphology, and organization, as well as the nature of the lamina propria and the location of the vascular innervation of the epithelium will influence the visual image observed through the colposcope (Fig. 8–2). Since Hans Hinselman in the early 1920s invented colposcopy, its major interest has been in the area of the cervix in relationship to finding the earliest origin of invasive squamous cell carcinoma. In recent years, its usefulness in investigating vaginal and vulvar lesions has been acknowledged. To understand its application to lesions of the lower genital tract, a thorough understanding of colposcopy of the cervix is necessary.

COLPOSCOPY OF THE CERVIX

Woman, when she is born, is endowed in the region of the vagina and cervix with two original epithelia. One is the original stratified squamous epithelium that lines the vagina and most of the portio of the cervix, and the original columnar epithelium lining the endocervix. The vagina is originally lined by columnar epithelium derived from the fused Müllerian ducts. This is replaced by the upward growth of a core of stratified squamous epithelium originating in the urogenital sinus. This core becomes vacuolated to form the vagina as the fetus grows cephalad. The vagina and the portio of the cervix thus become covered with stratified squamous epithelium (original or native stratified squamous epithelium). The original or native columnar lines the endocervical canal and sometimes part of the portio of the cervix and is contiguous with the endometrium at the internal cervical os. This single layer of tall columnar cells, mucus-secreting, occasionally ciliated, is derived from the Müllerian ducts. To the colposcopist, the area of interest is at the interface of these two epithelia, namely the squamocolumnar junction (Fig. 8–3). The interest is great because it is generally agreed that probably all stratified squamous carcinomas take origin from this area. This area lends itself to intensive examination by the colposcope.

Before any consideration of the interaction between the original epithelia in the development of neoplasia, understanding of the colposcopic appearance of the original epithelia and the changes that take place at their interface must be discussed.

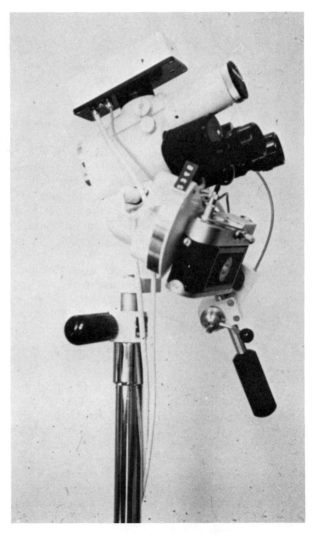

Figure 8–1. Leisegang IIIB colposcope with flash and camera attached.

Original Squamous Epithelium

Histologically, the mature stratified squamous epithelium of the cervix (and the vagina) presents a characteristic appearance of increased maturation from the base to the surface (Fig. 8–4). Several layers can be described from which various types of cells are seen on cytologic examination (Fig. 8–5). At the base is a zone composed of one or two layers of elliptic cells with scant cytoplasm and oval nuclei. This is called the basal or germinal cell layer. A second zone is the midzone from which the intermediate cells are seen on cytologic examination. The most mature cell population is seen at the surface and cytologically is represented by the superficial cells. This characteristic palisading of cells is also characterized by the presence of glycogen in the upper layers and thus the staining of the epithelium when subjected to the exposure of Schiller's or Lugol's iodine solution.

In 1960 Zinser and Rosenbauer[1] filled the vascular tree of the cervix with white latex and found that the terminal vessels that supplied oxygen to the epithelium

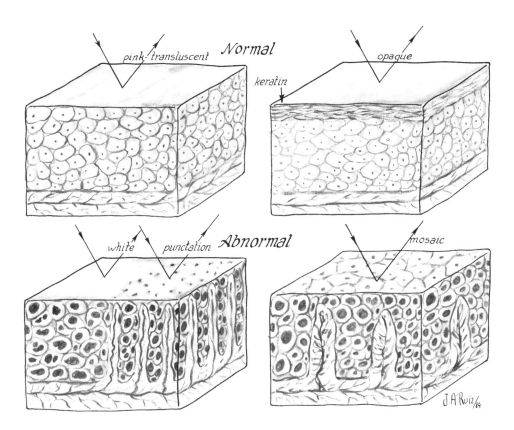

Figure 8–2. Tissue basis of colposcopy.

might be divided into four zones. The first zone is a plexus of relatively large, freely anastamosing vessels deep in the stroma. These continue into the second zone of palisade-like vessels running perpendicular or obliquely to the surface. These branch into the third zone of small vessels running parallel to the surface. This is called the basal network. From the basal network the fourth zone of terminal capillaries emerge (Fig. 8–6). Depending on the thickness of the surface epithelium, the basal network, and the subepithelial capillaries, terminal capillaries can be observed. The terminal capillaries can be divided into two types. The most common type are the network capillaries which form a dense and fairly regular network of fine capillaries (Fig. 8–7). These have an intercapillary distance of about 100 μ and are usually less than 200 μ. A second type, usually best seen around the os in the postmenopausal women, are the hairpin capillaries (Fig. 8–8). They have an ascending and descending branch of fine caliber vessels which are close together and form a loop at their interchange. Only the crests of the loops are visible appearing as a fine, regular punctate pattern. This pattern is very similar to that seen in the presence of a *Trichomonas* infestation.

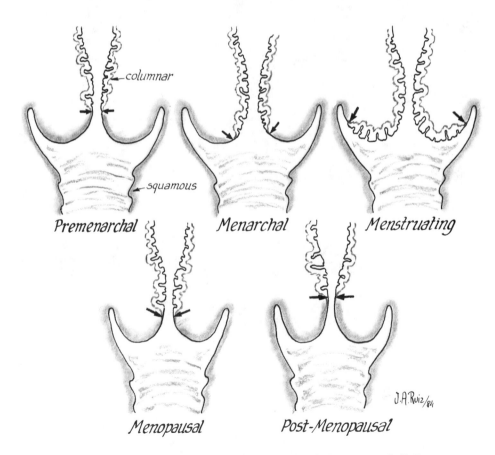

Figure 8–3. Location of squamocolumnar junction during a woman's lifetime.

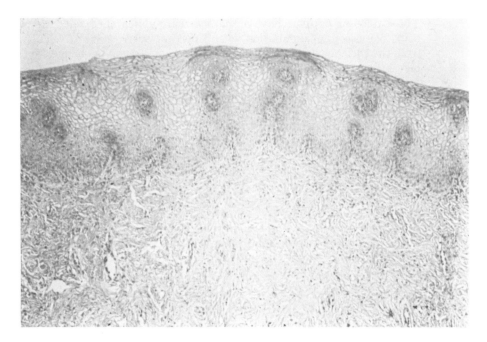

Figure 8–4. Biopsy of portio of the cervix. Normal stratified squamous epithelium with palisade effect of maturing cells. (Magnification × 350.)

When the original squamous epithelium is subjected to scanning electron microscopy, a characteristic appearance is seen. The superficial cells are flat and polygonal with a central raised area representing the nucleus. The cell borders are distinct and raised. At higher magnification numerous microridges are often seen within the cell boundaries (Fig. 8–9).[2]

Colposcopically, the original squamous epithelium appears pink and translucent. The network vessels can be seen. This is best viewed when the cervix is gently rinsed with a saline solution and the green filter of the colposcope utilized.

Original Columnar Epithelium

The original columnar epithelium, which is Müllerian duct derived, consists of a single layer of tall columnar cells with basal nuclei. These cells are mucus secreting and frequently have cilia (Fig. 8–10). Because of the single-layer nature of the columnar epithelium, when viewed through the colposcope after being washed gently with saline, the layer appears deep pink or red (Fig. 8–11, see Color Plate I*). This is the result of the strong light of the colposcope traversing the epithelium and impinging on the vascular presence in the lamina propria. The single layer epithelium is thrown up into numerous folds and crypts as described by Fluhmann (Fig. 8–12).[3] From many of these folds smaller folds are formed. This is especially prominent as one approaches the external os of the cervical canal.

*Color plates I and II appear following p. 177.

These folds or papillae have a characteristic appearance when subjected to the usual colposcopic examination with 3 percent acetic acid. The mucus is washed from the surface and between the clefts and some osmolar change swells the papillae so that they take on a characteristic grape-like appearance (Fig. 8–13).

The vascular network of the columnar epithelium is very complex. There is a network of uniform coiled vessels. Within each papilla there is an ascending and descending capillary. At the top of the papilla these two capillaries intertwine in a multichanneled network (Fig. 8–14).[4] Each papilla is separated from the next by an interpapillary or intervillus crypt. The terminal capillary loop in each papilla is easily seen colposcopically (Fig. 8–15, see Color Plate I).

The original columnar epithelium demonstrates its characteristic appearance when viewed by scanning electron microscopy. Finger-like villi with deep clefts are apparent. Each villus is covered by polygonal cells. They are about 4 μm in diameter. The cells tend to be uniform in size and closely packed. The surface is slightly raised. Ciliated cells may be seen in the cells located in the endocervix. When metaplasia occurs, a flattening and fusion of the cells can be seen occurring in a haphazard fashion on the villi (see section on Transformation Zone in this chapter) (Fig. 8–16).

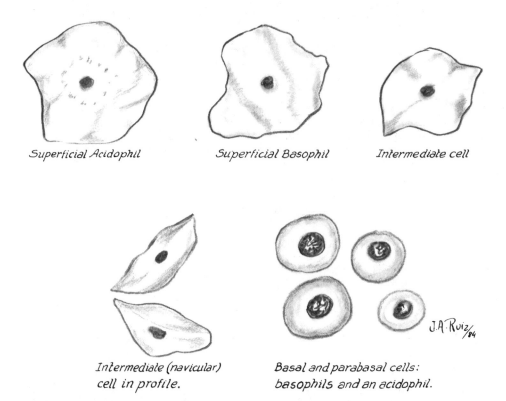

Superficial Acidophil   Superficial Basophil   Intermediate cell

Intermediate (navicular)   Basal and parabasal cells:
cell in profile.   basophils and an acidophil.

Figure 8–5. Cells seen on cytologic exam. Types of cells found in vaginal smears of a normal cycle.

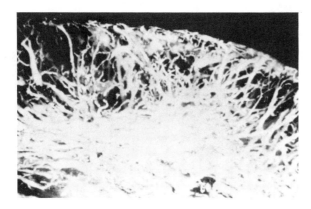

Figure 8–6. Latex cast of vascular tree of the cervix. *(From Zinser HK, Rosenbauer KA.[1])*

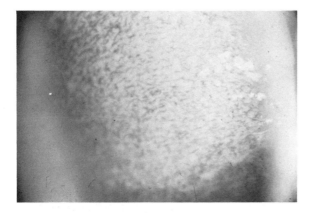

Figure 8–7. Colpophotograph of original squamous epithelium illustrating the arborizing network blood vessels. (Magnification × 2.)

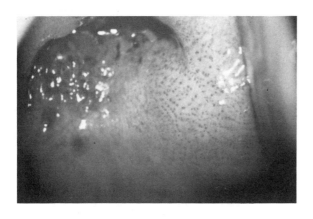

Figure 8–8. Colpophotograph of Trichomonas cervicitis. Hairpin type capillaries are very prominent. (Magnification × 2.)

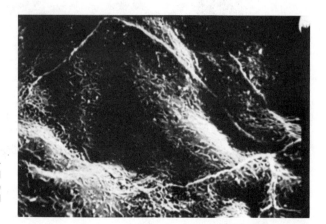

Figure 8–9. Scanning electro-microscopy of original stratified squamous epithelium. Note microridges and sharp cell boundaries. *(From Jordan JA.[2])*

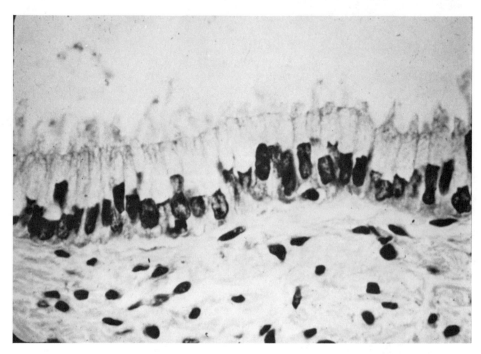

Figure 8–10. Biopsy of original columnar epithelium. Some of the tall columnar cells are ciliated. (Magnification × 40.)

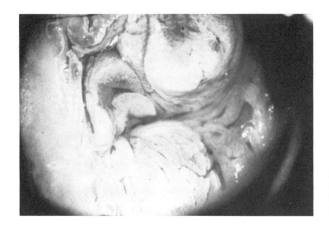

Figure 8–12 Colpophotograph of endocervix. Folds and papillae of columnar epithelium, are very prominent. (Magnification × 1.8.)

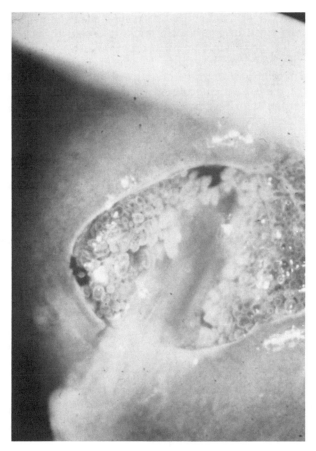

Figure 8–13. Colpophotograph of the cervix after the application of 3 percent acetic acid. Columnar epithelium has the typical "grape-like" appearance. Mucous coming from the endocervix is evident. (Magnification × 1.1.)

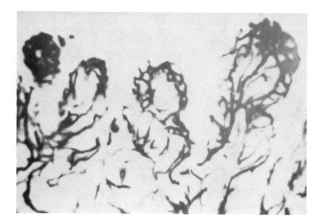

Figure 8–14. Alkaline phosphatase preparation of the complex vascular arrangement in columnar epithelium papillae. *(From Kolstad P, Stafl A.[4])*

Squamocolumnar Junction

The interface of these two original epithelia is called the squamocolumnar junction. As generally described in gynecologic texts, it is said to be located at the anatomic external os of the cervix. Examination of the cervices of women at different ages of their life, however, shows that the area of the squamocolumnar junction seems to move in relationship to the presence or absence of estrogen (see Fig. 8–3). Neonates will have the squamocolumnar junction more towards the portio of the cervix than within the canal due to the influence of intrauterine maternal estrogen. In the premenarchal stage, the squamocolumnar junction is more likely to be at the anatomic external os of the cervix. At menarche and first pregnancy,

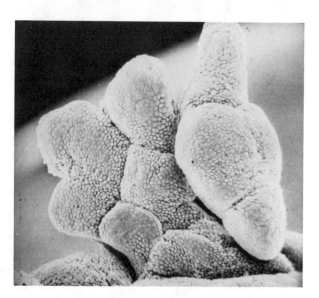

Figure 8–16. Scanning electron microscopy of papillae of the original columnar epithelium. Some areas have a flattened appearance. These represent areas of beginning metaplasia. *(From Jordan JA.[2])*

both of which are characterized by high estrogen levels, the squamocolumnar junction is usually on the portio of the cervix. It will stay in this area throughout the women's menstruating lifetime and then recede up the canal in the postmenopausal state. This deceptive movement of the squamocolumnar junction really does not occur. Instead, what the high estrogen levels do is to cause a rearrangement of the elements within the connective tissue of the cervix. This results in an eversion of the cervix so that the columnar epithelium is brought into contact with the environment of the vagina. With the withdrawal of this hormonal stimulus, the cervix inverts; the columnar epithelium and squamocolumnar junction recede into the endocervical canal. Accompanying the high estrogen level usually is a change in acidity of the vagina due to the emergence of the lactobacilli. The original columnar epithelium and its subjacent connective tissue stroma, when exposed to an acid media and in a background of high estrogen content, will produce just beneath the basement membrane a new cell called the reserve cell (Fig. 8–17). The reserve cell will then divide horizontally lifting off the original columnar epithelium and replacing it with a multilayered epithelium (Fig. 8–18). This multilayered epithelium will ultimately mature into a palisade-like epithelium, acquire glycogen, and for all intents and purposes will be identical to the original stratified squamous epithelium. The area in which this metaplastic process occurs is called the transformation zone. There are three periods during a woman's lifetime when this process of metaplasia is most active. First is during intrauterine existence, when the tissues are under the influence of the mother's estrogen, sec-

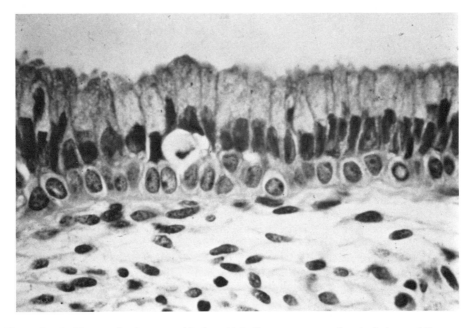

Figure 8–17. Biopsy of columnar epithelium. Note the appearance of a single layer of "reserve cells" beneath the original columnar epithelium. (Magnification × 400.)

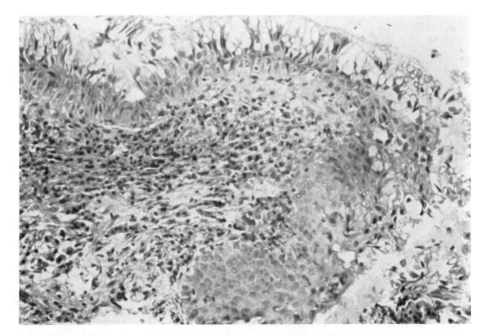

Figure 8–18. Biopsy of cervix showing papilla in various stages of reserve cell hyperplasia. In the upper part of the picture, the original columnar epithelium is being replaced by the reserve cells. In the lower part of the photo, the process is more advanced and a new multilayered epithelium is present. (Magnification × 350.)

ond is at the menarche, between the ages of 14 and 17 when estrogen levels are high, and third is in the first pregnancy when this eversion of the cervix is most acute by the end of the first trimester. If the concept that the initiation of neoplasia occurs with the onset of metaplasia is true, on a theoretic basis, the occasions that a woman may lay down the nidus for invasive squamous cell carcinoma can only occur during menarche and the first pregnancy.

The Transformation Zone

During the normal metaplasia, as the epithelium of the columnar layers becomes multilayered, the papillae fuse. This process is a haphazard one; the tips of the papillae which first come in contact with the acid media of the vagina will participate in the process (see Fig. 8–16). The various areas of metaplasia then expand and coalesce to finally form the transformation zone. The vascular structures of the individual papillae interconnect at the base. The growth of metaplastic tissue pushes the vessels down so that a vascular pattern, similar to that of the original squamous epithelium, occurs. If there is obstruction of the crypts by involvement only of their upper part in this metaplastic process, a Nabothian cyst will develop. If only the base of the crypts participates in the metaplastic process and the upper part remains open, a so-called "white-rimmed" gland opening will be present in

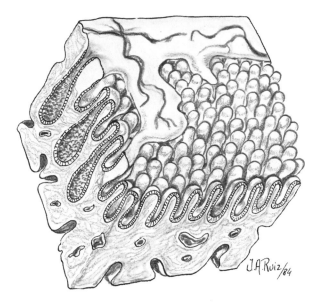

Figure 8–19. Diagram of the typical transformation zone.

the area of change. There also may occur islands of columnar epithelium which do not participate in this process. It is only by the recognition of these remnants of the original columnar epithelium are we able to identify the area of the transformation zone (Fig. 8–19). With the development of this zone, the original squamocolumnar junction (anatomic squamocolumnar junction) is replaced by a squamo-squamo junction, and a new squamocolumnar junction (physiologic squamocolumnar junction) develops.

Colposcopically, the early immature transformation zone reveals an opacity among the grape-like villi participating in the process (Fig. 8–20, see Color Plate I). The redness of the vasculature beneath the epithelium has a somewhat pale appearance. As the process matures, the villi fuse and give rise to at first an irregular surface which at a later date becomes smooth. Interspersed within the areas that form the transformation zone, the remnants of the columnar epithelium will be seen (Fig. 8–21, see Color Plate I). When this new epithelium becomes fully mature and fully glycogenated, it is no longer capable of developing cervical squamous neoplasia.

Atypical Transformation Zone

If during the process of metaplasia, the environment contains some oncogenic factor (herpes, DNA, human papillomavirus (HPV), sperm DNA), the metaplasing cells send out pseudopods and engulf the oncogenic factor incorporating it into its nucleus. The cell now takes on neoplastic potential (Fig. 8–22). These cells, instead of dividing and maturing in the usual palisade fashion, already described under normal metaplasia, will instead divide into blocks of tissue. There is a direct association between the growing mass and new vessel growth.[8] The population of potentially neoplastic cells stimulates the capillary endothelial cells of the nearby

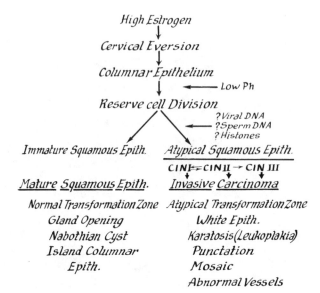

High Estrogen

↓

Cervical Eversion

↓

Columnar Epithelium

↓ ←—— Low Ph

Reserve cell Division

?Viral DNA
?Sperm DNA ←——
?Histones

Immature Squamous Epith.   Atypical Squamous Epith.

CIN I ⇄ CIN II → CIN III

Mature Squamous Epith.   Invasive Carcinoma

Normal Transformation Zone   Atypical Transformation Zone
Gland Opening   White Epith.
Nabothian Cyst   Karatosis(Leukoplakia)
Island Columnar   Punctation
Epith.   Mosaic
Abnormal Vessels

Figure 8–22. Allogram of the development of the transformation zone.

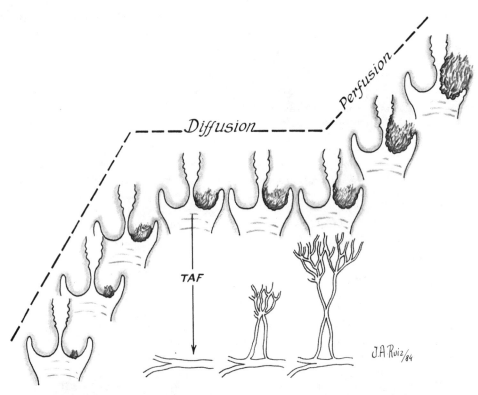

Figure 8–23. Diagram depicting Folkman's theory of tumor angiogenesis factor.

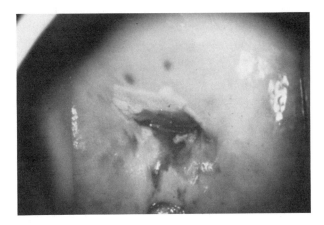

Figure 8-24. Colpophotograph after 3 percent acetic acid. Note red dots perforating acetowhite lesion. (Magnification × 1.1.)

capillaries so that there is marked alteration of the vascular network (Fig. 8–23). The vessels become tortuous and compressed vertically by the neoplastic epithelium and may extend close to the surface. When one looks on this epithelium with the colposcope, red dots will be seen, which is called *punctation* (Fig. 8–24). Further proliferation and interconnection of the proliferating dividing cells may result in the compression of the network into a basket-like structure around the neoplastic epithelium, producing the change which has a *mosaic* appearance (Fig. 8–25). Because of severe compression, some of the capillaries eventually disappear and result in an increase in the intercapillary distance. Thus, punctation and mosaic represent a remodeling of the preexisting vascular network of the columnar epithelium. The alterations in the terminal vascular network reflect the initial changes in the metabolism of the cells. At the same time that these cells are influencing the vascular pattern, they also are developing abnormal amounts of protein both within the cytoplasm and the nucleoplasm. This will impede the transmission of light from the colposcope and thus endow the tissue with varying degrees

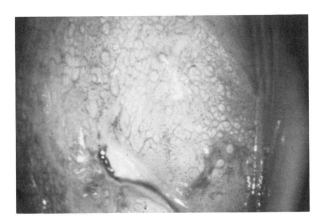

Figure 8-25. Colpophotograph of cervix after 3 percent acetic acid showing mosaic structure. Punctation frequently is intermixed with the mosaicism. (Magnification × 2.8.)

of opacity. If this tissue is washed with a dilute acetic acid solution, apparently the protein condenses and this opacity becomes more marked. This change of increased whiteness after denaturing with a mild acid is called an *acetowhite change* (Figs. 8–26, 8–27). This change is only transient; after a few minutes it will disappear. To see it again more dilute acetic acid must be applied. Another manifestation of the abnormal metabolic activity of the cells may be the development of excess amounts of keratin, which will appear as a plaque of intensely white change on the surface of the epithelium (Fig. 8–28). Unlike an acetowhite lesion this keratin, which is called *leukoplakia,* may be seen with the naked eye and does not require denaturing to manifest itself.

As the intraepithelial lesion develops, it may reach a stage where it will remain dormant for years. Finally it will stimulate new capillaries to appear. These are

8-26

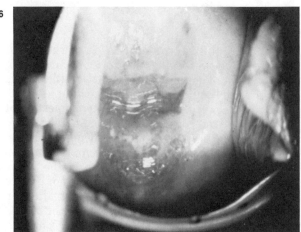

8-27

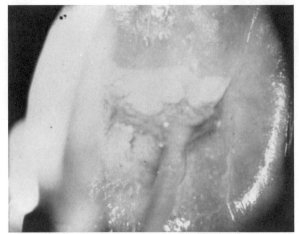

Figures 8–26 and 8–27. Colpophotograph of cervix prior to the application of acetic acid. No abnormalities are seen. (Magnification × 1.1.) After 3 percent acetic acid a sharply delineated acetowhite lesion with sharp margin is evident. (Magnification × 1.8.)

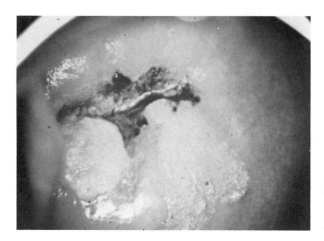

Figure 8–28. Cervix prior to acetic acid. Note white raised patches of leukoplakia on posterior cervical lip. (Magnification × 1.8.)

usually underneath the surface of the epithelium and parallel to it. They are usually nondividing vessels and have a variety of shapes and appearances, and are called *atypical blood vessels* (Fig. 8–29). With their appearance the increase in intercapillary distance may at first be somewhat decreased; as the tumor expands and compresses, the intercapillary distances will increase.

A transformation zone is said to be atypical, therefore, if any of the following are present when viewed through the colposcope: (1) acetowhite epithelium, (2) punctation, (3) mosaic, (4) leukoplakia, and (5) abnormal blood vessels. These areas of atypical colposcopic patterns may occur singly or in combination; they may be unifocal or multifocal, and are almost invariably sharply delineated from surrounding normal tissue. Their lateral margins rarely extend beyond the original squamocolumnar junction onto the native squamous epithelium.

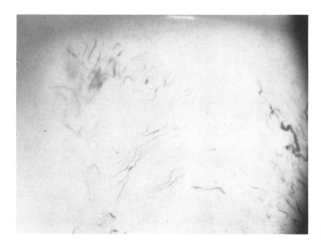

Figure 8–29. Cervix after being subjected to irradiation for invasive carcinoma. Note abnormal blood vessels (Magnification × 2.8.)

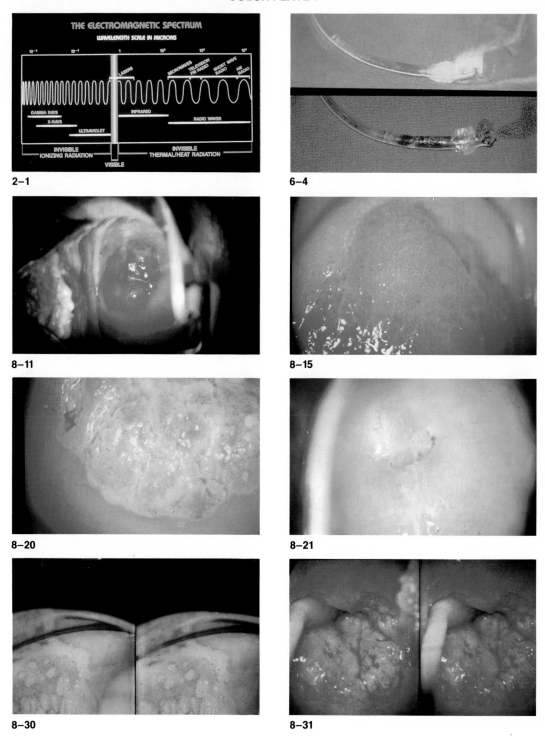

2–1

6–4

8–11

8–15

8–20

8–21

8–30

8–31

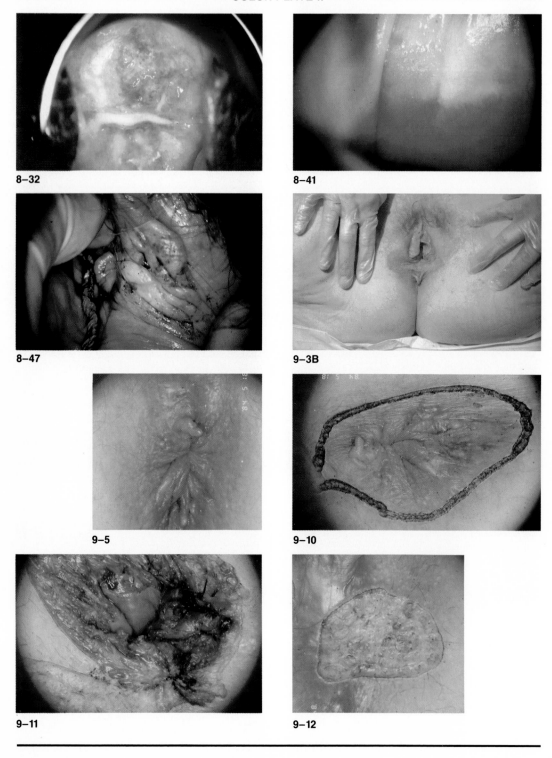

8-32

8-41

8-47

9-3B

9-5

9-10

9-11

9-12

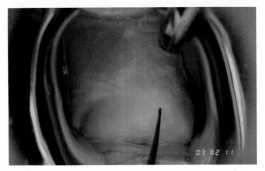

11–6

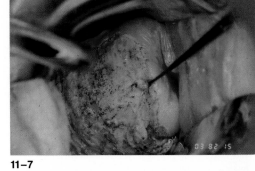

11–7

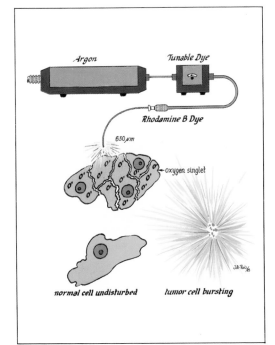

14–5

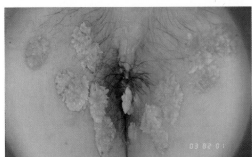

15–1

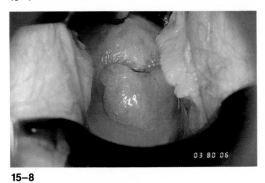

15–8

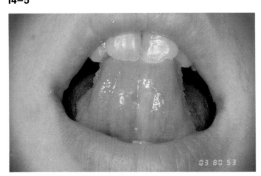

15–10

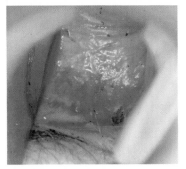

15–11

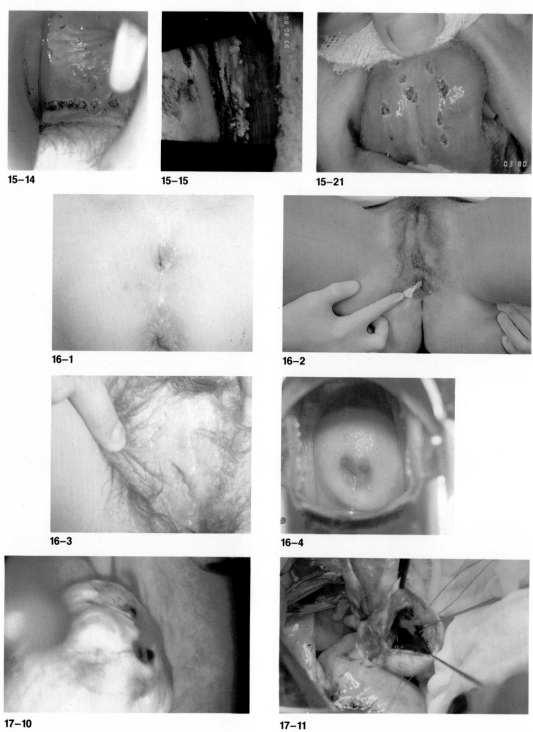

15–14

15–15

15–21

16–1

16–2

16–3

16–4

17–10

17–11

GRADING OF COLPOSCOPIC LESIONS

Although the atypical transformation zone identifies the site and extent of major intraepithelial neoplastic changes as well as true invasion, many atypical transformation zones demonstrate only minor histologic disturbances in cervical epithelia and are of no apparent clinical significance. All things being equal, the more abnormal the colposcopic appearance the greater the histologic abnormalities. It is possible for a colposcopist with vast experience to differentiate the various forms of cervical intraepithelial neoplasia from each other and from early invasive cancer on the basis of the colposcopic features. The features that are utilized are those of color, surface contour, vascular patterns, intercapillary distances, and the overall grade of the abnormality of the lesion.

The quality of the abnormal colposcopic lesion depends upon (1) the degree of whiteness of the epithelium, (2) the nature of the surface contour whether flat or irregular, (3) the fineness or coarseness of the caliber of the punctate vessels and their intercapillary distance, (4) the irregularity and pleomorphism of the mosaic pattern, and (5) the presence or absence of atypical blood vessels. The intercapillary distance is an extremely important indicator of the seriousness or severity of the atypicality of the colposcopic lesion. As shown by Kolstad,[5] when the intercapillary distance increases above 300 μ, the presence of this type of vessel is more likely to occur in the more serious cervical intraepithelial neoplasia (CIN) lesions (Table 8–1). The only place where this is less likely to happen is at the moment of microinvasion when new capillaries are produced and there may be a slight decrease in the intercapillary distance. Interpretation of the atypical transformation zone based upon these various features, are best graded by a modification of that originally suggested by Malcolm Coppelson[6] (Table 8–2). The color tone of a Grade I lesion is judged as normal or slightly whiter than normal, when viewed through the green filter. The surface is smooth; the border of the lesion tends to be somewhat diffuse. If there are any vascular changes present, it is characterized by a fine or regular punctate appearance, and/or mosaic; there is no increase in the intercapillary distance. These types of lesions may be seen in anything from flat condyloma, pregnancy, metaplasia, inflammation, regeneration and repair, and the milder degrees of CIN. A Grade II lesion has more intense whiteness and usually a sharp border from the surrounding normal epithelium. The surface is usually slightly raised and indeed may be granulated. There is usually some vas-

TABLE 8–1. INTERCAPILLARY DISTANCE AND HISTOLOGIC DIAGNOSIS

Histologic Diagnosis	Intercapillary Distance $> 300\ \mu$ (%)
Benign lesions	1.8
Dysplasia	14.6
Carcinoma in situ	57.1
Early invasive carcinoma	76.9
Invasive carcinoma	85.5
Normal mucous membrane of cervix = 50–150 μ	

(From Kolstad P.[5])

TABLE 8–2. GRADES OF ATYPICAL TRANSFORMATION ZONE

Grade	Surface	Margin	Color	Vessels
I	Flat	Indistinct	White	Fine; normal ICD
II	Flat	Distinct	Whiter	Dilated; slight increase ICD
III	Raised	Sharp	Whitest	Coarse; marked increase ICD; atypical vessels

ICD, intercapillary distance.

cular pattern in the form of an irregular punctation or mosaic and slight increase in the intercapillary distances. This may represent anything from CIN II to CIN III. The Grade III lesion is a lesion with definitely atypical vasculature combined with clearcut elevation of the surface pattern (Fig. 8–30, see Color Plate I). The vascular pattern is usually one of a coarse punctation or the presence of atypical blood vessels. The intercapillary distance may either be greatly increased or may be slightly decreased depending upon the nature of the underlying lesion. Frequently, in this type of lesion, when the acetic acid is applied, the epithelium may roll up like wet cigarette paper. This is especially true in the CIN III lesions, in which the intracellular bonds have been dissolved. In the microinvasion lesion the intercapillary distance, as already noted, may be slightly decreased (Fig. 8–31, see Color Plate I). In the invasive lesion, there is usually loss of the surface epithelium, there may be ulceration, and the atypical blood vessels may be bizarre (Fig. 8–32, see Color Plate II).

Thus, the Grade III lesion may represent anything from CIN III, microinvasion, or invasive cancer.

VAGINAL COLPOSCOPY

The colposcope is a valuable tool to evaluate vaginal lesions. Careful colposcopy of the vagina is indicated in the following situations: (1) in the presence of an abnormal cytologic smear following a hysterectomy, (2) in the evaluation of a patient who has no cervical lesion on colposcopy but has abnormal cytologic findings, (3) in the evaluation of patients with vulva or cervical carcinoma in situ and who are at risk for multifocal genital tract lesions, (4) in the presence of abnormal gross findings, and (5) in the women who have been exposed in utero to diethylstilbestrol (DES).

Although the colposcopic lesions observed in the vagina are basically the same as those observed on the cervix, namely acetowhite epithelium, punctation, leukoplakia, and atypical blood vessels, mosaic structure is rarely seen except in the DES-exposed patient. It should be recognized that the histology of the vagina is different from that of the cervix. The connective tissue of the vagina is loose and abundant as compared to the cervix, and vascular innervation is somewhat increased (Fig. 8–33). In addition, except in the DES-exposed female, there is no interface between columnar and stratified squamous epithelium and therefore no transformation zone. As a result, the colposcopic findings of lesions of the vagina

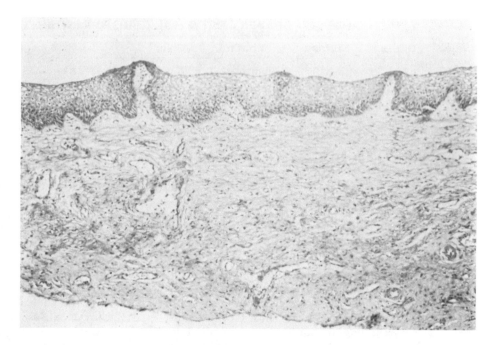

Figure 8–33. Histopathology of vaginal biopsy. Connective tissue stroma is loose and contains many blood vessels. (Magnification × 300.)

tend to be exophytic and tend to proliferate and produce large papillomatous projections with dilated vascular innervations. The grade of the lesion in the vagina always appears to be somewhat greater than that of the cervix for the same histopathology. Some of the conditions which are commonly seen during colposcopy of the vagina are described below.

Leukoplakia of the Vagina

Leukoplakia of the vagina is seen not infrequently with two common and a third less common condition. One of the most common causes of thickening of the vaginal epithelium is associated with the prolonged use of the diaphragm as a means of contraception (Fig. 8–34). Apparently, the acid nature of the jelly stimulates the epithelium of the vagina to become hypertrophied producing an appearance of thickened rugae with a somewhat opaque character to its coloration. No abnormal vascular changes are noted and on biopsy the report is usually acanthosis with or without hyperkeratosis.

The second most common thickening with a white papillary appearance is that associated with the human papillomavirus namely, condyloma acuminatum. This may be seen in two ways. First is the usual common exophytic papillary lesion characteristic of condylomata anywhere; the epithelium is thickened and the vessels are not too clear. Occasionally, the vessels may impart a red color to some of

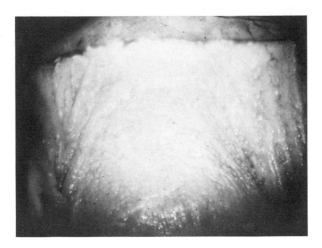

Figure 8–34. Anterior fornix of vagina of a patient with frequent diaphragm use. Note the rugae are thickened and white. (Magnification × 1.1.)

the condylomata (Fig. 8–35). The epithelium tends to be acanthotic and parakeratotic. A second form of condylomata is of greater import in that it is often confused with vaginal intraepithelial neoplasia. This is the so-called "flat condyloma" (Fig. 8–36). They are often multiple, raised, and white in character. They are ovoid in shape and usually occur on the crest of the vaginal ridges. They may have a diffuse even punctate appearance, which is often seen with vaginal intraepithelial neoplasia. Biopsy, however, will usually show the characteristics of human papilloma virus infection and thus distinguish them from true neoplastic lesions. The third less common cause of keratosis of the vagina is seen in women subjected to large doses of estrogen. These may be given either systemically or by means of local application of estrogen creams. These keratotic areas can be confused with condyloma (Fig. 8–37). Biopsy reveals hyperkeratosis.

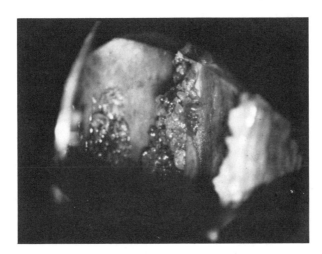

Figure 8–35. Condylomata of side wall of vagina. Papillary nature of lesion is prominent. (Magnification × 0.7.)

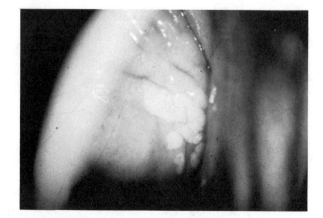

Figure 8-36. Left fornix of vagina after 3 percent acetic acid. Multiple raised white lesions resembling VAIN are seen. On biopsy, flat condyloma diagnosed. (Magnification × 1.8.)

Papillomatous Lesions

Colposcopy may be of aid in elucidating the nature of polypoid lesions that occur in the lateral vaginal fornices after hysterectomy. The appearance of granulation-like tissues in these areas always raise the question of fallopian tube prolapse. Granulation tissue, after total hysterectomy, may seem to have many atypical vessels; however, careful inspection of the vascular pattern will reveal tiny capillaries running in a smooth course and usually running parallel to the surface. Frequently, two or more vessels will run parallel and form a coil loop. Biopsy of these areas obviously will delineate the true nature of the lesion. The fallopian tube, on the other hand, frequently also will demonstrate on colposcopy the true Müllerian nature of the epithelium (Fig. 8-38). They may form somewhat papillary appearances after the application of 3 percent acetic acid. The vascular innervation tends to be very wide with an arborization pattern characteristic of normal vasculature

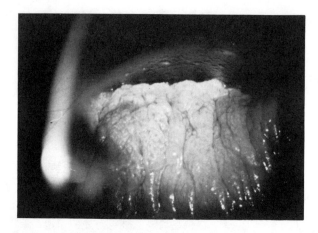

Figure 8-37. Anterior wall of vagina in patient on long-term estrogen therapy. Looks like condyloma. Biopsy reveals hyperkeratosis. (Magnification × 1.1.)

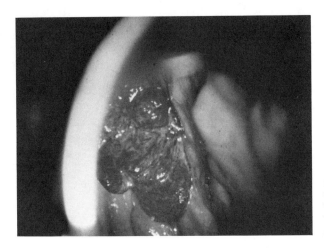

Figure 8–38. Colpophotograph of papillary lesion in left fornix of vagina. Note arborizing blood vessels. Biopsy revealed fallopian tube. (Magnification × 1.8.)

on the Müllerian duct derivatives of the lower genital tract. Again, biopsy reveals the true nature of the lesion.

Atrophy of the Vagina

The atrophic vaginal mucosa in the postmenopausal woman may frequently produce a cytologic report suggesting intraepithelial neoplasia or worse. On colposcopy the vasculature is very readily recognized as being normal and is very friable. Thus, when acetic acid is applied, subepithelial hemorrhages occur frequently producing a distorted appearance to the vagina (Fig. 8–39). However no abnormal vascular appearance or acetowhite lesions are seen. Estrogenation of the mucosa with local application of estrogen cream will revert the vaginal mucosa to its normal appearance. Following radiation, on the other hand, the atrophy due to the

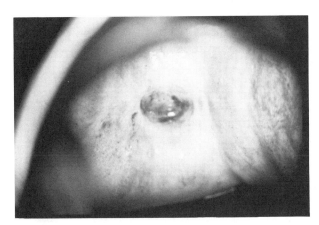

Figure 8–39. Atrophic cervix and vagina after saline. Blood vessels very prominent. Mucous membrane is very thin. (Magnification × 1.1.)

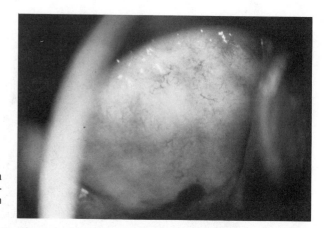

Figure 8–40. Apex of vagina following radiation. Note abnormal blood vessels. (Magnification × 1.8.)

use of this modality produces a thinned out friable epithelium with numerous atypical blood vessels (Fig. 8–40). These vessels are subepithelial and have all of the various shapes that are described for atypical vessels—"commas, tadpoles, spaghetti forms, and thick-thin-thick."

Vaginal Intraepithelial Neoplasia (VAIN)

The vaginal lesions of intraepithelial neoplasia tend to be multifocal. Prior to the application of acetic acid, they may be seen as slightly raised pinkish areas in the fornices of the vagina or adjacent to the edge of the cervix (Figs. 8–41, see Color Plate II; 8–42). Viewing at higher magnification, one will see punctation with varying degrees of increase in the intercapillary distances depending upon the severity of the lesion. The lesions tend to be raised with sharp borders. After the application of 3 percent acetic acid, they take on a Grade II-III acetowhite appearance interspersed with a coarse papillary punctation. The lesions of vaginal intraepi-

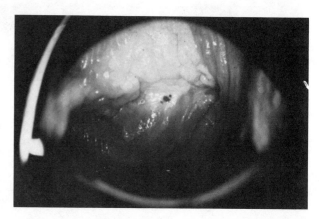

Figure 8–42. Apex of vagina of patient who underwent hysterectomy for CIS. Three percent acetic acid has been applied and sharply delineated acetowhite lesion develops. Biopsy reveals VAIN III. (Magnification × 1.1.)

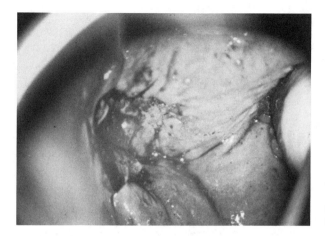

Figure 8–43. Right corner of vagina after 3 percent acetic acid. Acetowhite with abnormal vasculature can be made out. Epithelium is ulcerated. Biopsy revealed invasive disease. (Magnification × 1.1.)

thelial neoplasia rarely ever show a mosaic pattern. When true invasion occurs, a change in the vasculature occurs. The vessels become elongated and irregular within the papillary excrescences of the raised vaginal lesions (Fig. 8–43). Frequently, these lesions will be ulcerated as well. The presence of an invasive adenocarcinoma either as a metastasis or as a primary lesion, will take on the appearance of any invasive lesion with atypical blood vessels. Possibly the vasculature is somewhat more dilated and coarser than that seen in the invasive squamous cell lesion. Colposcopically, however, one cannot distinguish the nature of the invasive lesion based upon these vascular differences.

Vaginal Changes Associated with In Utero Exposure to DES

Unlike the lesions described above, the colposcopic appearances of in utero exposure to DES are determined by the relationship of an interface between stratified squamous epithelium and columnar epithelium.[7] Adenosis, the most common feature of in utero exposure to DES is merely the presence of Müllerian duct epithelium—columnar epithelium—in the vagina after birth. Thus all of the changes that take place at the interface during metaplasia of the cervix occur in the vagina; the appearances of the colposcopic lesions may be either columnar epithelium, acetowhite epithelium with or without punctation and mosaic structure (Fig. 8–44). These lesions usually are of a Grade I-II character and on biopsy will show varying degrees of metaplasia (Fig. 8–45). When the lesions take on a Grade III characteristic, then the possibility of squamous cell neoplasia should be entertained. The use of colposcopy in the diagnosis of clear cell adenocarcinoma has been helpful only if the lesion has reached the surface. Like cytology, many cases of clear cell adenocarcinoma have been missed on colposcopic examination. The lesion may be buried beneath normal-appearing epithelium. If the lesion is close to the surface, however, then one may see coarse punctation and atypical blood vessels suggesting the neoplastic process (Fig. 8–46). Obviously, if this is seen in an individual who is suspected of being DES exposed, biopsy is mandatory.

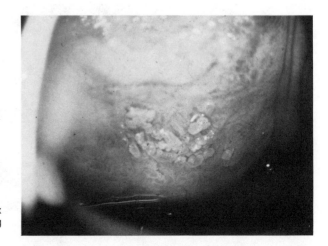

Figure 8–44A. Posterior fornix of DES-exposed patient showing columnar epithelium.

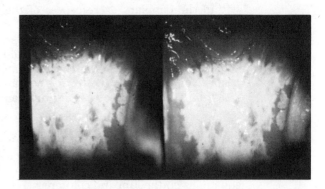

Figure 8–44B. Anterior fornix after 3 percent acetic acid. Grade II acetowhite change is present.

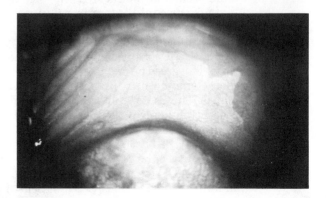

Figure 8–44C. Anterior fornix after 3 percent acetic acid. Grade I mosaic is present.

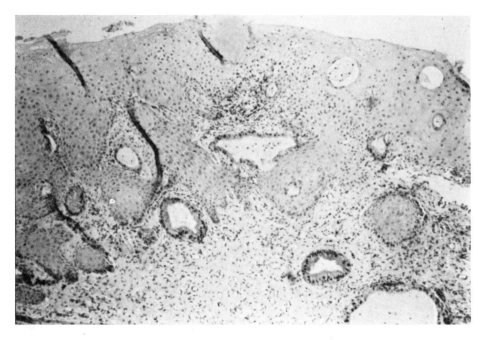

Figure 8–45. Biopsy of vagina. Endocervical glands can be seen in stroma. Some are completely replaced by metaplastic epithelium. Overlying epithelium is nonglycogenated. Biopsy characteristic of adenosis. (Magnification × 350.)

COLPOSCOPY OF THE VULVA

When abnormal-appearing vulva lesions are biopsied, they may include unimportant inflammatory dermatoses frequently encountered in extragenital skin, chronic vulva dystrophies, premalignant intraepithelial neoplasia, as well as invasive carcinomas. Recently, the international society for the study of vulva diseases adopted the classification noted below:

Classification of Vulvar Dystrophies

  I. Hyperplastic dystrophy
    Without atypia
    With atypia
 II. Lichen sclerosis
III. Mixed dystrophy—lichen sclerosis with foci of epithelial hyperplasia
    Without atypia
    With atypia

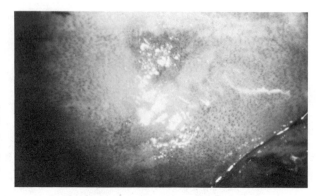

Figure 8–46. Nodule in anterior vaginal fornix of DES-exposed patient. Note coarse punctation. Above "highlight" abnormal vessels are present. Biopsy revealed clear cell adenocarcinoma. (Magnification × 1.8.)

This classification embraces the concept of vulva dystrophy which represents changes of the epithelium of the vulva to unknown etiologic agents. This classification is based on histopathologic features and emphasizes the importance of biopsies for accurate diagnosis. In the discussion of colposcopy of the vulva that follows, this classification of entities will be utilized. The colposcopic appearances of the inflammatory lesions and the various extragenital dermatoses that can occur on the vulva will not be alluded to. Even though colposcopy can be useful in the examination of the vulva, it is not as efficient as colposcopy of the cervix and the vagina. Although the normal thickness of the epithelium of the vulva averages 0.13 mm, the vascular changes of the stroma in the labia majora are hardly visible because the epithelium has a nontransluscent cornified characteristic. Application of oil to the skin may render the underlying terminal vessels visible. For this reason the usual features of punctation and mosaic are not seen readily in lesions of the labia majora. If persistent washing with dilute acetic acid is carried out, however, one may be able to bring out some of these vascular appearances. This is not quite as difficult as one approaches the labia minora where the cornification is less and the epithelium is somewhat thinner. In these areas the colposcopic images are much more likely to be similar to those seen in the vagina. The most frequent patterns encountered on the vulva is leukoplakia or acetowhite epithelium. Abnormal vessels will be seen when an invasive lesion is present.

In evaluating vulva lesions with the colposcope, two modalities aid in delineating the lesions. They are the use of acetic acid and the use of toluidine blue dye.

1. Acetic acid: Acetic acid will reveal acetowhite epithelium to aid in directing biopsies. This is especially true in the labia minora. Frequent washing with copious amounts, however, is necessary to bring out lesions in the labia majora. If this is done and subsequent evaluation with toluidine blue is desired, the latter may not be readily taken up by the acidified epithelium.
2. Toluidine blue: This dye is essentially a nuclear stain and when applied in vivo, becomes fixed to cell nuclei. Dye is applied in a 1 percent aqueous solution and allowed to stay on for 2 minutes. It is then decolorized with 1 percent acetic acid. In a normal keratin layer, there are no surface nuclei

and therefore the dye will be completely washed away. If nuclear material is present at the skin surface or if there is a break in the continuity of the epidermis, as in an ulcer, or when there are nucleated squamae present in the uppermost epithelial layer (parakeratosis), the dye will be picked up and will be seen as variation of blue staining (Fig. 8–47, see Color Plate II). The very fine spots will readily be picked out by colposcopic magnification. Parakeratosis alone does not denote neoplasia. It may be found in any benign conditions where there is a rapid turnover of cells, such as in condylomata acuminata. It is, however, a sign of abnormal squamous maturation and aids in directing one's biopsy. In doing the test the skin must be free of ointment or powders.

Condyloma Acuminatum

Like the cervix and the vagina, condylomata of the vulva is usually an obvious condition with the typical exophytic spiculed leukoplakic appearance (Fig. 8–48). Usually no vascular areas are noticeable when the lesion is on the labia majora. When it involves the labia minora, a diffuse, fine punctate appearance can be seen. Patients who have been treated repeatedly with podophyllin and who have persistence of their lesions, will frequently give an appearance that is somewhat darker than the typical condylomata. In addition, the lesion may be flatter and lack the spicules typical of the exophytic lesion. These lesions must be biopsied as they frequently will show atypicality of the nuclei suggesting a dysplastic process.

Hypertrophic Dystrophy

Colposcopically, the hypertrophic dystrophies are seen as thickened, white, keratinized areas with no vascular change. They are sharply delineated and raised. Isolated areas of vulva involvement are frequently seen (Fig. 8–49).

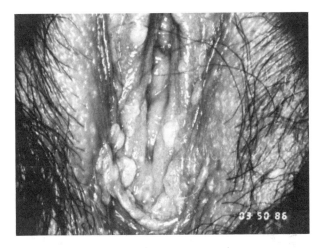

Figure 8–48. Cervicoscopy of vulva showing multiple condylomata. Diffuse punctation can be seen in lesion of inferior margin of right labium minus.

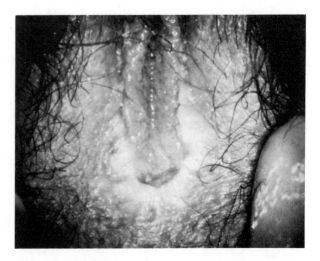

Figure 8–49. Perineum and vulva with raised white lesion of hypertrophic dystrophy.

Lichen Sclerosis

Lichen sclerosis is the thin kind of dystrophy in which a thin layer of white epithelium is seen. The surface very frequently is shiny; there is a crinkled appearance to the epithelium. There can be some degree of hyperkeratosis noted (Fig. 8–50).

Mixed Dystrophy

Both lichen sclerosis and hyperplastic dystrophy may be found on the same vulva and is called mixed dystrophy. This occurs in about 15 percent of all dystrophies of the vulva. Colposcopically, one may not be able to determine the differentiation

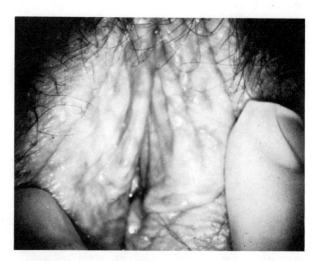

Figure 8–50. Vulva with white crinkly epithelium. Patient has marked pruritus. Biopsy consistent with lichen sclerosis.

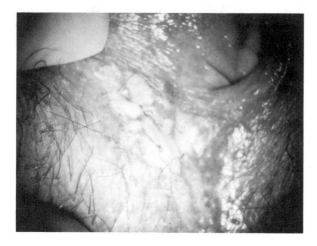

Figure 8–51. Raised white lesions of vulva. Biopsy revealed Bowen's disease.

between the two conditions, although there may be some raised plaques of white epithelium that suggest the underlying hyperplasia. The mixed dystrophies tend to have a higher incidence of atypia than do the hyperplastic lesions alone.

Carcinoma in Situ

The lesions of carcinoma in situ may be brown, red, white, or a combination. Their appearance depends upon the histologic make-up of the lesion. Many of the cases will have a superficial hyperkeratosis or parakeratosis and, therefore, have an intense appearance (Fig. 8–51). The lesions may or may not have vascular changes of punctation with increased intercapillary distances. Those lesions that are close to the labia minora are more likely to exhibit vascular changes (Fig. 8–52). The lesions of hyperplastic dystrophy and atypia (dysplasia) and carcinoma in situ (Bowen's disease) may appear to be identical. The lesions of both diseases may be single or multiple. They tend to be raised and frequently will have variation in

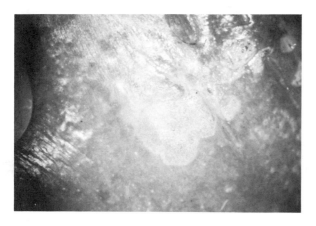

Figure 8–52. Area in right labia minora after 3 percent acetic acid. Lesion is raised with coarse punctation. Biopsy revealed VIN III. (Magnification $\times$ 1.8.)

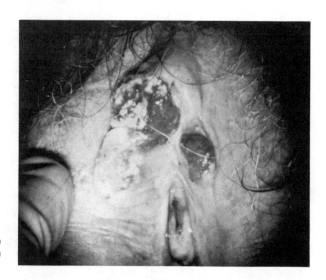

Figure 8–53. Obvious invasive carcinoma of vulva. Lesion raised and ulcerated.

color from the intense whiteness seen with condylomata or hyperplastic dystrophy.

Invasive Carcinoma

The usual invasive lesion of the vulva does not require colposcopic examination to make the diagnosis (Fig. 8–53). The lesions are usually raised, may be red or white, and frequently are ulcerated. Colposcopically, however, one can find the usual criteria of invasion, namely abnormal blood vessels, in these lesions. The value of the colposcope in identifying these lesions is most evident in the early stages of the disease when patients are frequently being treated for other entities with creams and emollients. Colposcopy at this time may identify areas which are different from the obvious and which on biopsy will show evidence of an invasive squamous cell carcinoma (Fig. 8–54). In addition, the colposcope when combined

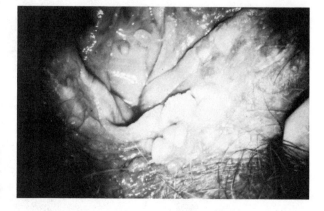

Figure 8–54. Lesion of vulva consisting of raised white lesions and reddish areas above. Biopsy of red areas revealed invasive carcinoma.

with toluidine blue may be helpful in delineating the extent of involvement of the epidermis of the vulva and thus aid in delineating the margins of the surgical specimen to be taken.

The basic evaluation of vulva lesions as described above is the biopsy. Inasmuch as many of the conditions may appear alike, even under the magnification of the colposcope, biopsy is mandatory to rule out neoplastic disease. This may be accomplished readily on an outpatient basis, either using the Keyes punch or an Eppendorfer biopsy forceps. Inasmuch as many of the vulva lesions are multifocal, magnification of the colposcope is needed for adequate identification. Biopsy will lead to correct diagnosis and proper therapy instituted.

REFERENCES

1. Zinser HK, Rosenbauer KA: Untersuchungen uber die angioarchitektonik der normalen und pathologisch veranderten cervix uteri. Arch F Gynak 194:73, 1960
2. Jordan, JA: Scanning electron microscopy of the physiological epithelium. In Jordan JA, Singer A (eds): The Cervix. London, WB Saunders, 1976, p 46
3. Fluhmann CF: The Cervix Uteri and Its Diseases. Philadelphia, WB Saunders, 1961, pp 30–102
4. Kolstad P, Stafl A: Atlas of Colposcopy. Baltimore, University Park Press, 1977
5. Kolstad P: The development of the vascular bed in tumours as seen in squamous cell carcinoma of the cervix uteri. Brit J Radiol 38:216, 1965
6. Coppleson M, Pixley E, Reid B: Colposcopy. Springfield, Ill., Charles C. Thomas, 1971
7. Burke L, Antonioli D, Knapp R, Friedman EA: Vaginal adenosis: Correlation of colposcopic and pathologic findings. Obstet Gynecol 44:257, 1974
8. Folkman J: Tumor Angiogenesis: Therapeutic Implications. N Engl J Med 285:1182, 1971

9

Laser for the Treatment of Vulvar Intraepithelial Neoplasia

Michael S. Baggish

INTRODUCTION

Carcinoma in situ of the vulva may be classified together with cervical intraepithelial and vaginal intraepithelial neoplasia to comprise a triad of disorders known as intraepithelial neoplasia of the lower genital tract. Although it has not been proven, substantial circumstantial evidence links the human papilloma virus (HPV)[1] and the herpes simplex virus (HSV)[2] to lower genital tract neoplasia. Recently data has been published which associates prior condylomata acuminata infections in one fourth of the women who subsequently developed vulvar intraepithelial neoplasia (VIN).[3,4] Baggish and Dorsey[5] reported a series of 35 cases of VIN of whom 43 percent (15) were under the age of 40 and 50 percent were multifocal. Although the natural history of this disorder, particularly its relationship to invasive squamous cell carcinoma, is by no means clear,[6] it is unlikely that the disease undergoes spontaneous remission, therefore all patients should be treated.

In past years the standard treatment of VIN was simple vulvectomy. This mutilating operation is not commonly performed any longer (Fig. 9–1). Skinning vulvectomy with split thickness grafting restores normal anatomy but requires hospitalization and a rather long recovery period.[7] The use of 5-fluorouracil cream or radiation have proven less successful than surgery and should not be used to treat this disorder.[8] The carbon dioxide (CO_2) laser has proved highly efficacious for the treatment of VIN and is particularly well suited to its multifocal geography and the superficial nature of the epithelial involvement.

BASIS FOR LASER TREATMENT

The stratified squamous epithelium of the vulva is less than 1 mm in thickness and the deepest rete peg rarely plunges more than 1 mm into the underlying dermis. Skin appendages are not commonly involved with the neoplastic process and

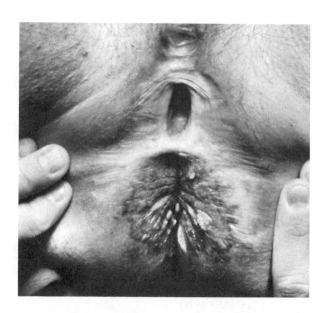

Figure 9–1. A patient with extensive perianal carcinoma in situ which also extended into the anal canal. Note: this woman had previous treatment by simple vulvectomy.

rarely exceed 3 mm in depth (Fig. 9–2). Treatment to a depth of 3 mm should eliminate intraepithelial disease and at the same time not result in scar formation.

All suspected neoplastic lesions of the vulva must be completely evaluated preoperatively by multiple biopsies, preferably performed with the dermal punch (Figs. 9–3A, 9–3B, see Color Plate II*; 9–4A, 9–4B). The dermal punch provides

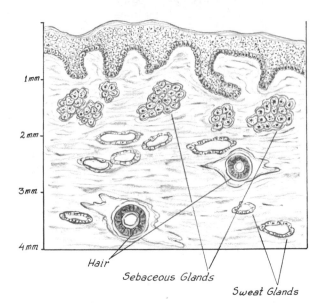

Figure 9–2. A typical section of vulvar skin showing surface stratified squamous epithelium and underlying skin appendages. The surface epithelium, deep rete pegs, and superficial appendages rarely extend beyond 3 mm depth.

*Color Plate II appears following p. 177.

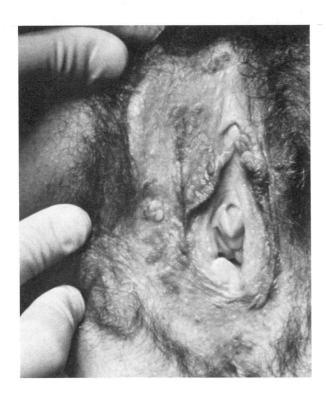

Figure 9–3A. Carcinoma in situ of the vulva is predominately a disease of women under 40 years of age. This 22-year-old woman with a condylomatous-type of carcinoma in situ had been mistakenly treated for benign warts for over 1 year.

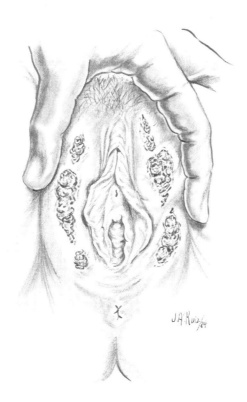

Figure 9–4A. Schematic drawing of extensive, multifocal vulvar carcinoma in situ.

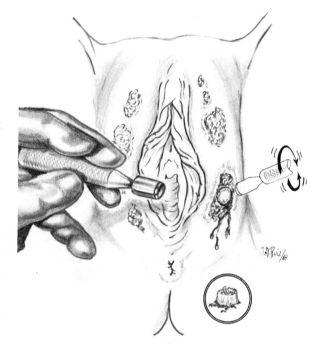

Figure 9–4B. The dermal skin punch provides the best specimen for the pathologist to orient. A circular piece of skin is obtained by twisting the punch in a "to and fro" circular motion. The piece of skin is then elevated with a fine forceps and cut off with Steven's scissors.

a circular sample which is easily oriented and which may be sectioned without tangential cutting. Since this disorder frequently presents as multifocal disease, several biopsies should be obtained to insure that one is dealing with intraepithelial rather than invasive disease.

I have found the colposcope particularly useful to localize these lesions. Magnification and the application of acetic acid helps to scrutinize lesions which would be otherwise missed by naked eye vision alone. Flat, warty lesions, pigmented warty lesions, red, eczematoid lesions, and hyperkeratotic lesions should all be biopsied (Fig. 9–5, see Color Plate II). Should any biopsy site suggest invasion, larger excisional samples must be submitted to rule out invasion. Invariably, treatment failures and discovery of invasion after treatment with the laser are due to inadequate preoperative diagnosis. To localize suspicious areas, complete biopsy-documented mapping of the vulva is required.

LASER SPECIFICATIONS

Anesthesia

All CO_2 laser treatment to the vulva requires anesthesia. For extensive disease that will be ablated at a single sitting, general anesthesia is indicated. For extensive disease that can be staged for treatment every 2 weeks, local anesthesia is very acceptable and treatment may be performed in the office setting. As a rule of thumb, I prefer to limit injection to 20 cc of 1 percent Xylocaine, a Carbocaine, or their equivalents at any one treatment. The main disadvantage to local anesthesia injection is the discomfort which the patient experiences due to the needle itself and to the burning sensation of the drug.

Mapping

Once the appropriate anesthetic has been administered, the laser beam is adjusted to deliver a 1.5 mm imprint, and trace spots outline the extent of the vaporization which is to be done (Fig. 9–6). For this, I have found it most convenient to gate the laser at 0.1 or 0.2 seconds and to set the power meter to 10 watts W. Either the free handpiece or the micromanipulator-directed laser may be utilized. I have found it most convenient to employ the free handpiece, defocused, to deliver a 1.5 mm spot. This methodology is rapid and when combined with eyeglass mounted magnification to 2.5 to 3 times is as accurate as the laser coupled to the microscope.

Prior to firing the laser onto the patient's tissues, calibration and adjustment of the spot on a moist wooden tongue depressor should be carried out.

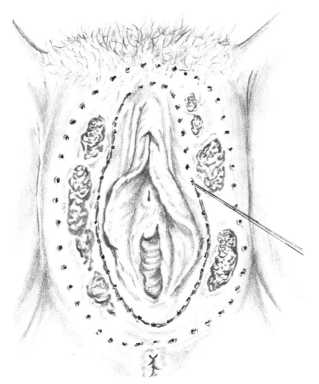

Figure 9–6. Initial laser mapping of lesions shown in Figure 9–4A. Initially the inner and outer margins of the tissue to be ablated are dot traced. Next the dots are connected with a tracing line made at low power density. A 2 to 3 mm peripheral margin is recommended.

Laser Vaporization

Since vaporization is to be performed to a depth of 3 mm only, high power densities are not necessary (Fig. 9–7). Power densities of less than 1000 W/cm^2 are most desirable because control is better and hemostasis is optimal. It is prefered to begin treatment at the lowest point of the field and work upwards. If local anesthesia is employed, a continuous dialogue with the patient is maintained throughout the operative procedure. As previously stated, a 1.5 to 2.0 mm spot is desirable; laser power is adjusted to 20 W continuous time. Vaporization is carried out employing a concentric circular motion, i.e., delivering the laser beam with small polishing-like circles with virtually all operator motion at the wrist joint (Fig. 9–8). Large tracts of skin may be vaporized in a very short period of time (Fig. 9–9). When the appropriate tissue has been removed, the char is wiped clean with a large cotton swab doused with 4 percent acetic acid (Figs. 9–10, 9–11, 9–12, see Color Plate II; Fig. 9–13) Ordinarily I do not prepare the vulvar skin preoperatively. If a skin prep is desired, however, Betadine or a suitable substitute is the solution of choice. Alcohol or other flammable materials should be avoided. When the neoplasia extends into the anal canal, a special laser speculum is inserted into the rectum and the microscopically directed laser is utilized to eliminate all visible disease to a depth of 1 mm. We have not hesitated to ablate circumferentially perianal intraepithelial neoplasia at one sitting. Troublesome bleeding is highly likely to occur with a tightly focused laser producing a 1 mm or less spot particularly with a transverse-electromagnetic (TEM_{00}) mode.

Laser Excision

When the sample obtained by the dermal punch biopsy indicates the possibility of stromal invasion, an excisional procedure is indicated. Under these circumstances, the suspicious portion of the neoplastic zone should be submitted for pathologic interpretation. For excision, small spots with TEM_{00} output are required. I prefer spot diameters of 0.5 to 1.0 mm and power outputs of 30 to 40 W. A 3 mm deep outlining cut is made, then a flap is developed by placing the

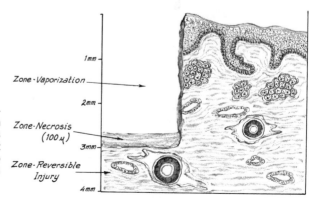

Figure 9–7. Microscopic drawing showing laser vaporization through the same skin section as shown in Figure 9–2. The defect produced by the laser extends to a depth of 3 mm. Deeper ablation is not necessary.

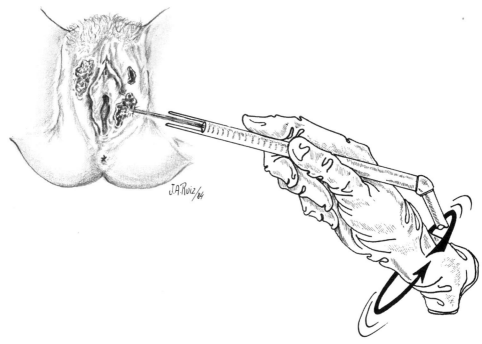

Figure 9–8. The technique for vaporization utilizing a laser handpiece. A circular, "polishing" motion is very easy to control. The motion is a fine wrist, finger/thumb movement, barely perceptible to the eye.

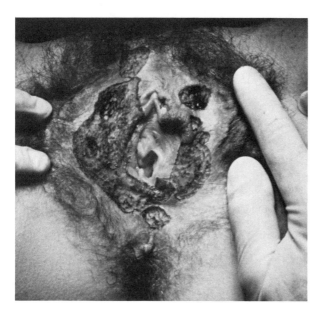

Figure 9–9. Laser vaporization of the 22-year-old women shown in Figure 9–3A. Intervening normal skin is preserved and healing will occur without scar formation.

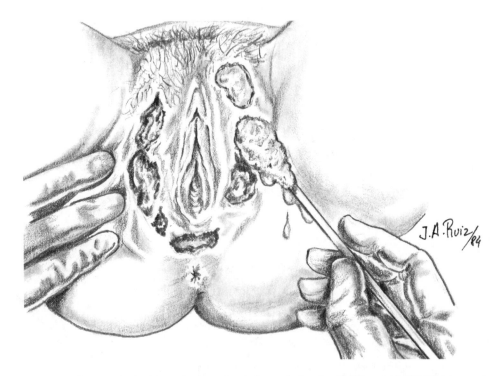

Figure 9–13. Schematic shows the laser treated area being thoroughly swabbed with 4 percent acetic acid. Light bleeding may occur occasionally but short bursts of the laser at 10 W/1.5 to 2 mm spot will seal these small bleeding vessels.

tissue on traction with a long-handled, fine skin hook. The tissue can then be cut away with little bleeding. When the specimen has been removed, the laser is defocused to a 2 mm spot, power is decreased to 15 W, and any bleeding vessels are coagulated (Fig. 9–14).

Accessories

Since the vulva is highly accessible, mirrors are usually unnecessary. To eliminate vapor and odor, a suitable evacuator is required. This equipment should be able to move large volumes of air and have suitable filters to trap debris. It is unwise to utilize wall suction because the debris present in the laser plume will inevitably clog up the wall suction necessitating costly repairs.

A 9 to 10 inch fine skin hook is the most facile tool to manipulate the labial and anal folds. (Titanium nonreflective hooks are currently available through the Codman Instrument Company.)

Perhaps the most useful accessories are small and large cotton-tipped applicators. When moistened with 4 percent acetic acid, they may be strategically placed

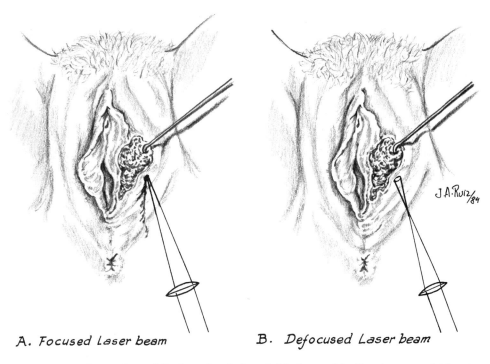

A. *Focused Laser beam*   B. *Defocused Laser beam*

Figure 9–14. Comparison of the laser hand piece tightly focused for fine deep vaporization or cutting versus the defocused handpiece. The latter is ideal for coagulating vessels and superficial vaporization.

to protect neighboring skin from the laser beam and prevent peripheral heat discomfort.

Postoperative Regimen

Undressed wounds invariably heal more slowly and with greater patient discomfort than wounds which are covered. "Bioclusive" (Johnson & Johnson) urethane dressings have recently been applied whenever possible following laser vaporization of the vulva. Such wounds when dressed are virtually painless. For undressed wounds it is recommended that patients utilize sea water sitz baths. Ocean water can be reconstituted by dissolving instant ocean (sea salts) in tap water. The ocean water is more comfortable for the patient than are saline sitz baths and the sea water debrides better while enhancing healing. Generally I recommend that patients take sitz baths at least four times per day. A 1:4 diluted solution of Betadine is squirted on the perineum following urination or defecation. Finally an electric hair dryer is employed to dry the vulva after sitz baths, showers, baths, or irrigations. This method of drying enhances healing and minimizes the chance of wiping away the delicate new epithelial covering cells. Healing progresses rapidly following the above regimen and is complete approximately 5 to 6 weeks following even extensive laser vaporization. When this routine is followed, laser wounds of the vulva heal without scar formation or retraction.

Follow-Up

The first scheduled visit after laser vaporization occurs at approximately 6 to 8 weeks. Patients are then followed at 3 months and 6 months thereafter. When patients are scheduled for staged laser treatment, it is most convenient to plan for repeat treatments every 2 weeks. For extensive lesions we have staged as many as five treatments under local anesthesia. When the last treatment has been completed, the patient is seen at 8 weeks, 12 weeks, then every 6 months.

Complications

Most women experience very little pain during the immediate postoperative period. The explanation for this relative analgesia relates to the nerve sealing action of the laser, resulting in a club-like nerve ending compared to the shaving brush pattern seen after a knife cut (Fig. 9–15). Delayed pain, however, especially in undressed wounds, can be expected to occur 7 to 10 days postoperatively.

Delayed bleeding which is more commonly seen after cervical vaporization is not usual after vulvar vaporization. This probably results because the vulvar wounds are much shallower than those on the cervix and the vessels are smaller.

In the reported series, no infections have been reported.[5,9]

When extensive areas of the vulva have been vaporized, coaptation of the labia may occur. During the postoperative period, the labia should be manually separated to avoid this problem.[10]

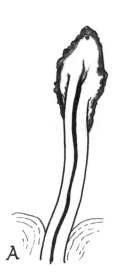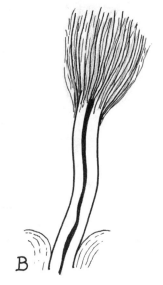

Figure 9–15. Schematic electron microscopic view of a nerve ending cut with the laser (A) versus a nerve ending following a sharp knife cut (B).

Results

The first report of the use of the CO_2 laser to treat vulvar intraepithelial neoplasia was published by Baggish and Dorsey in 1981.[5] Thirty-five women were treated, frequently staged for multiple treatments, with a failure rate of 3 out of 35. Our follow-up series of 48 women, followed for 12 months, produced only 4 failures (8.7 percent). Townsend et al.[9] reported 33 patients with VIN of whom 31 had their lesions eradicated—a 94 percent cure rate. In this series 85 percent of the women were treated as outpatients of whom 42 percent underwent multiple staged therapy.

CONCLUSION

Since vulvar carcinoma in situ is increasingly observed in a younger female population,[11] conservative methods of treatment that preserve functional anatomy must be offered to the patient. Even when lesions are extensive and have a tendency to recur, e.g., Paget's disease of the vulva, CO_2 laser results compare favorably to vulvectomy. When considered from the viewpoints of cost and time savings, convenience, and operative risk, the CO_2 laser is the treatment of choice for vulvar carcinoma in situ. The key to laser success is skilled and accurate diagnosis and the performance of equally skilled and precise surgery.

REFERENCES

1. Reid R, Stanhope CR, Herschman BR, et al: Genital warts and cervical cancer. Cancer 50:191, 1982
2. Aurelian L, Kessler I, Rosenshein NB, et al: Viruses and gynecologic cancers. Cancer 48:455, 1981
3. Buscema J, Woodruff JD, Parmley TH, et al: Carcinoma in situ of the vulva. Obstet Gynecol 55:225, 1980
4. Baggish MS: Carbon dioxide laser treatment for condylomata acuminata venereal infections. Obstet Gynecol 55:711, 1980
5. Baggish MS and Dorsey JH: CO_2 laser for the treatment of vulvar carcinoma in situ. Obstet Gynecol 57:371, 1981
6. Friedrich EG: Vulvar Disease. Philadelphia, WB Saunders, 1976, pp 80–87
7. Rutledge F, Sinclair M: Treatment of intraepithelial carcinoma of the vulva by skin excision and graft. Am J Obstet Gynecol 102:806, 1968
8. Forney JP, Morrow CP, Townsend DE, et al: Management of carcinoma in situ of the vulva. Am J Obstet Gynecol 127:801, 1977
9. Townsend DE, Levine RU, Richart RM, et al: Management of vulvar intraepithelial neoplasia by carbon dioxide laser. Obstet Gynecol 60:97, 1982
10. Baggish MS: Complications associated with carbon dioxide laser surgery in gynecology. Am J Obstet Gynecol 139:568, 1981
11. Hilliard GD, Massey RM, O'Toole RV: Vulvar neoplasia in the young. Am J Obstet Gynecol 135:185, 1979

10

Laser Vaporization of the Cervix for the Management of Cervical Intraepithelial Neoplasia

V. Cecil Wright

INTRODUCTION

Laser vaporization of ectocervical intraepithelial neoplasia was one of the first gynecologic applications of the carbon dioxide (CO_2) laser. It has been widely used to treat a large number of patients by colposcopists with varying degrees of expertise. Their methods and success rates have varied from marginal to excellent. The operative technique described in this chapter, one of three developed at St. Joseph's Hospital, London, Ontario, Canada following our adoption of laser surgery in 1977, has consistently yielded excellent results.[1,2]

Patients demonstrating abnormal cytology must be evaluated by an experienced colposcopist who consistently evaluates a large volume of patients to maintain expertise. The gynecologist must determine the location, extent, and severity of the diseased epithelium and take selected biopsies of the most suspicious areas under colposcopic guidance.

PREREQUISITES FOR CONSERVATIVE LASER SURGERY

The principles of conservative therapy must fulfill the following criteria:
1. The colposcopist must be certain from the qualitative assessment of the transformation zone that no invasive cancer is present.
2. The entire atypical transformation zone must be colposcopically defined.
3. Correlation must exist between cytology, colposcopy, and histology indicating only cervical intraepithelial neoplasia.

4. The cervical intraepithelial neoplasia (CIN) must occupy the ectocervix at or below the level of the external os with no extension into the endocervical canal (Fig. 10–1).

If disease extends into the endocervical canal or if the diagnoses are not consistent, the vaporization procedure is not applicable. In these instances, a cylindrical specimen of endocervical tissue (as opposed to the time-honored cone-shaped specimen) must be removed to evaluate the disease completely.[1] A cylindrical excision, performed with the laser, is recommended because the disease can extend into the endocervical crypts to a depth of 5 mm[3,4] and, with the usual conization procedure, disease is likely to be cut through and left behind undetected. The alternate procedures are described elsewhere.[1,5] It must be noted that the cervical crypts follow the distribution of columnar epithelium and carcinoma in situ usually follows the distribution of cervical crypts.[6]

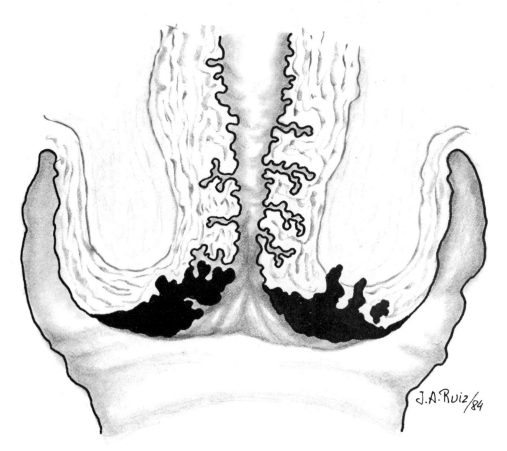

Figure 10–1. The typical candidate for laser vaporization. Disease is completely defined colposcopically with no extension into the endocervical canal.

RATIONALE FOR LASER VAPORIZATION

Employing the CO_2 laser with the operating microscope allows precision of application. The entire diseased area, transformation zone, and part of the area of susceptibility for squamous neoplastic change can be destroyed, the area of susceptibility being defined as that tissue lying between the original squamocolumnar junction and the internal histologic os.

Laser surgery is noncontact surgery as compared to other methods. It provides bloodless surgery frequently, depending upon the size and vascular pressure of the vessel. Thermal necrosis is less than 100 μ when the laser is properly employed. Healing is rapid, postoperative complications are negligible, and cure/success rates are high when compared to other methods of conservative therapy. With the cervical vaporization procedure, much of the volume of tissue removed becomes regenerated during the healing phase.

The actual vaporization procedure is brief and usually performed as an outpatient procedure. When coupled with the negligible morbidity and high cure rate, the laser provides a very cost-effective methodology for the patient.

OPERATIVE TECHNIQUE

The operative technique employed includes the following: A large, preferably dulled metal speculum is inserted into the vagina exposing the cervix. (Irregular surfaces reduce the potential of inadvertent reflection of the laser beam.) The transformation zone and area of pathology are again defined by washing the cervix with a 2 to 3 percent solution of acetic acid. This also removes any mucus.

A smoke-evacuating system is necessary to remove the vapor plume. A handheld suction tip can be positioned in the vagina by an assistant or the suction device can be attached to the upper blade of the speculum. Custom specula with attachments are commercially available. Prior to beginning surgery, the colposcopist must again assure himself that the CIN lesion occupies the ectocervix at or below the level of the external os with no extension into the endocervical canal. A calculated power density range of 750 to 2000 W/cm^2 can be easily employed. Very low power densities, i.e., below 350 W/cm^2, are not recommended because of increased time required to vaporized tissue. In general, the laser surgeon is encouraged to employ the highest power density for which he can maintain control and move the laser beam over the tissue surface as rapidly as possible. In calculating power density, the operator must take into consideration the transverse electromagnetic mode (TEM) of the laser, and the potential loss of power along the reflecting mirrors should an articulating arm be employed. The formula is adjusted accordingly. An effective laser beam diameter of 1.5 to 2 mm is mandatory for vaporization.

The entire transformation zone including the CIN lesion is first outlined with the laser beam. The marking with the laser beam must extend at least 3 or 4 mm beyond the diseased area and transformation zone. Beginning at the 6 o'clock position, the laser beam is moved quickly over the tissue to be destroyed. Rapid beam movement reduces thermal tissue conductivity and minimizes potential scarring.

Rapid movement of the beam also reduces heat build-up in the cervical tissue with a reduction in uterine cramping. It is essential to use the highest power density that the operator can maintain control. By doing this, heat conduction into surrounding normal tissue is minimized. The end result is rapid healing, minimal scarring, and reduced thermal necrosis. Beginning at the posterior area prevents obstructing blood and/or ooze from impinging upon the operative field. The laser beam is moved in multiple directions (diagonally, horizontally, and vertically) to prevent furrowing. With large surface areas, the site should be divided into smaller segments.

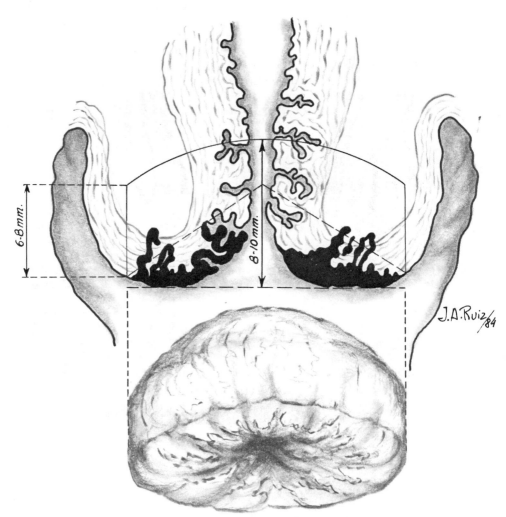

Figure 10–2. The ideal defect for laser vaporization of CIN. The slanted dotted line indicates line of typical resection for knife conization. Cylindrical based and dome topped defect is opposed to the cone-shaped specimen routinely obtained with a scalpel. Note that the scalpel cone can cut across disease lying within crypts resulting in persistent disease.

Vaporization of the entire transformation zone including the area of pathology must be performed to a minimum depth of at least 6 mm. This will ensure eradication of any CIN lesion extending into the cervical crypts. Also, part of the area of susceptibility for potential malignant change is reduced. Because of the anatomic topography of the cervix, it is important to dome the central area. Measurements from the most extreme plane of the ectocervix may extend 8 to 10 mm. A microruler can be employed to determine the depth of ablation. The end result should be a dome-topped cylindrical defect with straight sides and a curved apex (Fig. 10–2). The defect can be sizable but does not appear to affect the volume of tissue which is regenerated, the quality or duration of healing, or the postoperative complication rate. The entire process of vaporization when properly performed takes 2 to 12 minutes depending upon the extent of the disease. Healing is usually complete in 3 weeks after laser vaporization. The new squamocolumnar junction is almost always located at the level of the external os (Fig. 10–3). This makes follow-up colposcopy and cytology satisfactory.

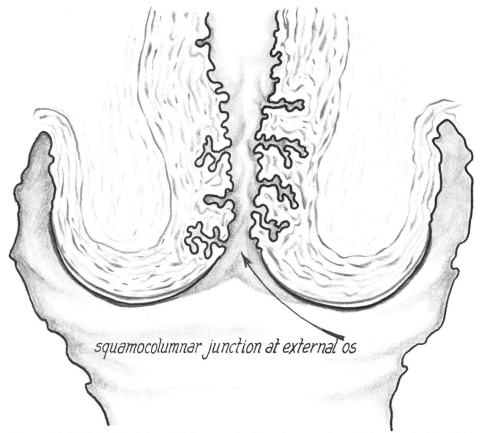

squamocolumnar junction at external os

Figure 10–3. Typical healed cervix after vaporization—the normal result after vaporization. Much of the vaporized volume of tissue regenerates and fills in the defect. In 90 percent of the cases, the new squamocolumnar junction relocates at the external os or lower into the ectocervix.

Persistent disease following laser surgery will occur if the initial marking beyond the lesion and transformation zone did not provide a 3 to 4 mm normal tissue buffer zone, or if a uniform measured minimum vaporization depth of at least 6 mm was not achieved at the periphery, or if the defect was not domed centrally incorporating frequently an 8 to 10 mm altitude. Usually the laser surgeon obtains a proper depth at the lateral margin but fails to achieve this at the central external os. It is most essential to dome the defect to match the anatomic topography of the cervix and assure adequate depth centrally.

MANAGEMENT OF INTRAOPERATIVE BLEEDING

The laser is noted for its hemostatic effect; blood vessels up to 2 mm in size may be sealed by lasing. Hemostasis results from the brief heat stimulation of the collagen within the vessel walls. At times, however, bleeding occurs during laser surgery which may be troublesome. There are several causes for this. A laser beam with a small spot size and high power density will sharply cut large vessels and reduce the coagulation effect. Low power density may provide insufficient heat conduction in time to coagulate the vessel before blood accumulates within the operative field. If sufficient power density is not employed, the beam's energy will be absorbed by the blood and the lasing action on the tissue will be nil. Also, rapid beam movement diminishes the heat conductivity and lessens hemostasis.

Therefore, the technique employed to control blood loss would depend upon the amount of bleeding and the power density employed at the time it occurs. Bleeding must be quickly and efficiently managed. Three points are crucial: thermal damage is time related and independent of power density, power density below $150 \ \text{W/cm}^2$ does not vaporize but creates a thermal effect only, and if the laser beam is in prolonged contact with the bleeding area, increased heat conduction in the normal adjacent tissue will occur. The zone of thermal necrosis will therefore be increased and healing will suffer.

The methods to control bleeding are the following:

1. Maintain the same power density. The blood is sucked from the operative site with nonflammable plastic or dulled metal suction devices and the blood vessels simultaneously are coagulated with the laser beam. This is very efficient and little time is lost. Use this method when bleeding occurs during moderate or high power density.
2. Decrease the power density. This decreases the rapid cutting effect. This is accomplished by enlarging the spot size (that is defocusing the laser beam) or by decreasing the watts of power on the laser. It is difficult to defocus the laser beam effectively with the laser attached to the operating microscope, since doing so makes the scope go out of focus. Therefore, decreasing the power is the preferable method. The beam is then applied to the bleeding site for sufficiently enough time to coagulate the vessel. Decreasing the power density produces more thermal conductivity, particularly if the time interval is increased, which will result in increased thermal damage. Therefore, this effort should not be prolonged.

3. Increase power density. Increasing the power density will allow the excessive blood in the field to be vaporized by the laser beam. This will then allow one to arrive at the base of the bleeding vessel efficiently and the brief thermal effect created may be sufficient enough to seal the blood vessel(s). Should the above methods fail, it may be necessary to inject a 1.5 percent pitressin solution into the cervical stroma. Pitressin decreases the size of the lumen of the vessels such that the brief thermal conduction of the beam in contact with these vessels will seal them easily.
4. Lastly, it may be necessary to place hemostatic sutures should blood loss become uncontrollable despite all recommended procedures.

POSTOPERATIVE CARE, MANAGEMENT OF COMPLICATIONS, AND THERAPEUTIC EFFECTIVENESS

Postoperative care is minimal. Pain is usually not a problem, but patients with discomfort should be advised to take a mild analgesic. They should be instructed to refrain from intercourse, douching, and using tampons for a suggested period of at least 3 weeks. Postoperative complications are not common. Patients experiencing brisk delayed bleeding should be colposcopically examined in the clinic or office setting. Employing the colposcope can easily differentiate bleeding related to a general ooze or an arterial pumping vessel. Should the bleeding occur, the usual time is between 5 and 10 days from the time of laser vaporization. Bleeding, which occurs within the first 24 hours, can be somewhat more severe since it may result from a very diffuse ooze caused by blood vessels opening up for some reason. This type of bleeding area may require suturing. Such a complication, however, is very unusual. Bleeding that occurs between 5 and 10 days can be managed in the following ways: Frequently nothing is required except to assure the patient that no definitive therapy is necesary. For a general ooze, a tight vaginal pack placed against the area for a period of 24 hours frequently suffices. Focal cautery to an arterial bleeder is necessary on occasion. Should these methods fail, the individual placing of a suture may be required to stop persistent bleeding. Less than 1 percent of all patients will be admitted to hospital to control bleeding. Postoperative infection is rare. This is most likely related to the fact that the blood vessels and lymphatics become sealed at the time of laser surgery. Secondly, if the laser is properly employed, very little thermal conductivity occurs, thus thermal necrosis and tissue sloughing with delayed healing should not occur. Patients

**TABLE 10–1. CURE RATES AFTER ONE
LASER SURGERY**

Disease	Vaporization	No. Cured	(%)
CIN I	124	121	97.6
CIN II	160	152	95.0
CIN III	230	218	94.7
Total	514	491	95.5

TABLE 10–2. OVERALL SUCCESS OF LASER VAPORIZATION

	No.	%
Cases cured by 1 or 2 laser treatments	512	99.6
Hysterectomy required	2	0.4

treated by laser vaporization for CIN disease should be seen for the first visit 3 months after laser surgery. It is recommended that during the first year after laser vaporization, the patient should have three follow-up examinations. Such examinations should consist of cytology and colposcopic evaluation. Removing the recommended domed cylindrical defect as described will result in cure rates that exceed 95 percent after the first laser (Table 10–1). Any suspicious areas seen at colposcopy should be biopsied. Should cytology be reported as abnormal, histologic confirmation is mandatory. Therefore, reassessment with colposcopy may locate the lesion and if not the area should be excised.[1] Most patients, after establishing the severity of disease, will respond to a second laser surgery (Table 10–2). If the three examinations within the first year are normal, it is recommended that the patients have yearly Pap smears. It is necessary to have a thorough discussion with the patient pertaining to the disease which has been treated.

Vaporizing a central cylinder with a domed top as described herein removes three times the volume of tissue achieved with scalpel conization. Follow-up, however, indicates that the tissue removed with a scalpel appears to be permanently removed and therefore reduces tissue volume permanently. This has been associated with pregnancy loss.[7,8] Healing following laser vaporization is different. Despite the volume of tissue removed as recommended with laser vaporization, much of this volume regenerates and fills in the defect. Tables 10–3 and 10–4 reflect the number of pregnancies and the outcome after laser vaporization. This demonstrates that pregnancy loss was not increased after laser vaporization.

In conclusion, removing a planned dome-topped cylindrical tissue volume employing the carbon dioxide laser with the operating microscope, assuming a basic understanding of laser physics and disease distribution, can result in a supe-

TABLE 10–3. PREGNANCY FOLLOWING LASER SURGERY FOR CIN

Total pregnancies	61
Term deliveries	46
Delivery before 37 weeks	2
Spontaneous abortion before 13 weeks	6
Therapeutic abortion	1
Extrauterine pregnancy	3
Cesarean section	5
Presently pregnant	3
Perinatal deaths	0

**TABLE 10–4. INDICATIONS FOR
CESAREAN SECTION**

Breech presentation	3
Fetal distress	1
Failure to progress in labor	1

rior treatment success rate with minimal complications when compared to other conservative therapeutic modalities.

REFERENCES

1. Wright VC, Davies E, Riopelle MA: Laser surgery for cervical intraepithelial neoplasia: Principles and results. Am J Obstet Gynecol 145:181, 1983
2. Wright VC, Riopelle MA: The management of cervical intraepithelial neoplasia: The use of the carbon dioxide laser. Laser Surg Med 2(1):59, 1982
3. Anderson MC, Hartley RB: Cervical crypt involvement by cervical intraepithelial neoplasia. Obstet Gynecol 55:546, 1980
4. Przybora LA, Plutowa A: Histological topography of carcinoma in situ of the cervix uteri. Cancer 12:268, 1959
5. Wright VC, Riopelle MA: Gynecological Laser Surgery: A Practical Handbook. Houston, Biomedical Communications, 1982
6. Kaufman C, Ober KG: Cancer of Cervix. Ciba Foundation Study Group No. 3. London, Churchill, 1959, p 60
7. Jones J, Sweetman P, Hibbard BM: The outcome of pregnancy after cone biopsy of the cervix: A case-control study. Brit J Obstet Gynecol 86:913, 1979
8. Larsson G, Grundsell H, Gullberg H, Svennerud S: Outcome of pregnancy after conization. Acta Obstet Gynecol Scand 61:461, 1982

11

Laser Treatment of the Vagina

Duane E. Townsend

INTRODUCTION

The extension of laser therapy to the field of gynecology has added a new dimension in the treatment of premalignant as well as benign diseases of the vagina. Irradiation and extensive surgery for preinvasive vaginal neoplasia has been essentially eliminated. Multiple condylomata, particularly in the pregnant patient, are easily managed by vaporization. Moreover, other benign conditions, such as endometriosis, vaginal cysts, and scarring, can be removed with little side effects. Paramount to the use of laser therapy is the pretreatment evaluation. In this chapter, the essential parameters in the evaluation of women with premalignant disease will be reviewed and then the technique of laser therapy will be presented in depth.

VAGINAL INTRAEPITHELIAL NEOPLASIA

The neoplastic lesions of the vagina account for 1 to 4 percent of all gynecologic malignancies. The overwhelming number of these are preinvasive and squamous cell in type. The incidence of vaginal intraepithelial neoplasia (VAIN) is increasing along with cervical intraepithelial neoplasia (CIN) and vulvar intraepithelial neoplasia (VIN). Moreover, many of these lesions are associated with the papilloma virus infections which are also common for the CIN and VIN lesions.

The cause of VAIN is unknown, but it will be found in 1 to 3 percent of patients with CIN.[1] In a publication of 66 cases, Hummer[2] noted that for carcinoma in situ of the vagina, the interval from a previous diagnosis of CIN III was less than 2 years in two thirds of the cases and the longest interval 17 years. The patient's ages ranged from 24 to 75 with a mean age of 52. More recently, there has been an increasing incidence of this disease in the younger population. Radiation therapy is probably a predisposing factor due to the low dose radiation that causes a sublethal injury to the tissue.[3] Women receiving chemotherapy and immunosuppressive therapy have an increased incidence of VAIN. Postmenopausal atrophy of the vagina may be an associated factor, as many women in the postmenopausal age group will have an abnormal Papanicolaou smear due to estrogen deficiency. Generally these patients can be managed with the intravaginal application of estrogen cream.

As mentioned previously, many of the VAIN lesions are associated with a papilloma virus which may be a major predisposing factor.

Detection and Evaluation of VAIN

As with CIN, VAIN is an asymptomatic lesion usually brought to the attention of the physician by an abnormal Pap smear. In many cases, women have had a prior hysterectomy for CIN, but a surprisingly high number of patients with VAIN have an intact uterus. Unfortunately, in many instances, women will be subjected to cervical cone and even hysterectomy before the vagina is thoroughly investigated. Since a woman who has had CIN is at increased risk for having VAIN, a Papanicolaou (Pap) smear should be taken annually after a hysterectomy has been performed for CIN. However, vaginal intraepithelial neoplasia does occur spontaneously, and a woman who has had a hysterectomy performed for benign disease should be cytologically tested every 3 years.

Cytologic sampling of the vagina is different than the method for cervical lesions. The entire mucosa must be sampled. Although the majority of VAIN lesions are found at the apex, a third are found in the mid and lower third of the vagina. A cotton-tipped applicator or wooden spatula moistened with saline to prevent the adherence of cells to the surfaces is recommended. Circumferential sampling is performed as the speculum is withdrawn and rotated.

As with CIN and VIN, the colposcope has revolutionized the evaluation of women with VAIN. In the past, extensive strip biopsies were carried out. Because of this imprecise method of evaluation, therapy was often radical. With colposcopy, lesions are easily located so that therapy is precise and conservative. For those women who have an intact cervix and where an abnormal smear is present, a thorough colposcopic inspection and tissue sampling of the cervix, which includes an endocervical curettage if the patient is not pregnant, is necessary. With a negative evaluation of the cervix, the vagina as well as the vulva must be carefully scrutinized.

Colposcopic evaluation of the vagina tube requires more time than cervical colposcopy. The Pap smear is always repeated. Once the vagina has been cytologically resampled, the vaginal mucosa is thoroughly moistened with white vinegar delivered by cotton-soaked balls, and the speculum is withdrawn and rotated. White vinegar is equivalent to 5 percent acetic acid and is preferable since it makes the lesion turn white quickly and with greater intensity. Women who have a vaginal infection should always be treated for that infection prior to colposcopic inspection. This is necessary to lessen the chance of burning from the vinegar as well as to avoid the confusion that occurs from the punctation due to inflammation. Once the infection is cleared and in those who have no infection, the mucosa is thoroughly moistened with vinegar and the speculum is reinserted and again withdrawn and rotated as colposcopic inspection is performed. By withdrawing and rotating the speculum, the mucosa will fold down over the ends of the speculum blade permitting an end-on view of the tissue. Most of the VAIN lesions,

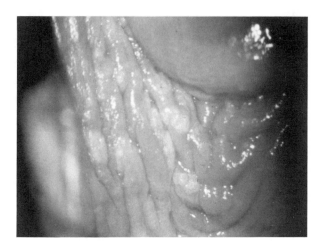

Figure 11–1. Multifocal vaginal intraepithelial neoplasia in the upper one third of the vagina.

when stained with vinegar appear white, are sharply bordered and granular (Figs. 11–1, 11–2). In over half the cases, fine punctation is present with mosaic a rare finding. If a patient appears to have invasive cancer, i.e., atypical vessel and irregular surface contour, biopsies are immediately taken. When invasive cancer is not present, the tissues are then stained with one half strength of aqueous Lugol's solution. Lesions will stain a pale yellow contrasted with the mahogany of normal epithelium.

After staining with Lugol's solution in a manner similar to that with vinegar, the speculum is reinserted after moistening the blades with lubricating jelly or water. This is necessary because of the drying effect caused by the vinegar and

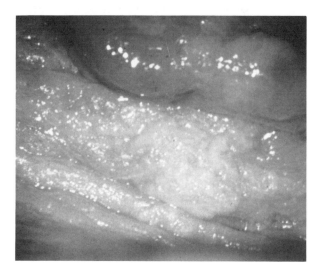

Figure 11–2. Close-up of vagina in Figure 11–1 after acetic acid 4 percent has been applied. The condylomatous pattern is very apparent.

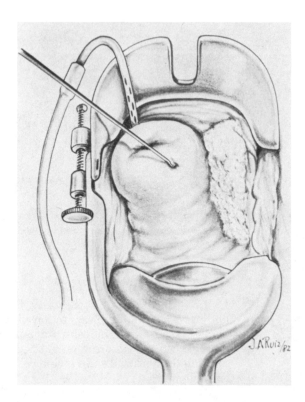

Figure 11–3. Drawing of the case shown in Figures 11–1 and 11–2 illustrating the use of the long handled hook to expose the lateral fornix and the lesion.

Lugol's solution. Again, the speculum is withdrawn and rotated, and the site or sites of lesions are noted. Biopsies are taken at this time. Bleeding is controlled by the application of Ferric Subsulfate (Monsel's solution; Mallinckrodt, Paris, Ky.). Painful areas are noted which will influence laser therapy. If pain is a problem, the mucosa can be injected with a local anesthetic using a small gauge spinal needle.

All postmenopausal patients in whom invasive cancer has been excluded should be reevaluated after they have used intravaginal estrogen cream for at least 3 weeks. The application of the hormone cream will make the lesions more apparent and will negate the false-positivity due to the deestrogenized mucosa.

Most lesions will be multifocal and located in the upper one-third of the vagina (Fig. 11–3). Rarely is the entire mucosa involved. In some instances after hysterectomy, lesions will be found within the folds at the 3 and 9 o'clock positions. In these cases, it is necessary to evert the folds with an Iris hook or use an endocervical speculum to investigate the tunnels (Fig. 11–4).

The frequency of VAIN progressing in invasive cancer is unknown. Because of the lack of current methods to determine the true premalignant lesion, however, all epithelial abnormalities should be eradicated. A variety of treatment techniques have evolved over the past half century[4] with most recent being laser therapy.

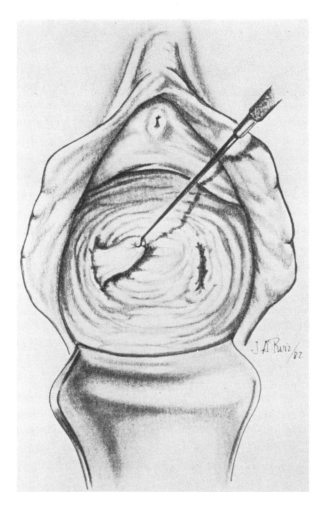

Figure 11-4. Long handled iris hook constructed of titanium exposes the mucosa within vaginal tunnels. These tunnels are common after hysterectomy.

Excision Biopsy

Office excision is useful in patients who have only one or two small lesions in the vagina. In most cases an 80 percent cure rate can be achieved; however, lesions that recur require an alternative method of therapy.

Intravaginal 5-FU

Woodruff[5] introduced the use of topical 5-fluorouracil (5-FU) for VAIN disease. He noted that the cytotoxic antimetabolite was successful in eight of nine patients. His single failure was in a woman who had hyperkeratosis overlying her preinvasive lesion. We have investigated the use of 5-FU for the past dozen years and find it very successful in many instances.[6] With laser therapy, however, 5-FU is used less frequently. This is primarily due to the unpleasant side effects that are associated with 5-FU treatment.

Cryosurgery

Cryosurgery therapy has not been reported to be useful in VAIN lesions. The major drawback with the freezing technique is the lack of suitable probes and the problem of depth control.

Electrocautery

Electrocautery has been utilized sparingly. Again, the lack of depth control and the large area of tissue necrosis due to cautery are the major drawbacks of this method.

Radiation Therapy

Radiation therapy has been used commonly for many years and is still suggested by some even today. Radiation therapy, however, has major side effects, such as diarrhea and nausea, and causes stricture and shortening of the vagina. It may also initiate new lesions. With the advent of laser vaporization, radiation has been virtually eliminated as a legitimate treatment technique.

Surgical Excision

The use of surgical excision, even partial or complete vaginectomy with graft, is the most common method of therapy. The recurrence rate with this technique is very high and often results in a shortened and narrowed vagina. Surgical excision should be utilized only in those patients in whom there is difficulty in deciding if there is an invasive component.

Intravaginal Estrogens

In the postmenopausal patient, as mentioned previously, intravaginal hormone cream should be utilized. In a surprisingly high number of cases, i.e., approaching 30 to 40 percent, the Pap smear will often revert to normal. This is probably the result of maturing the vaginal epithelium that was being misinterpreted when it was so atrophic. In these patients, careful follow-up is necessary to make certain they do not have a VAIN lesion which could be readily detected at a future date. When there is persistence of VAIN after the use of estrogen cream, additional therapy is initiated.

LASER THERAPY

Stafl[7] was the first to report on the use of laser for VAIN. His success in six patients was excellent. Petrelli[6] from our own clinic reported on a slightly larger series of patients, again with a high success rate. We recently reported the largest series of VAIN lesions treated by laser.[8] The 52 patients managed had a success rate of 90 percent. Most treatment was carried out in the office. The latest report was by Jobson and Homesley.[9] In their series, the entire vaginal tube was vaporized. They reported an 84 percent success rate after a single treatment session and a 100 percent success rate after a second treatment session. Their method required anesthesia, virtually total ablation of the vaginal mucosa, and 1 or 2 days in the hospital often with an indwelling catheter. The patients required many office visits for vaginal dilations.

Whether to treat focally, as we have done, or extensively, as in Jobson's method, is not settled. However, it is certainly less traumatic, less expensive, and safer to ablate individual lesions in the office even though it may take extra therapeutic sessions. The technique of individual laser ablation is prefered by this author and will now be detailed.

The technique of laser therapy is somewhat different for VAIN than for CIN. Generally, lower power densities are utilized and local analgesics are injected into the tissue to serve both as a protective barrier from vaporizing too deeply as well as provide pain relief. Therapy, in most cases, can be performed in the office except in those patients who have extensive involvement of the vaginal mucosa. In these cases, light anesthesia on an outpatient basis is suggested. With office therapy, the technique of colposcopic inspection using acetic acid and Lugo's solution is meticulously repeated to reconfirm the sites of the lesions. With laser therapy, a special aluminum oxide-coated laser speculum (this reduces the chance of laser beam reflection) equipped with a special evacuation tube for the fumes is utilized. Therapy is initiated at the apex of the vagina after injecting the area with analgesic solution. A power density in the range of 400 to 500 W/cm^2 is selected. A spot the size of at least 1.5 to 2 mm is preferred. The larger spot size reduces the chance of deep penetration and provides better hemostasis. Initially a 2 mm border of normal tissue around the lesion is vaporized down to a depth of approximately 2 mm. During vaporization of the vagina, the contrast between the mucosa and submucosal tissue is particularly easy to recognize. In virutally all cases, a 1 mm depth will remove almost all of the mucosa, however, a 2 mm depth is recommended to insure complete vaporization of abnormal tissue (Figs. 11–5; 11–6, 11–7, see Color Plate III*). Since glands in the vagina are seldom more than a few millimeters deep, it is not necessary to treat to the same depth that is carried out for cervical disease. Measuring is carefully performed to insure proper depth. After outlining the lesion by vaporizing the border of normal tissue, the intraepithelial disease is removed using a circumferential or cross-hatch method down to the depth that was initially achieved when the lesion was outlined. Should bleeding be a problem, hemostasis can be achieved by using a defocused beam or Monsel's solution. Lesions that are present within the recesses, folds, and tunnels at the apex of the vagina present a special problem. These patients should be treated under light anesthesia. An endocervical speculum may be used to expose the lesion for vaporization. An alternative method is to evert the lesion with an Iris hook and then perform the treatment. When the disease is off the apex or in the middle third of the vagina, vaporization is performed as the tissue folds down over the

---

*Color Plate III appears following p. 177.

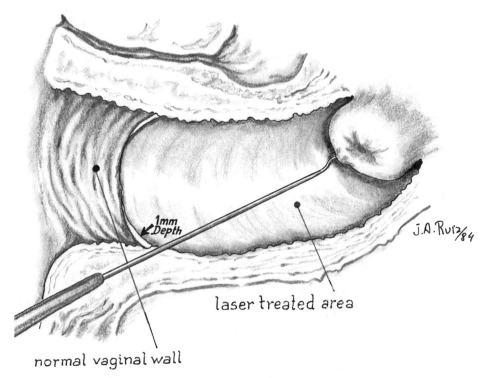

1mm
Depth

laser treated area

normal vaginal wall

Figure 11–5. Schematic view of the lateral vaginal wall immediately after laser vaporization of neo-plastic lesion. Note the wide peripheral margin.

end of the speculum blades permitting an end-on ablation of the lesion. Because it is difficult to outline the area in this manner, individual lesions are vaporized as they come into view. For extensive disease, it is recommended that the patients have outpatient anesthesia. Anesthesia is necessary in these cases due to the extensive rotating of the speculum that is carried out in order to eradicate the disease. Lesions in the lower third of the vagina and at the introitus can be treated by passing the beam between the blades of the speculum (Figs. 11–8A, 11–8B).

Over 90 percent of patients can be treated in the office with a high degree of success. Tranquilizers an hour prior to the office treatment is probably of benefit in order to alleviate the anxiety which is often associated with laser therapy. When extensive areas are treated, vaginal dilations are recommended to reduce the chance of stenosis. An occasional patient will complain of pain following therapy but it is seldom a problem. Mild analgesics are usually sufficient. Discharge is slight, usually blood tinged, and may be odorous. Douching is not recommended nor is sexual activity for at least 3 weeks because of the possibility of contact bleeding. Systemic infections have not occurred following laser ablation of the vagina. Urinary catheterization is not necessary unless extensive ablation is performed. No major side effects have been noted following laser therapy for VAIN,

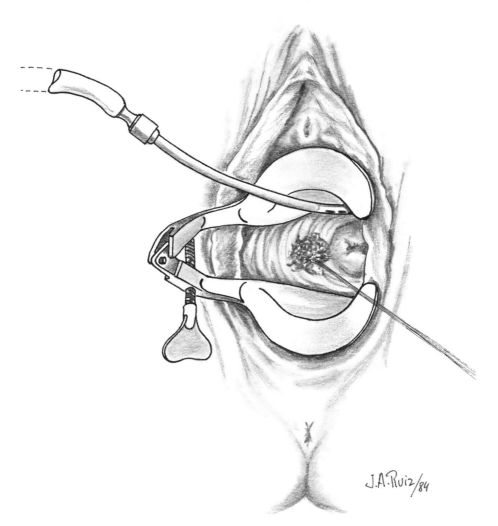

Figure 11–8A. Schema of the single-hinged laser speculum in place. The front view shows the laser angulated to one side.

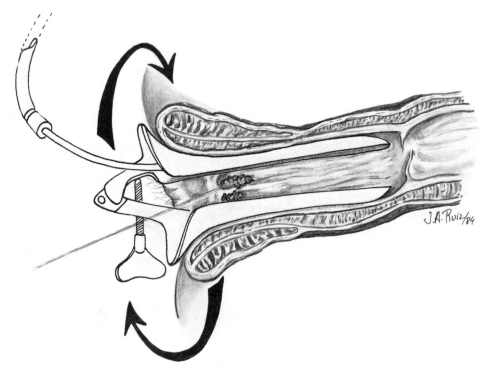

J.A.Ruiz/84

Figure 11–8B. The side view shows the beam directed between the speculum blades and striking the vaginal lesion.

but there is one unreported case of vesicovaginal fistula which was repaired without incident. The case points out the importance of *not treating too deeply.*

Follow-Up

Patients are generally seen at 6 weeks after laser therapy unless there has been extensive ablation which necessitates more frequent examinations. At the 6-week examination, the extent of healing is noted and in most cases will be complete. When extensive areas of ablation are performed, healing may not be complete until 8 weeks. The next examination is performed 3 months after treatment. At this time, a Pap smear and colposcopic examination is performed. If no suspicious areas are noted and the Pap smear is normal, patients are seen 6 months after treatment for another Pap smear and colposcopic exam. If this examination is normal, patients are then followed every 6 months by cytology. Those patients in whom persistent disease is found are retreated by laser therapy. Postmenopausal patients are instructed to insert intravaginal estrogen cream every third night beginning 3 weeks following therapy. Once healing is complete, estrogen cream application is strongly recommended indefinitely to maintain a healthy tissue.

Benign Disease

Baggish was the first to report on the use of laser therapy for genital tract condyloma acuminatum.[10] He reported a high success rate and pointed out that most cases could be treated in the office. The elimination of condyloma acuminatum in pregnancy is important to avoid infant contact with the lesion which could cause laryngeal warts. Laser therapy is particularly attractive in pregnancy since it permits the avoidance of potentially teratogenic chemicals such as podophyllin, trichloroacetic acid, 5 percent fluorouracil cream, or bleomycin. Conventional methods of treating genital warts, such as electrocoagulation, cyrosurgery, and electrodesiccation, are typically followed by a disappointing high recurrence rate. Surgical excision is associated with excessive bleeding.

The method of laser beam vaporization for condyloma acuminatum is somewhat different than that for the VAIN lesion. The depth of vaporization is less, and it is important to treat several millimeters of surrounding normal tissue because of the finding that the papilloma virus often exists in normal tissue around the proliferative lesion. The central area of proliferative tissue is initially vaporized to a depth of 1 mm and then shallow "brushing" of less than 1 mm in depth for a distance of 3 to 5 mm surrounding the lesion follows (Fig. 11–9). When vaginal lesions are extensive, a high rate of recurrence is common. Patients must be

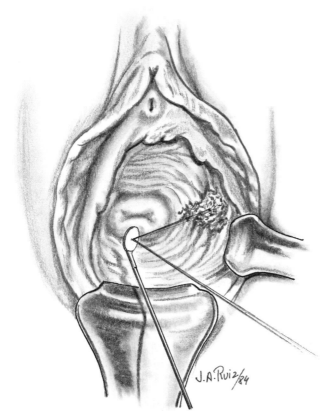

Figure 11–9. A thin-coated, long handled mirror can be used to reflect the laser beam to a lesion that is otherwise difficult to view.

informed that additional therapeutic sessions will be necessary. As pointed out in previous chapters, the examination of the male is critical in those patients who have recurrent lesions.

Granulation tissue following hysterectomy can be a very stubborn lesion. Laser vaporization after biopsy to exclude a neoplastic component is performed easily and simply. Local anesthesia is recommended because of the proximity of the peritoneal lining.

Endometriosis of the vagina is frustrating to the patient and physician because of the pain it causes with sexual activity as well as its resistance to therapy. In treating half a dozen patients, I have found that the lesions are easily vaporized and the recurrence rate is small. Since many of these lesions are found at the apex of the vagina following hysterectomy, great care must be taken not to vaporize too deeply. The use of local anesthetics, again, is strongly recommended to avoid vaporizing too deeply as well as to provide pain relief.

Cases of prolapsed fallopian tube have been treated with laser beam vaporization, again, with a high degree of success, minimum morbidity, and no recurrences.

Vaginal scarring as well as vaginal cysts are amenable to laser vaporization with virtually no recurrence.

SUMMARY

The extension of the carbon dioxide laser for vaginal disease is rapidly expanding. Without question, the undesirable side effects of major surgery have now been eliminated. Laser therapy is highly cost effective but does require a great deal of training and experience before it can be used in a beneficial and safe manner.

REFERENCES

1. Graham JB, Meigs JV: Recurrence of tumor after total hysterectomy for carcinoma in situ. Am J Obstet Gynecol 64:1159, 1962.
2. Hummer WK, Mussey K, Decker DG, Dockerty MB: Carcinoma in situ of the vagina. Am J Obstet Gynecol 108:1109, 1970
3. Novak ER, Woodruff JD: Postirradiation malignancies of the pelvic organs. Am J Obstet Gynecol 77:667, 1959
4. Hernandez-Linares W, Puthawala A, Nolan JF, et al: Carcinoma in situ of the vagina: Past and present management. Obstet Gynecol 56:356, 1980
5. Woodruff JD, Parmley TH, Julian CG: Topical 5-fluorouracil in the treatment of vaginal carcinoma in situ. Gynecol Oncol 3:124, 1975
6. Petrilli ES, Townsend DE, Morrow CP, et al: Vaginal intraepithelial neoplasia: Biologic aspects and treatment with topical 5-fluorouracil and the carbon dioxide laser. Am J Obstet Gynecol 138:321, 1980
7. Stafl A, Wilkinson EJ, Mattingly RF: Laser treatment of cervical and vaginal neoplasia. Am J Obstet Gynecol 128:128, 1977
8. Townsend DE, Levine RU, Crum CP, Richart RM: Treatment of vaginal carcinoma in situ with the carbon dioxide laser. Am J Obstet Gynecol 143:101, 1982
9. Jobson VW, Homesley HD: Treatment of vaginal intraepithelial neoplasia with carbon dioxide laser. Obstet Gynecol 62:90, 1983
10. Baggish MS: Carbon dioxide laser treatment for condyloma accuminata veneral infections. Obstet Gynecol 55:711, 1980

12

Excisional Conization of the Cervix by CO₂ Laser

James H. Dorsey

INTRODUCTION

A number of different surgical procedures performed on the cervix have been described in the literature under the general title of "Cervical Conization." Lisfrac reported an operation similar to the modern cold knife conization in 1815 and suggested that it be applied in the treatment of invasive cervical cancer.[1] It soon became apparent that a more radical approach was necessary to effect a reasonable cure rate, and cervical conization was seldom mentioned in the literature until the concept of premalignant and early invasive cervical neoplasia was introduced into gynecology.[2,3] At that time cervical conization became a diagnostic procedure used to accurately assess presence or absence of malignant disease.[4] Until very recently in the United States, hysterectomy has been considered the treatment of choice for cervical carcinoma in situ. As a better understanding of the nature of intraepithelial neoplasias developed, however, and the colposcope became widely used as an instrument for identifying the site and the extent of the cervical disease, more conservative operations proved to be therapeutic.[5–7] There are now many large series of patients with cervical intraepithelial neoplasia treated by conization procedures and excellent results have been demonstrated.[8] It must be remembered that hysterectomy does not guarantee the eradication of intraepithelial neoplasia since the disease may reoccur in the vaginal vault or indeed may be multifocal. Invasive vaginal vault cancer has also been demonstrated following hysterectomy for cervical carcinoma in situ, and in one large European series, the incidence of invasive cancer following hysterectomy exceeded that following therapeutic conization.[9–11] Since conization for cervical intraepithelial neoplasia (CIN) produces cure rates in excess of 95 percent, it becomes difficult to justify the more serious operation of hysterectomy except in unusual circumstances.

INDICATIONS FOR EXCISIONAL CONIZATION

In the majority of patients with CIN, cervical colposcopy identifies the transformation zone and locates the neoplastic process and its borders. In this situation, the lesion can be extensively biopsied and the intraepithelial nature of the neo-

TABLE 12–1. INDICATIONS FOR EXCISIONAL CERVICAL CONIZATION

Incompletely visualized neoplastic lesion
Incompletely visualized transformation zone
Cytology not compatible with pathology
Microinvasion on directed biopsy

plastic process established with certainty. An ablative procedure that destroys the lesion and the transformation zone to an appropriate depth may then be performed with the expectation of cure rates equivalent to those achieved by excisional conization.[12–15] In 10 to 20 percent of the patients, however, the transformation zone cannot be visualized in its entirety or the lesion may disappear into the canal. It is obviously impossible to take an adequate directed biopsy in this circumstance, and an excisional conization must be performed to ensure accurate diagnosis. Occasionally, a cytologic examination shows more severe dysplastic cells than can be demonstrated by colposcopically directed biopsy of the cervix. This discrepancy becomes an indication for conization if a source for the cells cannot be found in another location such as the vagina or the vulva. Although "skip" lesions, areas of intraepithelial neoplasia located in the canal and completely separate from the visible lesions, are thought to be exceedingly rare, there are some who believe that all patients with CIN should have excisional conization. Burghart argues that the original squamous epithelium is not invulnerable to the development of neoplasia, and challenges the postulate that squamous carcinoma arises only in the transformation zone.[16] If one accepts this tenet, then excisional conization should be used to establish the true extent of the disease and its site or sites of origin as well as for therapy. Most colposcopists however feel that ablative procedures can be effectively used in the therapy of visible intraepithelial lesions, and the accepted indications for excisional conization are given in Table 12–1.

2 mm.
500 w/cm2

1 mm.
2000 w/cm2

Figure 12–1. For any given power setting, the density of the energy distributed increases as the surface area of the spot decreases.

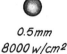

0.5 mm
8000 w/cm2

●

0.1mm.
20000 w/cm2

THE LASER AS AN EXCISIONAL INSTRUMENT

The carbon dioxide (CO_2) laser is a surgical instrument that can be used for either ablative or excisional operative procedures.[17] When an ablative procedure is done, a relatively large focal spot is selected so that the energy may be evenly spread or "painted" over the volume to be vaporized. By utilizing a smaller focal spot and turning up the power, the laser beam becomes a cutting instrument rather than a brush with which to paint (Fig. 12–1).

GENERAL THEORY OF LASER EXCISIONAL CONIZATION

The use of the laser beam as a knife for performing excisional conization procedures was first reported from our clinic in 1979.[18] Although the operation had previously been attempted,[19] the lack of hemostasis associated with the use of the laser beam as a scalpel seemed to make the operation excessively difficult. Much of the hemostatic property of the beam is lost when high power density and small spot size are used for cutting, because the lateral heat lost to the tissue is small and the beam slices through the smaller blood vessels without sealing them. There was also the fear that the thermal artifact produced in the cone specimen would make it impossible for the pathologist to properly evaluate the margins of the cone specimen. The problem of bleeding is easily solved by injection of a dilute solution

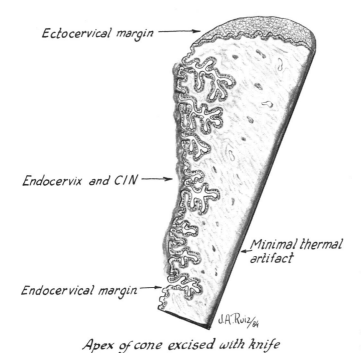

Ectocervical margin

Endocervix and CIN

Minimal thermal artifact

Endocervical margin

J.A. Ruiz/84

Apex of cone excised with knife

Figure 12–2. The thermal artifact produced in the cone biopsy specimen is minimal because of the rapidity with which the high power density laser beam cuts and because the endocervical margin is cut with a knife.

of Pitressin (1:30 dilution) into the cervical stroma. Small blood vessels are thus constricted and do not bleed when sealed by the cutting laser beam. When the cone specimen is removed, a lower power density and larger spot size are used to go back over the cervical stroma to more thoroughly seal or coagulate possible bleeding points. By the same token, the thermal artifact produced in the cone biopsy specimen is minimal because of the rapidity with which the high power density beam was able to cut (Fig. 12–2).

THE TECHNIQUE OF LASER EXCISIONAL CONE

Excisional laser conization is usually performed in the outpatient surgical suite under light general anesthesia. We have also successfully performed the procedure in the clinic using local anesthesia or paracervical block. It is certainly more convenient, however, in the major of incidences to administer a general anesthetic since the patient may experience significant discomfort if the cone is large or deep. This also gives the surgeon the opportunity to perform a pelvic examination under anesthesia.

With the patient in the lithotomy position, colposcopy using 4 percent acetic acid is again performed. A weighted posterior retractor and a single tooth tenaculum applied to the anterior portio vaginalis of the cervix produce excellent visualization and bring the cervix down to the vaginal outlet where the cone specimen can be more easily handled (Fig. 12–3A). The ectocervical limits of the lesion are identified and the incision outlined by short bursts of laser energy leaving a margin of 2 to 3 mm of normal cervical tissue (Fig. 12–3B). The cervix is then gently blotted with povidone-iodine solution. No further cleansing is necessary. A dilute solution of Pitressin is prepared by adding 10 units (one half ampule) to 30 cc of sterile water for injection; 10 cc of this preparation is then injected in 1 cc increments into the stroma surrounding the external os. A spot size of 0.2 to 1 mm and a power setting of 20 to 50 W are appropriate depending upon the type of equipment available and the preference of the surgeon. Remember that the laser incision will have a width equal to the spot size diameter and incisions much narrower than 0.5 mm are more difficult to deepen since tissue edges are close together.

The colposcope is always used to visualize the cervix when excising a laser cone biopsy. Though some surgeons favor using the handheld laser, we prefer to use a micromanipulator for a number of reasons:

1. It enables the operator to direct the beam at the cervix from outside the operative field, whereas the handpiece introduces another instrument into the operator's field of vision.
2. The micromanipulator produces a more accurate incision than a handheld laser since it is not as cumbersome to move.
3. The beam is always in focus when the colposcope is focused. It is not always possible to use the focal spot of the handpiece for cutting in the depths of the incision as the hand piece will not fit into the incision itself.

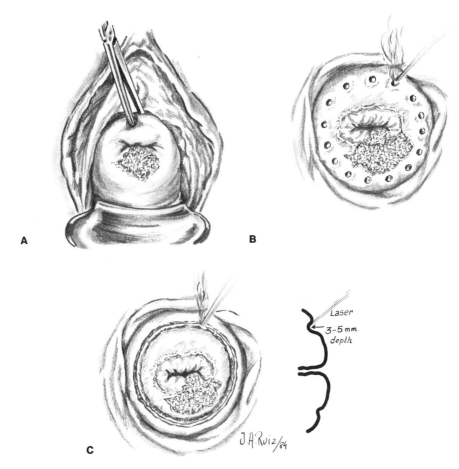

Figure 12–3A. A retractor is placed into the posterior vagina and the ectocervical limits of the lesion and outlined by a series of lower power density imprints. **B.** A dilute solution of Pitressin, 1:30 is injected into the cervix. **C.** Spot size is reduced to 0.5 mm and power turned up to 20 to 50 W. An incision traces the previously placed imprints.

4. Combination procedures, i.e., vaporization and excisional procedures, are often done on the patient as one operative procedure and the micromanipulator provides a much more accurate tool for volumetric ablation.

It is not difficult to direct the laser beam toward the apex of the cone. The original incisions must be deepened to at least 3 to 5 mm straight into the stroma so that the cone can be easily grasped with forceps or a hook (Fig. 12–3C). Traction on the cervix with the tenaculum or traction on the cone specimen with the iris hook enables the beam to be angled towards the endocervical canal (Figs. 12–3D, E, F). Often, the apex of the cone is severed with a knife in order to avoid any

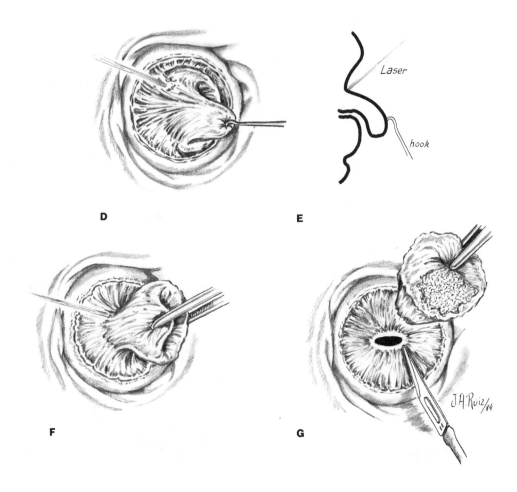

Figure 12–3D. The stroma of the cervix is placed on traction by means of a fine, long-handled hook as the beam cuts deeply into the cervical connective tissue. **E** and **F.** The hook or forceps enables the beam to be angulated toward the endocervical canal. **G.** The apex of the cone is cut with a sharp knife.

thermal artifact in this region. The pathologist can then accurately determine if the apical margin is free of disease (Fig. 12–3G).

THE GEOMETRY OF THE CONE BIOPSY SPECIMEN

It is easier for the surgeon to decide upon the diameter of the base of the cone than it is to rationally select the length of the endocervical canal to be removed. Obviously, the diameter of the base of the cone varies directly with the size of the T zone and the lesion to be excised. A very small base results if there is no lesion visible and the T zone is located within the external os (Fig. 12–4A). The endo-cervical canal cannot be visualized, and therefore, the surgeon must attempt to make an accurate estimate of the length of the endocervical canal to be removed. We have had some success in determining the length of the endocervical canal to be removed by identifying the uppermost extent of the lesion in the endocervical canal with a contact endoscope. This instrument accurately locates the internal cervical os and the exact length of the cone apex can be calculated. If this tech-nique is not available, the internal os can be located with a uterine sound and the surgeon makes a decision as to the appropriate length of the cone (Fig. 12–4B).

Not all conization specimens are truly cone shaped. The geometric form of the specimen to be removed must always be tailored to fit the case. The large irregular lesion will have a large irregular ectocervical base while some smaller specimens will appear more cylindric than cone shaped (Figs. 12–4C, D). No matter what the shape may be, the term conization has been used for many years and will continue to identify an operation performed for the diagnosis and therapy of intraepithelial neoplasia.

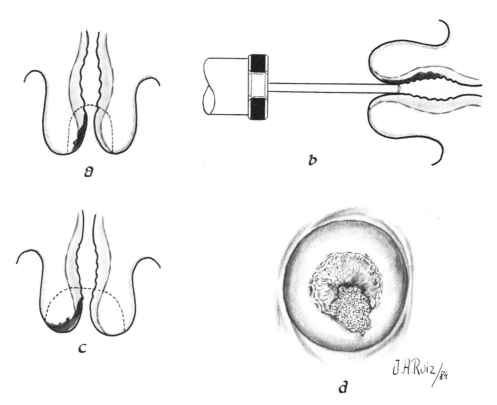

Figure 12–4. A lesion high in the canal, predicates that the base of the cone have a small diameter (**a**). The 6 mm contact hysteroscope can be utilized to determine the apex of the cone (**b**). A large lesion extending into the canal necessitates a large based cone (**c**). The shape and extent of the cone specimen varies with the configuration of the lesion (**d**).

HEMOSTASIS

Though bleeding is minimized by the combination of Pitressin injection and laser coagulation, occasional larger vessels are severed by the beam and brisk bleeding results. It is difficult to coagulate an actively bleeding vessel in a pool of blood since laser energy is absorbed by a very thin layer of blood itself. To seal the vessel, active bleeding must be controlled by tamponade and laser energy used to coagulate the cut end of the vessel. A cotton tip applicator is used to apply pressure directly over the bleeder to stop the blood flow. The applicator is then gently rolled away from the area as the laser beam is applied with a circular motion around and over the vessel. The cotton tip applicator can also be placed within the endocervical canal and pressure directed toward the bleeder to effect the tamponade (Fig. 12–5).

Occasionally, when the combination of laser energy, tamponade and Pitressin, does not yield adequate hemostasis, we utilize conventional methods such as suture, electrocautery, or ferric subsulfate solution. Postoperatively, the defect in the cervix is painted with a latter solution even if completely free of bleeding as this seems to form a protective coagulum and reduce the instance of delayed hemorrhage.

Patients who are on oral contraceptives often have a large everted cervix that appears chronically infected and bleeds readily when biopsies are taken. It is wise to have this patient stop the pill for the cycle prior to the procedure as it is our impression that this definitely reduces the possibility of both intraoperative and postoperative bleeding.

Conization of the cervix during pregnancy is seldom necessary. Most pregnant patients with CIN can be safely followed by colposcopy at regular intervals during pregnancy. Directed biopsy may be taken if absolutely indicated. The pregnant

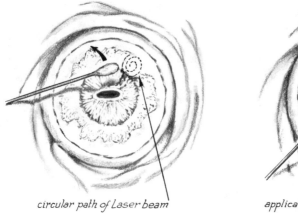
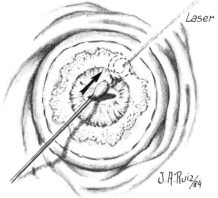

circular path of Laser beam   *applicator exerting pressure toward bleeding*

Figure 12–5. A bleeding vessel must be tamponaded with a dry cotton tipped applicator. With a power setting of 10 W and a 1.5 mm spot the peripheral feeding vessels are coagulated. The swab is rolled off the bleeding point. The central area is coagulated.

cervix can pose a formidable problem for hemostasis. In the rare instance in which invasive cancer is suspected, but not visible because of endocervical involvement, or if microinvasion is present on directed biopsy, laser conization may be safely performed. We take the additional steps of placing lateral sutures in the cervix at 3 and 9 o'clock in order to further ensure hemostasis. Additionally, any vessel of significant size that is visualized colposcopically in the stroma is also sutured with 000 Vicryl swaged on a fine gastrointestinal needle. Any pregnant patient undergoing conization should be admitted to the hospital where the operation is performed under general anesthesia with blood available for immediate transfusion.

PATHOLOGIC INTERPRETATION

The colposcopist must have a thorough working knowledge of the pathology of intraepithelial neoplasia of the lower reproductive tract and must communicate often with the pathologist. A cone specimen that has not been properly oriented is of very little use in determining the adequacy of margins. The colposcopist should explain the technique of laser excisional conization so that the pathologist is able to section the specimen correctly. We prefer to open our cones and pin them out on a piece of cardboard with the stromal side down (Fig. 12–6).

There are other ways in which to effectively section the specimen and the pathologist and colposcopist should agree on the technique and inspect the pathology slides together.

RESULTS OF LASER CONIZATION

In a series of 138 laser excisional conizations performed during the years 1978 through 1982, overall results have been excellent. There has been no intraoperative hemorrhage. Average blood loss has been approximately 2 cc. Six patients (4.3 percent) required emergency visits for vaginal bleeding heavier than a period, but

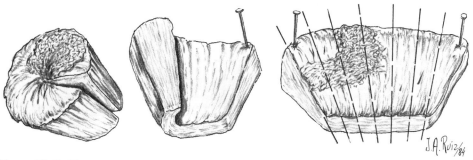

Figure 12–6. The cone specimen is opened and pinned to cardboard with the stromal side down. Appropriate sections are taken to establish whether or not the margins are clear.

only one patient in this series required suturing under anesthesia, because of post-operative hemorrhage (0.7 percent).

Over 100 patients have been followed for more than a year with colposcopy and cytology at 6-month intervals. The overall "cure rate" has been 96 percent. Four patients have demonstrated CIN in repeat biopsies and one of these was discovered within the first 6 months following surgery and thus had persistent disease.

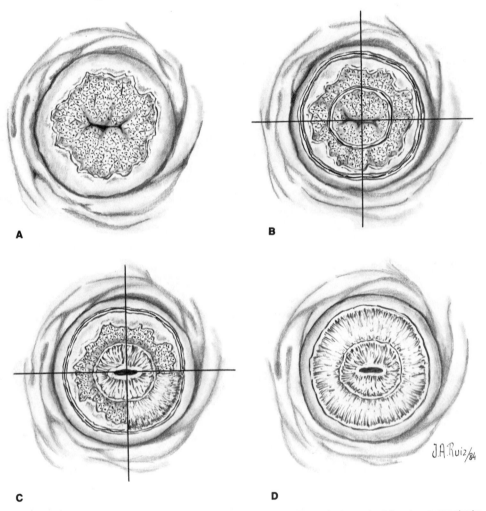

A   **B**

C   **D**

Figure 12–7. (A) A large lesion (CIN) extends into the endocervical canal while also extensively involving the ectocervix. **(B)** A central excisional cone is outlined and will provide the specimen to determine endocervical involvement. The peripheral areas, previously biopsied, are outlined. **(C)** Central cone is completed. Incremental vaporization begins in a lower quadrant and extends to a depth of 5–7 mm. **(D)** Vaporization of CIN is completed to a depth of 7 mm removing the entire atypical transformation zone with a 3 mm peripheral margin.

COMBINATION CONIZATION

The term "combination conization" is used in our clinic to describe laser procedures that involve both excision and vaporization of large CIN lesions that are removed in a single operation.[20] Often, a large area of intraepithelial neoplasia may involve the endocervical canal, the peripheral areas of the cervix and may even spread out into the vagina. These peripheral areas can be visualized and adequately biopsied with the aid of the colposcope thus proving their intraepithelial nature of this portion of the disease. The rule of excisional conization for lesions disappearing into the canal must be followed, however, and the central portion of the cervix should be excised using the technique just described. The end result is a cone biopsy specimen which is hopefully therapeutic as well as diagnostic for the canal lesion and a more moderate vaporization of the peripheral areas of the intraepithelial neoplasia (Fig. 12–7).

The vaporization procedure of these peripheral areas is carried out in the same manner as described for routine vaporization conization and this is done after the excisional portion of the operation is completed. Vaporization to 7 cm is necessary in order to destroy endocervical crypt disease. In the most peripheral portions of the cervix, beyond the last endocervical gland as well as in the vaginal portion of the disease, there is obviously no reason to vaporize so deeply and destruction to 3 mm should be adequate.

The benefit to the patient of this combination procedure over traditional cold knife excision is that a much more conservative operation has been performed. It is far easier to maintain normal cervical architecture using this microsurgical technique of vaporization to minimal but adequate depth and excision of a small cone biopsy than to attempt total excision of the lesion with a knife when one is almost certain to take larger amounts of stroma.

SUMMARY

Excisional conization of the cervix by CO_2 laser is a safe and effective method of performing this operation for both diagnosis and therapy. The benefits of the procedure are ease and accuracy of performance, rapid healing, low complication rate, excellent patient acceptance, and a very high rate of success. Often, excisional and vaporization procedures are utilized in the same patient and the combination of these microsurgical techniques provides the most conservative approach to the theory of CIN.

REFERENCES

1. Lisfrac J: Memoire sur une nouvelle methode de practique l'operation de la taille chez les femmes. Gaz Med France 2:835–846, 1815
2. Galvin FA, TeLinde RW: The present-day status of noninvasive cervical carcinoma. Am J Obstet Gynecol 57:15–36, 1949
3. Galvin GA, Jones HW, TeLinde RW: Significance of basal-cell hyperactivity in cervical biopsies. Am J Obstet Gynecol 70:808–821, 1955

4. TeLinde RW: Hysterectomy for carcinoma in situ. In Meigs (ed): Surgical Treatment of Cancer of the Cervix. New York, Grune & Stratton, 1954, pp 130–136

5. Schiffer MA, Greene HJ, Pomerance W, et al: Cervical conization for diagnosis and treatment of carcinoma in situ. Am J Obstet Gynecol 93:889, 1965

6. Richart RM, Sciarra JJ: Treatment of cervical dysplasia by outpatient electrocauterization. Am J Obstet Gynecol 101:200, 1968

7. Ostergard DR, Gondos B: Outpatient therapy of preinvasive cervical neoplasia: Selection of patients with the use of colposcopy. Am J Obstet Gynecol 115:783, 1973

8. Coppleson M: Management of preclinical carcinoma of the cervix. In Jordan, Singer (eds): The Cervix. London: WB Saunders, 1976, pp 453–474

9. Kolstad P: Diagnosis and management of precancerous lesions of the cervix uteri. Int J Gynaecol Obstet 8:551, 1970

10. Kolstad P, Klem V: Long-term followup of 1121 cases of carcinoma in situ. Obstet Gynecol 48(2):125–129, 1976

11. Kolstad P: Conization treatment of cervical intraepithelial neoplasia. Obstet Gynecol Surv 34(11):827, 1979

12. Baggish MS: High power density carbon dioxide laser therapy for early cervical neoplasia. Am J Obstet Gynecol 136:117, 1980

13. Baggish MS: Management of cervical intraepithelial neoplasia by carbon dioxide laser. Obstet Gynecol 60:379, 1982

14. Chanen W, Rome RM: Electrocoagulation diathermy for cervical dysplasia and carcinoma in situ: A 15-year survey. Obstet Gynecol 61:673, 1983

15. Burke L: The use of the carbon dioxide laser in the treatment of cervical intraepithelial neoplasia. Colp Gynecol Laser Surg 1:41, 1984

16. Burghardt E, Ostor AG: Review: Site and origin of squamous cervical cancer: A histomorphologic study. Obstet Gynecol 62:117, 1983

17. Dorsey JH: Excisional conization of the cervix. In Andrews AH, Polanyi TG (eds): Microscopic and Endoscopic Surgery with the CO_2 Laser. Boston, John Wright, 1982, p 231

18. Dorsey JH, Diggs ES: Microsurgical conization of the cervix by carbon dioxide laser. Obstet Gynecol 54:565–570, 1979

19. Toaff R: The carbon dioxide laser in gynecological surgery. In Kaplan I (ed): Laser Surgery I-II. Jerusalem, Jerusalem Academic Press, 1976

20. Baggish MS, Dorsey JH: The laser combination cone. Am J Obstet Gynecol 151:23, 1985

13

Invasive Gynecologic Cancer Treated by Laser

Helmut F. Schellhas

SURGICAL LASERS APPLIED IN ONCOLOGY

Significant advances in oncology have been made by the use of surgical laser systems. Lasers presently used in clinical oncology include the carbon dioxide (CO_2) laser, the neodymium-yttrium-aluminum-garnet (Nd:YAG) laser and hematoporphyrin derivative (HpD) laser photoradiation therapy which utilizes a tunable dye laser system. These various lasers have different physical properties and beam characteristics. The biophysical effects in tissue are quite different and therefore applicable in different clinical situations (Table 13–1).

CO_2 Laser

The CO_2 laser is used for tissue vaporization and incisional surgery. The CO_2 beam has a high absorption coefficient in organic tissue and is ideally suited for tissue vaporization. Tumors can be vaporized to any depth with precision. A limiting factor is bleeding since a thin layer of fluid absorbs the laser beam and renders it ineffective for tumor destruction. The CO_2 laser beam can also be used as a cutting instrument. Since the edges of the incised tissue develop a very small zone of thermal damage, small vessels are sealed causing a hemostatic effect and probably avoidance of intraoperative seeding of malignant cells and postoperative oozing of blood, serum, and lymphatic fluid.

Nd:YAG Laser

The Nd:YAG laser is clinically used as a coagulator. The beam emits in the near infrared portion of the electromagnetic spectrum at 1060 nm. The absorption coefficient in biologic tissue is low. The beam has a high scatter effect in tissue which includes backscatter of a large portion of the beam on the tissue surface. Forward scatter is observed when a hollow organ such as stomach or bladder is irradiated. A large portion of the beam penetrates beyond the organ wall.[1] The beam causes a wide zone of tissue coagulation and necrosis. When used with a very high power density, the Nd:YAG laser beam can also vaporize tissue. Necrotic tissue scatter-

TABLE 13–1. BIOLOGIC EFFECTS OF LASERS USED IN ONCOLOGY

	CO_2 Laser	Nd:YAG Laser	HpD-Laser Photoradiation Therapy
Wavelength (nm)	10,600	1060	630–640
Absorption coefficient	High	Low	Absorbed by photosensitized cells only
Backscatter	Low	High	—
Internal scatter	Low	High	—
Tissue vaporization	Good	Poor	—
Tissue coagulation	Poor	Good	—
Tissue necrosis	Marginal	Good	Very good

ing has been found to be reached with an enhanced vaporization effect.[2] The coagulation effect achieves excellent control of bleeding.

Compared with the CO_2 laser, the tissue effect of the Nd:YAG laser beam is not immediately visible. The extensive tissue necrosis results in postoperative tissue slough. While the surgeon can observe the effectiveness of the CO_2 laser beam in tissue immediately, he has to use a very careful irradiation dosimetry for the Nd:YAG laser beam because of the late tissue effects. The penetration depth of the Nd:YAG laser beam is predictable and controllable. Both the CO_2 and the Nd:YAG laser are used in oncologic surgery with high power and continuous wave. The CO_2 laser is mainly used as a scalpel and vaporizer. The Nd:YAG laser is applied as a coagulator to control bleeding or destroy tumor tissue. The CO_2 laser beam is delivered through a mirror system while the Nd:YAG laser is transmitted through fiberoptics.

Laser Photoradiation Therapy

Photoradiation therapy of malignant tumors using photosensitizing HpD systemically is a method in which a laser system is used to activate the selective cytotoxic effect of the HpD for malignant cells which produces their immediate necrosis.[3] The laser is used for photoactivation and destruction of sensitized tissue and not as a primary surgical instrument. A dye laser is used which emits at 630 to 640 nm which is a bright red light. The effective tissue penetration of the incident light is 0.5 to 1.5 cm and depends on the tissue structure. Singlet oxygen is generated in malignant cells which destroys them. This system can also be used for diagnostic purposes since the HpD retained in malignant cells fluoresces.[4]

Clinical cancer institutes will require the availability of an institutional comprehensive laser center which includes both surgical and diagnostic laser systems and an active laser laboratory for clinically applied research. Many medical centers have different surgical laser systems in various departments. A cooperative approach in the utilization of this equipment will be mutually very beneficial.

Choice of Instruments

The main interest for the surgical oncologist in these three different laser systems is the established fact that these instruments can be effectively used for the control of isolated tumors which have not responded to radiation therapy and which cannot be surgically resected by conventional means. Which one of the three laser systems is preferable over the others for certain clinical situations might perhaps be determined after the study of the following paragraphs. A combination of two or all three laser systems for the treatment of a particular tumor problem might be necessary.

CO_2 LASER SURGERY

Power, Beam Spot Size, and Power Density

For tumor volume destruction a laser beam is required which has a high absorption in tissue which is characteristic for the CO_2 laser. In addition, a high volume absorption and high tissue penetration is desired which, however, the CO_2 laser beam does not provide. To compensate for this inadequacy, both a large beam spot size and a high laser power are needed. The power density of the beam is inversely proportional with the square of the diameter of the incident beam. A commercially available surgical laser operating with a maximum power of 30 W and the minimal beam diameter of 0.2 mm achieves the very high power density of 95,500 W/cm^2. Such a high power density is very adequate for deep penetration of tumor tissue. The small beam size of 0.2 mm makes it, however, most tedious to destroy a large tumor volume of several cm^3 and viable tumor cells probably will remain unaffected. A spot size of 2 mm is more practical for tumor volume destruction. The 30 W power laser, however, provides only a power density of 955 W/cm^2 for this spot size which is inadequate for tumor volume destruction. To achieve the power density of 95,500 W/cm^2 with a beam spot size of 2 mm, the laser would require a power output of 3000 W. The tube of such a powerful laser would hardly fit in an operating room. For tumor volume vaporization, a modest power density of 4000 W/cm^2 would be adequate if a beam spot size of 2 mm could be provided. This, however, requires a surgical laser system with the power output of 125 W which is not commercially available.

This example demonstrates the inadequacy of presently commercially available surgical laser systems for tumor volume vaporization. Tumor tissue vaporization is possible under the present circumstances but very tedious and not exact resulting more in palliation than cure. An automatic scanning device has recently been introduced which programs the laser to move the focused beam precisely over an outlined area for tissue vaporization. This device is very elegant and renders a medium or high power commercial surgical laser more useful in surgical oncology. For surgical cancer centers, it is advisable to have a powerful CO_2 laser custom built for multidisciplinary use.[5]

Laser Beam Delivery System

Surgical CO_2 lasers utilize a multiarticulated arm in which the beam is reflected by a mirror system from the point of exit at the cavity to the focusing lens of the "hand piece." The length of the arm, which is also called "manipulator," varies in different laser instruments. For abdominal and also for vulvar and transvaginal surgery, it is important to have adequate distance between the laser console and the operative field. This distance is too short to be practical in several commercial instruments. The power of the laser is measured in some instruments at the beam exit from the cavity and is attenuated as it passes to its focal point. In other instruments the power is read at the terminal part of the beam. The laser surgeon should be aware of this difference. The multiarticulated arm is preferable in surgical oncology for tissue vaporization and the cutting mode over the beam delivered through a surgical microscope. The spot diameter of the focused beam can be altered by interchangeable lenses with different focal distances.

Cancer of the Cervix

Primary Carcinoma of Cervix
The laser has no role in the primary treatment of diagnosed invasive carcinoma of the cervix. The conventional treatment with radical surgery or radiation therapy is not replaced by any laser treatment. Indirectly, the CO_2 laser might have some effect in the natural history of early or occult cervical carcinomas. A diagnostic cervical conization procedure with the CO_2 laser seals the vascular spaces and might have a lesser tumor cell embolizing effect than cold knife surgery. The tissue margins remain adequate for diagnosis if a "bloodless" technique is used with the local injection of vasoconstrictors, a very small spot size of the beam which vaporizes only a very narrow marginal incisional zone, and a high power density of the incident beam which allows a speedy incision and results in minimal thermal tissue damage.[6]

Recurrent Carcinoma of Cervix
Selective unresectable pelvic tumors postradiation therapy can be vaporized with the CO_2 laser. Limitless amounts of tissue can be removed with great precision. Since the beam penetrates bone, one of the absolute indications for laser surgery is recurrent pelvic tumor attached to bone. Such a clinical indication is seen in Figure 13–1. The pelvic sidewall tumor can be surgically approached extraperi-

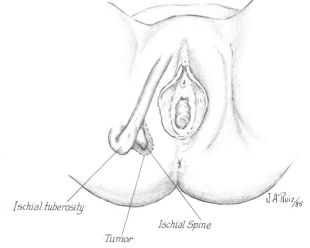

Figure 13–1. Isolated recurrent tumor (dark field) developed on the posterior ischial spine following previous surgery and radiation therapy. Laser vaporization is the best surgical means of removing tumor tissue attached to bones. *(From Schellhas HF.[7])*

Ischial tuberosity

Ischial Spine

Tumor

toneally or transperitoneally through the abdominal wall or transvaginally by dissecting the perivaginal tissue which might also require transection of the rectum in a patient who already has a colostomy or requires one for different reasons. Once the tumor has been surgically exposed the laser beam is directed against the pelvic sidewall. The tissue will become charred after the tumor surface has been vaporized which will stop the beam. Further vaporization attempts of the carbonized tissue layer will result only in a heating of the underlying tissue and its thermal damage without further vaporization. Constant debridement of the charred tissue is necessary. The wound bed of the tumor should be checked by multiple biopsies and frozen section examination to determine the completeness of the procedure. Indications for vaporization of recurrent unresectable pelvic tumors postradiation therapy have to be individualized and are relatively few. In addition to pelvic sidewall recurrences, we have utilized the CO_2 laser on metastatic malignancies to the vagina, a tumor attached to the os sacrum, and a groin tumor.[7,8] Hemorrhaging tumors are difficult to treat with the CO_2 laser alone and will be discussed in another paragraph.

Primary Carcinoma of the Vulva and Vagina

With the availability of new CO_2 lasers which provide power densities of 100 kW/ cm^2 and a spot diameter of 0.2 mm, our interest in incisional surgery for primary vulvar and vaginal malignancies has been renewed. Older laser systems providing a maximal power density of 4 kW/cm^2 with a 1 mm spot diameter have been too slow in radical surgical procedures. Especially fat layers took too long to cut. Clinically it was not important whether a groin dissection had a blood loss of only 10 ml with laser resection or 100 ml with the scalpel.[9] The scalpel dissection was much faster and was therefore preferred. The superior speed of the cold knife for radical vulvectomy justified its preference over the laser. The electrosurgical knife is much handier than the cumbersome laser arm though the author prefers cold knife tissue resection over the "Bovie" knife. The presently available very high power densities of 50 to 100 kW/cm^2 render carbon dioxide CO_2 laser surgery attractive again for radical vulvar and vaginal surgery. A long articulated surgical arm is practical for vulvar surgery. Tissues to be incised should be held in good tension. Finger pressure lateral to the incisional line applied with moist laps compresses the blood vessels and results in good hemostasis. Dryness of the surgical field is important for adequate absorption of the beam.

The following are at present two important indications for the use of the CO_2 laser in surgery for vulvar and vaginal malignancies.

Lymph Node Involvement or Extensive Tumor
The CO_2 laser beam seals capillaries and lymphatics. Groin dissection with the CO_2 laser appears to be advantageous when lymph nodes appear to be clinically involved. Skin flaps were dissected with a power density of 2500 W/cm^2. Along the femoral vessels the tissue was dissected with a power density of 600 W/cm^2. Tumors extending into the ischiorectal fossa or fixed to the pubic bone were resected with the maximum available power density. In the presence of infiltrating tumor, decreased instrumentation and minimal touch laser beam incision enhance the surgical technique.

Vaginectomy "From Below"

A good vaginectomy depends on the identification of the paravaginal tissue planes. With the surgical principles important for CO_2 laser surgery, optimal tissue tension is supplied for adequate incision, the surgical field is kept dry to avoid absorption of the beam by blood. These careful measures help greatly to identify the required planes for dissection and the laser incision keeps the blood loss small.[8]

Disseminated Ovarian Carcinoma

Generalized carcinomatosis of the peritoneal and serosal surfaces so typical for ovarian carcinoma is for the surgeon a most frustrating situation because he cannot resect it all. Especially in a second-look operation after previous adjuvant application of chemotherapy or radiation therapy or both, complete surgical eradication of diffuse carcinomatosis is desirable. The hope to accomplish this task with a surgical laser has been expressed many times. Presently available CO_2 or Nd:YAG laser systems are not suited for the performance of such an operation. The beam size is too small and the radiation dosimetry is too difficult for safe application on bowel surfaces. The HpD-laser photoradiation therapy might be applicable in the future if the proper beam wavelength can be delivered over the enormously large peritoneal and serosal surfaces for the time period required. A beam scanner or a strobe flash with high light intensity might facilitate this endeavor in the future.

Any small metastatic disease confined to isolated areas could of course be approached like any benign endometriotic foci for tissue vaporization. The surgeon has to secure a tissue diagnosis first. This situation is, however, not often encountered. Isolated tumor nodules are probably better surgically excised than vaporized.

CO_2 Laser Vaporization of Vascular Tumors

Power Density, Focused and Unfocused Beam

A low power density will have a better hemostatic effect than a high power density. A large capillary hemangioma of the cervix, for instance, was successfully treated by Bellina and associates with power densities of 100 to 150 W/cm^2.[10]

A high power density vaporizes a larger tissue volume. The choice of power density depends on the vascularity of the individual tumor. It is advantageous to apply a focused laser beam rather than a defocused or unfocused beam. The latter will cause more thermal tissue damage and carbonization of tissue. The carbonized layer will stop the beam and requires debriding. The speed of the beam movement is also important because the longer the beam remains directed against one spot the deeper is the marginal damage of tissue dehydration and carbonization.[11]

Cryosurgery and CO_2 Laser Surgery in Combination

A bleeding malignant tumor will be difficult to treat with the CO_2 laser alone because the beam is quickly absorbed by a layer of blood before the incident beam can have any effect on the tumor tissue. The tissue thickness (layer of blood) which will absorb 95 percent of the light energy of the CO_2 laser which has an absorption coefficient in tissues of about 20/cm is 150 μm according to Verschueren.[11]

We have frozen bleeding tumor tissue with a liquid nitrogen spray before tissue vaporization with the CO_2 laser (Fig. 13-2). The ischemic frozen tissue absorbs the focused laser beam and is then vaporized. The depth penetration of the cryogen is deeper than that of the laser beam. Continuous lasing will eventually open intact vessels below the frozen zone which then will require refreezing. We use the highest available power density for volume reduction of vascular tumors in conjunction with the freezing technique.[12]

For the vaporization of frozen tissue, full advantage of the thermal properties of the CO_2 laser beam should be taken. A laser beam with high power density should be focused on the tissue for optimal destruction. The intra- and extracellular fluid will boil and evaporate and develop the plume which consists of the steam and dehydrated tissue particles. An unfocused laser beam would only gradually increase the tissue temperature and cause dehydration and slow tissue vaporization. Further dehydration of tissue will result in the formation of a layer of carbonized tissue which will stop the laser beam and cause further thermal damage in the adjoining tissues. The layer of carbon requries debridement before further tissue vaporization can be continued. Debridement of charred tissue is also necessary with the optimal tissue vaporization technique but it will be a lesser problem.

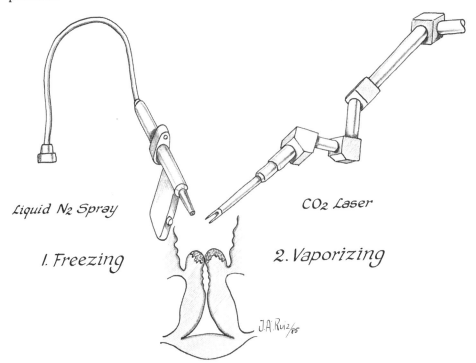

Figure 13-2. A combination of cryosurgery and laser surgery is used for hemostasis and vaporization of vascular tumors. *(From Schellhas HF.[12])*

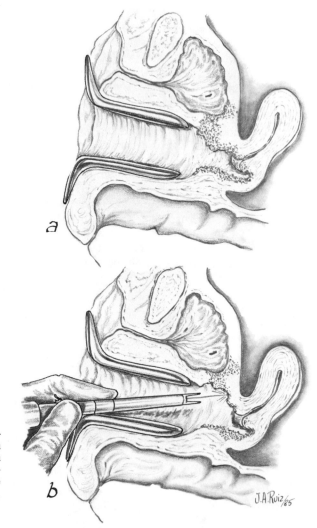

Figure 13–3. Metastatic squamous carcinoma to the vagina and bladder vesicovaginal fistula (**a**). The handpiece of the Sharplan laser is inserted into the vagina for tumor vaporization (**b**). (*From Schellhas HF.*[12])

The combined cryogen and CO_2 laser technique was clinically applied in patients with hemorrhaging metastatic carcinoma of the cervix to the vagina and vulva and to carcinoma of the cervix metastatic to the pelvic bone (Fig. 13–3).[8]

ND:YAG LASER SURGERY

The Biologic Effect in Tissues

The invisible beam emitting at 1060 μm in the near infrared portion of the electromagnetic spectrum provides a high tissue penetration which is approximately 10 times deeper than the tissue penetration of the CO_2 laser.[11] The marked beam scatter within the tissue produces a high volume absorption. A large tissue volume is heated up and causes tissue coagulation and hemostasis without its removal. Additional ND:YAG laser irradiation of coagulated and desiccated tissue causes tissue vaporization if high energy densities are used. The Nd:YAG laser appears, therefore, ideal for the surgical destruction of recurrent gynecologic tumors especially when they are hemorrhagic. Back scatter of the beam results in the loss of a large part of the laser energy which, however, is dependent on the quality of tissue irradiated. Since beam absorption was found to be enhanced in necrotic tissue, it can be assumed that tumor tissue is an optimal medium for Nd:YAG laser beam irradiation.[2]

The Nd:YAG Laser System

Like the surgical CO_2 laser systems, the Nd:YAG laser consists of a mobile console which consists of the electric system, an open water cooling system, and the control unit. The laser tube is contained within the console or attached outside the console and supported by an adjustable arm. The beam is transmitted through a fiberoptic system. A pilot light is either provided by a coaxial He-Ne laser (red light) or a xenon lamp (white light). A gas or air flow system is provided to clear the operative field. The system can, however, be used without the gas or air flow. The surgical probes are devised for use through an endoscope. A handheld device allows open laser surgery. The power output at the treatment site can be continually adjusted from 10 to 70 or 100 W in the various laser systems.

Clinical Application

Government regulations have classified the Nd:YAG laser as an investigational device. An approved Investigational Device Exemption (IDE) must be obtained before the laser can be used clinically. The IDE requires a protocol which is approved by the Institutional Review Board. Investigators can be added to the IDE of the laser company from which the system has been purchased which simplifies the administrative process.

Clinically the Nd:YAG laser is very established in the field of gastroenterology where its application has been life saving in patients hemorrhaging from ulcers or varices. For tumor control the laser has been used in urology, neurosurgery, gastroenterology, and thoracic surgery (tracheobronchial lesions). Goldrath coagulates the endometrium of patients with functional uterine bleeding.[13] The indications for surgery are not very frequent in gynecologic oncology. An institutional laser should be shared by all interested departments.

We have used Nd:YAG laser coagulation in patients with recurrent squamous carcinomas of the cervix and the ovary to the lateral pelvic sidewall and vagina.[14] Vascular tumors are treated best with this laser system. The previously described combination of cryosurgery and CO_2 laser surgery has been replaced by the Nd:YAG laser beam.

Against vaginal cuff lesions, we utilized laser energies of 600 to 5000 W. Against the pelvic sidewall we utilized 10,000 to 13,000 W. Forward scatter is an important consideration when the laser beam is directed against the vaginal cuff because bladder and bowel can be thermally damaged.[1]

REFERENCES

1. Halldorsson T, Langerhole J: Thermodynamic analysis of laser irradiation of biological tissue. Appl Optics 17:3948–3958, 1978
2. Buchholz J, Haverkamf K, Meyer HJ, et al: Scattering effects in laser surgery. In Kaplan I (ed): Laser Surgery II. Jerusalem, Jerusalem Academic Press, 1978
3. Dougherty TJ, Kaufman JE, Goldfarb A, et al: Photoirradiation therapy for the treatment of malignant tumors. Cancer Res 38:2628–2635, 1978
4. Lipson RL, Baldes EJ, Olsen AM: Hematoporphyrin derivative for the detection of cervical cancer. Obstet Gynecol 24:78–84, 1964
5. Muckerheide MC, St. Mary's Hospital, Milwaukee, Wisconsin: Personal Communication, 1982
6. Larsson G: Conization for preinvasive and early carcinoma of the uterine cervix. Acta Obstet Gynecol Scan (Supp) 114:1–40, 1983
7. Schellhas HF: Laser surgery in gynecology. Surg Clin North Am 58:151–166, 1978
8. Schellhas HF, Barnes AE: Indications for laser surgery in gynecologic oncology. Int Adv Surg Oncol 5:365–384, 1982
9. Schellhas HF, Fidler JM, Rockwell MJ: The carbon dioxide laser scalpel in the management of vulvar lesions. In Kaplan I (ed): Laser Surgery I. Jerusalem, Jerusalem Academic Press, 1978
10. Bellina JH, Gyer DR, Voros JI, Rariotta JJ: Capillary hemangioma managed by the CO_2 laser. In Bellina JH (ed): Gynecologic Laser Surgery. New York, London, Plenum Press, 1981
11. Verschueren R: The CO_2 laser in tumor surgery. Van Gorcum. Amsterdam, Assen, 1976
12. Schellhas HF: Cryogens and carbon dioxide laser in cyclic combination for volume reduction of vascular tumors. In Kaplan I (ed): Laser Surgery III, Part I. Tel Aviv, OT PAS, 1977
13. Goldrath MH, Fuller TA, Segal S: Laser photovaporization of endometrium for the treatment of hemorrhagia. Am J Obstet Gynecol 140:14–19, 1981
14. Schellhas HF, Weppelmann B: The neodymium:YAG laser in the treatment of gynecologic malignancies. Lasers in Surgery and Medicine (submitted for publication)

14

Photoradiation Therapy in the Treatment of Gynecologic Tumors

Thomas J. Dougherty

INTRODUCTION

Photoradiation therapy (PRT) is a novel approach to the treatment of a variety of solid, malignant tumors in man and animals. This therapy, while still in early stages of clinical application in many areas, is being found to be particularly useful in treatment of cancers of the bronchus, [1-6] bladder, [7-10] skin, [11-15] esophagus, [16-18] and as an adjunct to surgery.[3] Application of PRT to treatment of gynecologic tumors has not been extensive but has demonstrated considerable promise, especially in cases difficult to treat by other means.[19,20]

Photoradiation therapy involves the use of a relatively selective tumor photosensitizer, hematoporphyrin derivative (HpD) or its tumor-active component (DHE), which appears to be an ether formed by covalently linking two hematoporphyrin moieties.[21] Following systemic injection and allowing time for serum and most normal tissues to clear the drug (2 to 3 days), the porphyrin is activated photochemically in situ by means of visible light generally delivered from a dye laser system emitting near 630 nm (Fig. 14-1). It is known that in addition to tumor, liver, kidney, spleen, and to a lesser extent, skin, retain HpD and DHE. Most normal tissues clear the drug over a period of a few days.[22,23] This allows for a relatively selective effect on the tumor following the porphyrin activation. Singlet oxygen produced by energy transfer from the light-activated porphyrin to endogenous oxygen is the likely cytotoxic species. In in vitro experiments, when this singlet oxygen is quenched[24] or enhanced,[27] tumor cell destruction is quenched or enhanced accordingly. Vascular effects are clearly important in destroying the tumor. Fluorescence and radiographic studies indicate a concentration of the porphyrin around the vascular stroma.[23] Following light treatment, tumors become devoid of blood often within a few hours after treatment. Histologically, the earliest changes seen in tumors following HpD or DHE + light are red cell coagulation within the vessels, at which time the tumor cells show no obvious degeneration. Within a few hours, complete vascular collapse and rupture occurs with

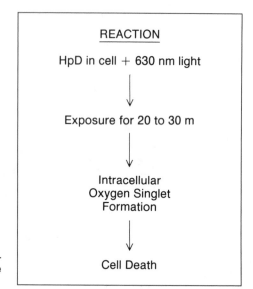

REACTION

HpD in cell + 630 nm light

↓

Exposure for 20 to 30 m

↓

Intracellular
Oxygen Singlet
Formation

↓

Cell Death

Figure 14–1. General scheme for photoradiation therapy using hematoporphyrin derivative (HpD) and dye laser light.

concomitant tumor cell destruction to depths of 5 to 15 mm. The exact details of this overall process are under investigation. A review[26] and two recent workshop proceedings are available.[27,28]

CLINICAL RESULTS

To date approximately 2000 patients with a variety of cancers have been treated by PRT in approximately 30 centers throughout the world. While the greatest number of patients have had either skin tumors (primary, recurrent, metastatic) or bronchial tumors, other types demonstrating complete or partial responses include cancers of the bladder, esophagus, stomach, eye, peritoneal cavity, and gynecologic tract.[1–20,27,28] The vast majority of the patients had advanced tumors recurrent after conventional therapies. A recent compilation of the early and carcinoma in situ cases of the bronchus, bladder, and skin treated by PRT, showed a complete response in 42 of 51 cases.[28] No untoward complications were reported in these cases. It is likely that the effectiveness and selectivity of PRT in early stage cancers will make it a treatment of choice in some cases. A further advantage of PRT is that prior therapy such as chemotherapy and radiation therapy, as well as prior PRT generally are not contraindications, although there is some evidence that patients on Adriamycin may overreact to treatment.[27,28] Further, there is no evidence to indicate that it in any way jeopardizes subsequent surgery, radiation, or chemotherapy.

In addition to potentially curative treatment, PRT is effective in palliation for advanced bronchial and esophageal tumors. In a recent study of 22 patients with bronchial obstructions, Balchum and Doiron[29] report complete response in 20, 15 of whom returned to work. Follow-up has ranged to approximately 1 year.[29] In this group, complete response has meant complete opening of the bronchus to the wall. These investigators have selected patients who were not in acute respiratory distress prior to treatment. Those who demonstrate such respiratory distress can be at high risk after PRT due to occasional heavy secretions and necrotic debris which can further block an airway.[29]

METHODOLOGY

Patients receive intravenous injection of 2.5 to 3.0 mg/kg HpD (Photofrin) (or 1.5 to 2.0 mg/kg DHE—Photofrin II, trade name of Photofrin Medical Inc., Cheektowaga, N.Y.) which immediately renders them photosensitive for 30 days or more. This necessitates remaining out of sunlight or any other bright light whether indoors or outside. Ordinary room light has not presented a problem. At the end of 30 days, patients test their sun sensitivity by cautiously exposing a small area to the sun for 5 minutes. An advantage of DHE is that this photosensitivity problem appears to be minimized, although not eliminated. Three days following injection—a time interval generally found to be optimal for normal tissue clearance, the lesion, with an appropriate margin, is exposed to 630 nm light generally delivered from a dye laser source. In some cases it is feasible to demonstrate the red fluorescence of the tumor indicating porphyrin uptake (Figs. 14–2, 14–3, 14–4; 14–

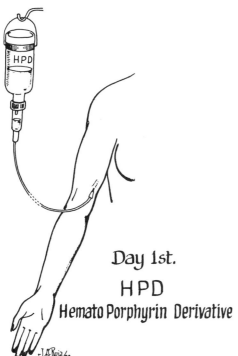

Day 1st.

HPD

Hemato Porphyrin Derivative

Figure 14–2. On day one of treatment, HpD is administered intravenously.

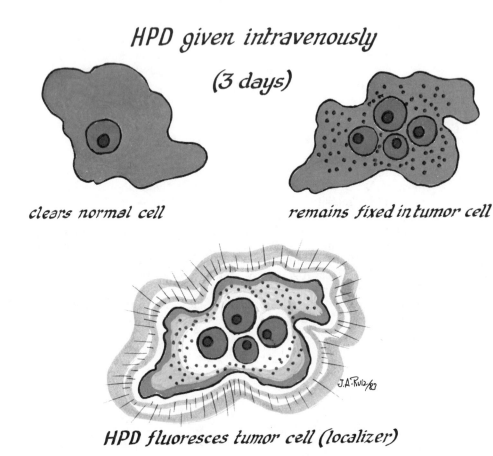

HPD given intravenously

(3 days)

clears normal cell   *remains fixed in tumor cell*

HPD fluoresces tumor cell (localizer)

Figure 14–3. Schematic drawing which shows HpD clearing normal cells but remaining fixed to neoplastic cells. The interaction of HpD and light produces tumor localization by fluorescence.

5, see Color Plate III*). For exposed tumors, this can be easily accomplished by using a Wood's lamp and observing the porphyrin fluorescence through appropriate filters, e.g., argon laser goggles. For some inaccessible tumors, special scopes have been devised to observe the porphyrin fluorescence which, in some cases, can be used as a means of locating occult tumors.[5,30] Quartz glass fibers, 200 to 600 μ m in diameter, are used for light delivery. These fibers can be efficiently coupled into the laser and provide convenient means to deliver the light to almost any site either by directing at the surface of the tumor (1 cm or less) or by interstitial methods. In most cases one of several special ends are used on the fibers (Fig. 14–6). For surface treatment a small convex lens is used to provide a uniform light area. Within a lumen, e.g., bronchus, trachea, esophagus, or sometimes within the

---

*Color Plate III appears following p. 177.

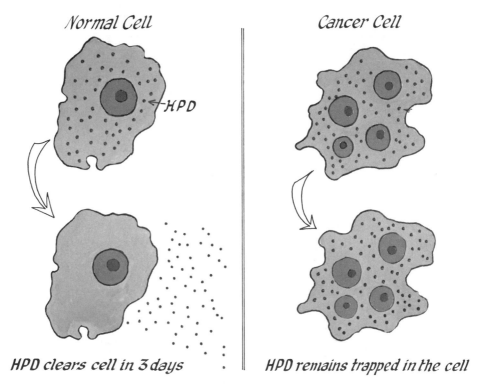

Normal Cell

Cancer Cell

←*HPD*

HPD clears cell in 3 days

HPD remains trapped in the cell

Figure 14–4. The HpD clears normal tissues 3 days following injection, but remains at tumor sites.

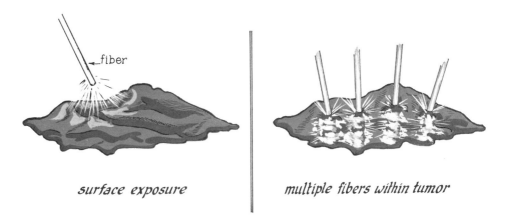

←fiber

surface exposure

multiple fibers within tumor

Figure 14–6. Fine quartz fibers deliver the dye laser light to the tumor site.

vagina, a diffuser is used on the fiber which provides peripheral light distribution over a distance of 0.5 to 3 cm at the end of the fiber. Such fibers are also recommended for interstitial light delivery. These fibers provide sufficient illumination interstitially to cause tumor necrosis to a radius of approximately 10 mm from the point of insertion. The larger tumors require multiple fibers (provided sufficient power is available) or multiple insertions. The wavelength for in situ activation of the porphyrin is generally at 630 nm to take advantage of the greater tissue penetration of this wavelength compared to the shorter wavelengths which could also be used to activate the porphyrins. For superficial tumors, power densities range from approximately 20 to 120 mW/cm^2 to deliver typically, 20 to 100 J/cm^2 over 5 to 30 minutes. The lower dose range is limited to the more superficial tumors. For the larger tumors and for obstructing tumors, the light diffusion fibers are imbedded into the lesion either directly or through 18-gauge needles. The power density is 300 to 400 mW for each centimeter of diffuser to deliver 200 to 300 J/cm over 5 to 15 minutes. Thus, a 3-cm diffuser would require an output from the fiber of up to 1.2 W which would require approximately 1.5 W from the dye laser for each fiber considering coupling efficiencies of 70 to 80 percent. Current laser systems typically produce approximately 1.5 W with a 5 to 6 W argon laser pump and up to 4 W with the 18 to 20 W argon pump lasers.

APPLICATION TO GYNECOLOGIC TUMORS

In the 1960s, Lipson et al. demonstrated HpD uptake in malignant tumors of the cervix[31] as well as those of the bronchus [32,33] and other sites.[34] The first reports of the therapeutic use of Hpd to treat gynecologic tumors were in 1982 by Ward et al. [19] and Forbes et al. from Australia, [12] and Soma et al. from Japan.[20] Recently Rettenmaier et al. have reported early results of PRT for a number of gynecologic tumors including carcinoma in situ.[28] Soma's group has extended their study more recently.[35] A summary of results appears in Table 14–1.

TABLE 14–1. SUMMARY OF RESULTS OF PRT FOR GYNECOLOGIC TUMORS[a]

	Response			Follow-Up
	CR	PR	NR	
Primary cancers				
Vagina	2	1	—	2 yr
CIS, cervix	3	2	—	1.5 yr
CIS, vulva	1	—	—	<1 yr
Recurrent/metastatic cancers				
Vagina	4	4		2 yr
Cervix	1[b]	1[b]	1[c]	<1 yr
Total	10	10	1	

[a]Power densities ranged from 50 to 500 mW/cm^2.
[b]Light dose = 40 joules/cm^2.
[c]Light dose = 20 joules/cm^2.
(Data from Forbes I et al.[12] and Soma H et al.[20])

The tumors ranged from carcinoma in situ to large invasive tumors in some cases exceeding 6 cm in diameter. The cervical tumors recently reported by Rettenmaier received 40 J/cm^2 at 630 nm except for one case, which received 20 J/cm^2, a dose causing no response. The larger tumors reported by Forbes were treated by interstitial methods using fibers without diffusers delivering approximately 400 mW at 630 nm. To adequately cover the entire lesion with light, multiple placements were used (in some cases more than 20). The use of diffusers in the fibers greatly reduces the number of individual placements required since the light covers a linear length slightly longer than the length of the fiber and allows input of a much higher power density without introducing adverse thermal effects.[36] The intraepithelial tumors received 60 J/cm^2 (complete response) to >500 J/cm^2 of 630 nm light.

In these preliminary studies obviously a wide range of light doses have been used by the investigators. While large tumors will require fairly aggressive treatment in order to achieve complete regression, the smaller lesions are likely to be adequately treated by 100 to 200 J/cm^2 of 630 nm light, a dose which has proven sufficient to cause complete necrosis of large (>1 cm) endobronchial tumors.[30] It is perhaps noteworthy, however, that no complications of treatment were found in this group of patients even for those receiving the highest light doses. In all cases complete healing occurred without severe damage to normal epithelium. The only toxicity reported was the usual generalized photosensitivity resulting from systemic HpD. While generally persistent for approximately 30 days, this condition can last for several months. Early evidence indicates that this condition is reduced by using the purified material, DHE.[21]

The power densities of 630 nm light used in some cases were sufficiently high where thermal effects were likely to contribute to the overall response. It has been shown by Svaasand et al.[37] that power densities at 630 nm exceeding 100 mW/cm^2 at the surface can cause hyperthermic effects up to 3 mm for treatment of 30 minutes or more in tumors of moderate blood flow. The exact role of thermal effects in conjunction with PRT are under investigation but early results indicate that synergistic effects can be expected for temperatures of 40.5 to 44.5°C or higher.[38]

Case Reports

Case 1: Recurrent Serous Crypt Adenocarcinoma.[19] A 56-year-old patient who had undergone total abdominal hysterectomy, bilateral salpingo-oophorectomy and postoperative external radiation therapy 16 years earlier, presented with a fungating vaginal vault tumor, 4 × 3 cm in diameter and estimated to be 3 cm in depth. Recurrence 2 years earlier was treated by cyclophosphamide and 5-fluorouracil. She received 5.0 mg/kg HpD and received interstitial PRT (regular fiber without diffuser) using a single fiber on days 3, 4, and 15 following the injection of HpD for a total of 11 separate 20-minute treatments. Fibers were inserted approximately 1 cm into the lesion. Within a month the lesion had completely regressed leaving an epithelialized cavity 4 × 3× 2 cm. Follow-up to date is reported up to 1 year during which time no tumor has recurred within the treated area, but she has developed other lesions outside the vagina.

Case 2: Primary Vaginal Carcinoma.[20] A 77-year-old patient was found to have a 4 × 3 cm nodule on the right side of the vaginal wall diagnosed as moderately differentiated squamous cell carcinoma, State I. She received 2.5 mg/kg Photofrin (HpD, Oncology Research and Development, Cheektowaga, N.Y.). Two days later the lesion was illuminated with 630 nm light at a power density of 250 mW/cm^2 for 20 minutes (300 J/cm^2). The same procedure was followed at 3 weeks and 6 weeks following the first treatment. The patient was treated without anesthesia. One month later the tumor had regressed. Histology showed necrotic cells and karyorrhexis. No complications from treatment were observed. Five months after treatment the tumor had completely regressed and remains so at 2 years with negative vaginal smears.

Case 3: Intraepithelial Cancer of the Uterine Cervix.[28] A 51-year-old woman was detected in a mass screening program to have Class IV cells and a small erosion on the external orifice of the uterus. Biopsy indicated carcinoma in situ. She received 2.5 mg/kg HpD and 2 days later the surface of the lesion was illuminated with 630 nm light at 400 nW/cm^2 for 30 minutes (720 J/cm^2). The erosion disappeared and showed negative biopsies with Class II cells. Follow-up to date has been 1.5 years without recurrence and without complications.

CONCLUSION

Photoradiation therapy for treatment of gynecologic lesions requires a large controlled study to properly define adequate light doses and to assess long-term results. The preliminary studies reported to date, however, indicate a role for PRT in treatment of recurrent or primary tumors of the vagina even those heavily treated by prior therapies. The treatment appears to be devoid of major toxicity and complications such as bladder or rectal damage and no systemic effects have been found in spite of the excessively large light doses used in some instances. The role of PRT in treatment of carcinoma in situ (CIS) lesions remains to be determined, but it may offer a convenient nontraumatic method for both CIS and dysplasia. The main drawback in these cases may be the induced photosensitivity requiring patients to protect themselves from bright light for 30 days or more. Two approaches to solving this problem are the use of the purified HpD preparation Photofrin II now available and possibly topical application of the porphyrin being explored by several groups.

Improvement in light delivery systems is necessary. Since the reports of the studies cited here, considerable improvement in light delivery systems and methodology has occurred as have improvements in laser systems for clinical PRT studies.[28]

REFERENCES

1. Hayata Y, Kato H, Konaka C, et al: Fiberoptic bronchoscopic laser photoradiation for tumor localization in lung cancer. Chest 82:10, 1982
2. Kato H, Konaka C, Ono J, et al: Effectiveness of hpd and radiation therapy in lung cancer. In Kessel D, Dougherty TJ (eds): Porphyrin Photosensitization. New York, Plenum Press, 1983, pp 23–40
3. Kato H: Lung cancer. In Hayata Y (ed): Laser Photoradiation for Tumor Detection and Treatment. Tokyo, Igaku-Shoin, 1983, pp 39–56
4. Vincent RG, Dougherty TJ, Rao U, et al: Photoradiation therapy in the treatment of advanced carcinoma of the trachea and bronchus. In Doiron D, Gomer C (eds): Porphyrin Localization and Treatment of Tumors. New York, Alan R. Liss, 1984, pp 759–766

5. Balchum OJ, Doiron DR, Profio AE, Huth GC: Fluorescence bronchoscopy for local-izing early bronchial cancer and carcinoma in situ. In Recent Results in Cancer Research, vol. 82. Berlin-Heidelberg: Springer-Verlag, 1982, p 90

6. Cortese DA, Kinsey JH: Endoscopic management of lung cancer with hematopor-phyrin derivative phototherapy. Mayo Clin Proc 57:543, 1982

7. Benson RC Jr, Farrow GM, Kinsey JH, et al: Detection and localization of in situ carcinoma of the bladder with hematoporphyrin derivative. Mayo Clin Proc 57:548, 1982

8. Hisazumi H, Misaki T, Miyoshi N: Photodynamic therapy of bladder tumors. In Hay-ata Y (ed): Laser Photoradiation for Tumor Detection and Treatment. Tokyo, Igaku-Shoin, 1983, pp 85–87

9. Ohi T, Tsuchiya A: Superficial bladder tumors. In Hayata Y (ed): Laser Photoradia-tion for Tumor Detection and Treatment. Tokyo, Igaku-Shoin, 1983, pp 79–84

10. Benson RC Jr, Kinsey JH, Cortese DA, et al: Treatment of transitional cell carcinoma of the bladder with hematoporphyrin-derivative phototherapy. J Urol, 130:1090–1094, 1983

11. Dougherty TJ: Unpublished results

12. Forbes I, Cowled PA, Leong AS-Y, et al: Phototherapy of human tumors using hae-matoporphyrin derivative. Med J Aust 2:489, 1980

13. Kennedy J: HpD photoradiation therapy for cancer at Kingston and Hamilton. In Kessel D, Dougherty TJ (eds): Porphyrin Photosensitization. New York, Plenum Press, 1983, pp 53–62

14. Tokuda Y: Primary skin cancer. In Hayata Y (ed): Laser Photoradiation for Tumor Detection and Treatment. Tokyo, Igaku-Shoin, 1983, pp 88–96

15. Wile AG, Dahlman A, Burns RG, Berns MW: Laser photoradiation therapy of cancer following hematoporphyrin sensitization. Lasers Surg Med 2:163, 1982

16. Aida M, Hirashima T: Cancer of the esophagus. In Hayata Y (ed): Laser Photoradia-tion for Tumor Detection and Treatment. Tokyo, Igaku-Shoin, 1983, pp 57–64

17. McCaughan, JS: Unpublished results

18. Nava H: Unpublished results

19. Ward BG, Forbes IJ, Cowled PA, et al: The treatment of vaginal recurrences of gyne-cologic malignancy with phototherapy following hematoporphyrin derivative pre-treatment. Am J Obstet Gynecol 142(3):356, 1982

20. Soma H, Akiya K, Nutahara S, et al: Treatment of vaginal carcinoma with laser pho-toirradiation following administration of haematoporphyrin derivative. Report of a case. Ann Chirurg Gynaecol 71:133, 1982

21. Dougherty TJ, Potter WR, Weishaupt KR: The structure of the active component of hematoporphyrin derivative. In Doiron D, Gomer C (eds): Porphyrin Localization and Treatment of Tumors, New York, Alan R. Liss, 1984, pp 301–314

22. Gomer CJ, Dougherty TJ: Determination of ^{3}H and ^{14}C hematoporphyrin derivative distribution in malignant and normal tissue. Can Res 39:146, 1979

23. Bugelski PJ, Porter CW, Dougherty TJ: Autoradiographic distribution of hemato-porphyrin derivative in normal and tumor tissue of the mouse. Can Res 41:4606, 1981

24. Weishaupt KR, Gomer CJ, Dougherty TJ: Identification of singlet oxygen as the cyto-toxic agent in photoinactivation of a murine tumor. Can Res 36:2326, 1976

25. Weishaupt KR, Dougherty TJ: Unpublished results

26. Dougherty TJ: Photodynamic therapy (PDT) of malignant tumors. CRC Crit Rev Oncol/Hematol, 2(2):83–116, 1984

27. Kessel D, Dougherty TJ (eds): Porphyrin Photosensitization. New York, Plenum Press, 1983

28. Doiron D, Gomer C (eds): Porphyrin Localization and Treatment of Tumors. New York, Alan R. Liss, 1984

29. Balchum OJ, Doiron DR, Huth GC: HPD photodynamic therapy for obstructing lung

cancer. In Doiron D, Gomer C (eds): Porphyrin Localization and Treatment of Tumors. New York, Alan R. Liss, 1984, pp 727–746

30. Hayata Y, Kato H, Ono J, et al: Fluorescence fiberoptic bronchoscopy in the diagnosis of early stage lung cancer. In Recent Results in Cancer Research, vol. 82. Berlin-Heidelberg, Springer-Verlag, 1982, p 121

31. Lipson, RL, Pratt JH, Baldes EJ, et al: Hematoporphyrin derivative for the detection of cervical cancer. Obstet Gynecol 24:78, 1964

32. Lipson RL, Baldes EJ, Olsen AM: Hematoporphyrin derivative: A new aid of endoscopic detection of malignant disease. J Thor Cardiovasc Surg 42:623, 1961

33. Lipson RL, Baldes EJ, Olsen AM: A further evaluation of the use of hematoporphyrin derivative as a new aid for the endoscopic detection of malignant disease. Dis Chest 46:676, 1964

34. Lipson RL: The photodynamic and fluorescent properties of a particular hematoporphyrin derivative and its use in tumor detection. Master's Thesis, University of Minnesota, 1960

35. Soma H, Nutahara S: Cancer of the female genitalia. In Hayata Y (ed): Laser Photoradiation for Tumor Detection and Treatment. Tokyo, Igaku-Shoin, 1983, pp 97–109

36. Svaasand LO, Ellingsen R: Calibration of application of nonionizing radiation. Part 2. Experimental Results. Report #RB/PE029, Division of Physical Electronics, University of Trondheim, Norwegian Institute of Technology, 1983

37. Svaasand LO, Doiron DR, Dougherty TJ: Temperature rise during photoradiation therapy of malignant tumors. Med Phys 19(1):10, 1983

38. Dougherty TJ: An overview of the status of photoradiation therapy. Clayton Foundation Symposium on Porphyrin Localization and Treatment of Tumors, Santa Barbara, Calif. 1983

15

Condylomata Acuminata Genital Infections Treated by the CO$_2$ Laser

Michael S. Baggish

INTRODUCTION

Genital tract infections caused by the human papillomavirus (HPV) are occurring with increasing frequency in the United States and elsewhere.[1,2] To date these infections have proved resistant to successful treatment by conventional techniques.[3] If one were to judge the importance of a disease based on the number of cases seen in practice, the economic impact, and the degree of vexation created in the afflicted women, genital warts would clearly be on the top rung of the rating scale. Furthermore, not only are these warts ugly and irritating, but they may well be causative to the initiation of incipient neoplasia in the cervix, vagina, vulva.[4,5] Although a definite relationship between HPV infection of the newborn, exposed during vaginal delivery, and the subsequent development of vocal cord papillomas is uncertain, its importance is highly significant.[6] Circumstantial evidence points to HPV type 11 which has been isolated from both genital condylomata acuminata and vocal cord warts.[7]

Typically condylomata acuminata exhibits erratic and often unpredictable growth patterns. Depending on their location, the lesions may be polypoid, flat, papillomatous, fleshy, white, or pigmented (Fig. 15–1, see Color Plate III*). They may occur singly, in clusters, or in confluence (Fig. 15–2). These lesions may appear in all sizes, ranging from microscopic to very large. Although symptoms may be totally lacking, warts may produce pain, irritation, itching, discharge, or malodor. The lesions grow most rapidly during periods of altered immunity, e.g., pregnancy, oral contraceptive intake, cancer chemotherapy, transplant suppression, and acquired immune deficiency (Fig. 15–3).

---

*Color Plates III and IV appear following p. 177.

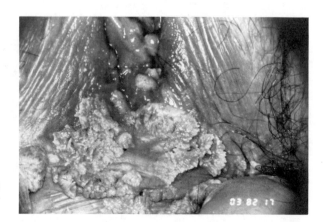

Figure 15–2. Clusters of warts extend downward from the posterior fossette.

Podophyllin, trichloracetic acid, and 5-fluorouracil cream (5-FU) have been extensively prescribed. The above agents generally have yielded poor clinical results and frequently are associated with unpleasant side effects.[8] Other methods of therapy such as cryosurgery, electrocautery, and knife excision are either impractical or result in scarring.

The carbon dioxide (CO_2) laser is well suited as a method to eradicate condylomata acuminata. Not only can the laser reach most sites of possible wart involvement, but the heat of the beam destroys the virus. Additionally, the precision of the technique promotes rapid healing. By varying power and spot size, the laser is useful to treat surrounding skin harboring the virus, but which shows no overt manifestations of the disease.

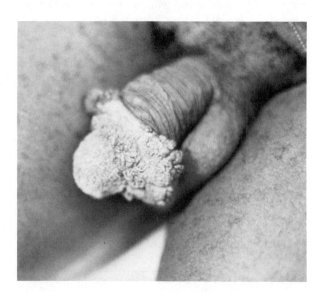

Figure 15–3. Massive condylomata acuminata are frequently associated with altered immune conditions.

BASIS FOR LASER USE

The CO_2 laser eliminates condylomatous lesions to a depth of 1 mm or less. Since the virus proliferates in the prickle and basal cell layers of the epithelium it is not necessary to ablate deeper[9] (Fig. 15–4). The instantaneous heat created by the impinging laser beam raises the temperature within the cell to 100°C; subsequent heat of carbonization creates even higher temperatures resulting in destruction of the virus. This action contrasts with viral survival following cryosurgical treatment. Superficial destruction does not produce scarring, therefore, even extensive laser vaporization will not eventuate in vulva, vaginal, or cervical scar formation.

Since warts may be distributed throughout the lower genital tract, e.g., extending into orifices such as the anus or urethra, methodology which allows reliable entry into such small operative fields renders the laser unique especially when it is coupled to the microscope (Fig. 15–5). Microwarty changes in the epithelium, not visible to the naked eye, are seen through the colposcope. Such abnormalities can be destroyed accurately with the laser using microsurgical techniques.

Condylomata acuminata, especially during pregnancy are highly vascular lesions. The CO_2 laser especially at lower power densities seals vascular channels as it vaporizes. Since treatment is superficial, only small vessels, e.g., less than 0.5 mm in diameter, are encountered and are easily sealed off.

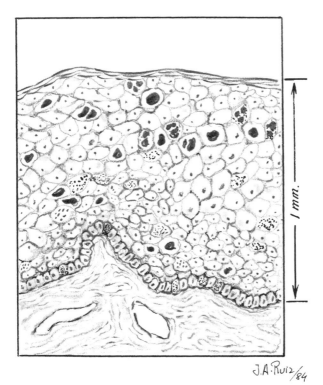

J.A.Ruiz/84

Figure 15–4. This drawing schematically shows human papilloma virus (dots) proliferating in cells of the basal and prickle layers. Note the bizarre cells with multiple nuclei in the upper layers, e.g., koilocytoses.

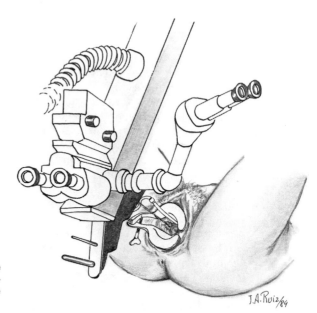

Figure 15–5. The laser may be coupled to a teaching microscope and fired between the blades of a vaginal speculum.

SPECIFICATIONS FOR LASER SURGERY

Vaporization will eliminate surface epithelium only, i.e., 1 mm or less, so low power densities are advantageous. Large spots are virtually always indicated, i.e., measuring 1.5 to 2.0 mm in diameter. Power densities should rarely exceed 600 to 700 W/cm^2. For very extensive disease, even larger spots may be utilized, e.g., 3.0

LESION	SPOT SIZE (mm)	POWER (watts)	MODE	TIME (sec)	VELOCITY
Vaporization Individual warts	1.5	15	defocus MULTI	continuous	slow
Excision Individual or Clusters	0.5	20-30	focus TEM 00	continuous	rapid
Vaporization Clusters	2-3	40-50	defocus MULTI	continuous	rapid
Brush	2-3	10-15	defocus MULTI	continuous	rapid
Strategic site Vaporization	0.5-1.0	5 or <5	focus TEM 00	0.2	slow

Figure 15–6. Specifications for treating various categories of human papillomavirus infections with the CO_2 laser.

mm combined with power settings of 50 to 60 W. The major advantages of these settings obtained with high power lasers relate to the speed with which vaporization can be done. Under such circumstances, the articulated arm and free hand-piece of the laser are most valuable especially when the vulva and lower vagina are involved. For laser vaporization of the rectum, urethra, oral cavity, upper vagina, or cervix, the laser microslab coupled to a variable magnification micro-scope provides the best delivery system (Fig. 15–6).

ANESTHESIA

For laser vaporization of the vulva and lower half of the vagina, either local injec-tion or general anesthesia is always required. When warts are extensive, I have found it advantageous to put the patients to sleep and eliminate all the disease during one operation. General anesthesia is needed when anorectal laser surgery is performed since this entails the insertion of a laser speculum and substantial manipulation.

For minimal wart disease or when staging therapy for moderate disease, local anesthesia can be employed. The primary disadvantages of local anesthesia center on the discomfort it produces and the pesky bleeding at the injection site. Approx-imately one half the patients in our series received local anesthesia.

Preparation

Ordinarily no skin or mucous membrane preparation is done.

OTHER SITE INVOLVEMENT

If condylomata acuminata are to be eliminated, a compulsive examination is abso-lutely necessary to determine the extent of extragenital involvement. Warts have been found in the anus, mouth, nose, eyes, on the hands, feet, legs, and scalp. It is our policy to always explore and treat these extragenital sites (Figs. 15–7; 15–8, see Color Plate III; 15–9; 15–10, 15–11, see Color Plate III).

TECHNIQUE OF LASER VAPORIZATION

The treatment program calls for the vaporization of warts from outside inwards and the reduction of the lesions to the level of surrounding normal skin surface (Fig. 15–12). There is no advantage to treating deeply since the virus does not penetrate into the deeper tissues. I introduced the technique of "brushing" skin between confluent warts and similarly treating skin or mucous membrane surfaces showing pebbly or warty change when viewed via the colposcope (see Brushing section.)

Our usual plan is to ask patients to shave the perineum since warts are other-wise difficult to localize in the dense hair growth (Fig. 15–13). All external warts are vaporized and neighboring skin brushed. Next, a laser speculum (Codman) is

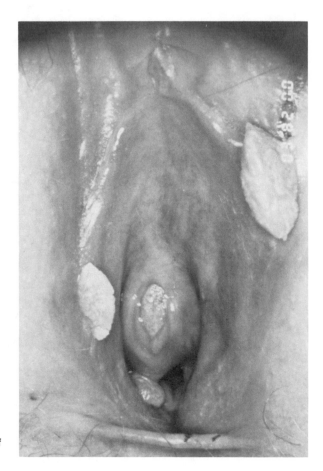

Figure 15–7. Warty lesions of the labia and urethra.

lubricated and placed into the anus (Fig. 15–14, see Color Plate IV). The blades are gently opened and the mucosa is inspected and any visible warts are vaporized utilizing low power densities 300 to 400 W/cm². The speculum is rotated clockwise to cover the entire anus. A wet sponge is usually placed above to seal the rectum and a vacuum hose is attached to the laser speculum to automatically effect smoke evacuation. When anal treatment has been completed and a second speculum is placed in the vagina (Fig. 15–15, see Color Plate IV). The cervix is exposed and any warty lesions are vaporized. Next, using a long-handled fine hook to manipulate the cervix, the vagina fornices are exposed and treated. Then the remaining vaginal walls are examined and treated. Frequently, microwarty changes are noted on the lateral vaginal walls; these are brushed by angulating the laser and shooting between the blades of the speculum or the laser beam is reflected from a specially coated, long handled mirror.

The hymenal ring and vestibule are favorite sites for proliferating condylomata

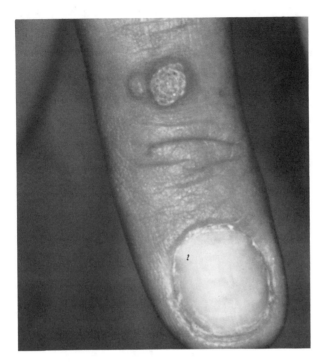

Figure 15–9. Persistence of genital warts will occur if other sites are not treated. Here the patient has a wart on her index finger.

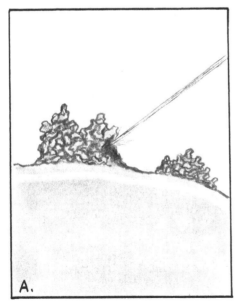

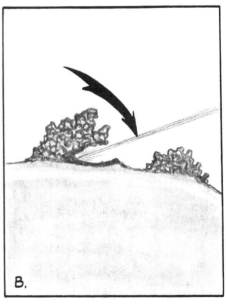

Figure 15–12. Striking the wart on one side, from "outside-in", causes the lesion to collapse on itself towards the impinging laser beam. This maneuver spares surrounding skin.

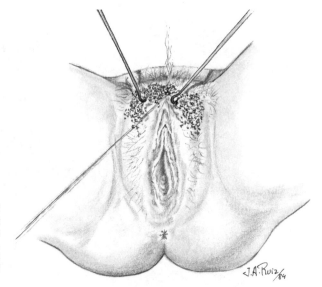

Figure 15–13. In areas of dense hair growth, the patient should be encouraged to shave the area prior to laser treatment. This will eliminate the fire hazard as well as diminishing the risk of leaving warts behind.

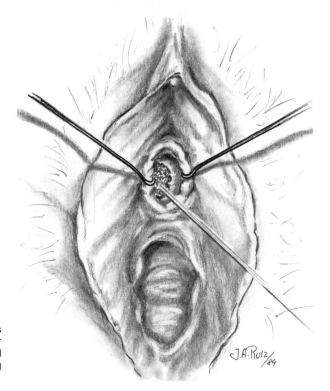

Figure 15–16. Two iris hooks expose a urethral wart. Laser vaporization is the only practical and safe method for eliminating warts in this location.

acuminata. The warty change may not be apparent until after the application of 4 percent acetic acid; loop capillaries highlight true condylomatous tissue.

The urethra is inspected by exposing it with two long-handled skin hooks and moist cotton-tipped applicators. Warts are treated in this location in a fashion similar to anal warts (Fig. 15–16).

EXCISIONAL

When large warts or clusters of warts are located on a pedicle, it is frequently expeditious to excise the cluster. Using small spots, i.e., 0.5 mm diameter and high power density (1000 W/cm^2), excision is rapidly carried out. Brisk bleeding is encountered when an arteriole is traversed. Rather than damage the skin excessively by attempting to control the bleeding by laser coagulation, the placement of a stitch will actually save time (Fig. 15–17).

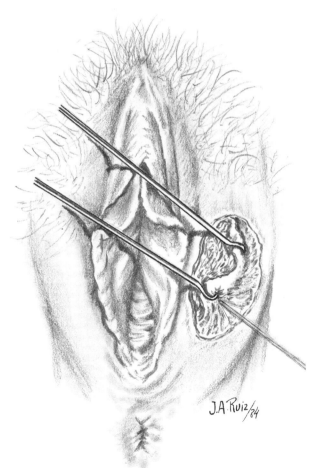

Figure 15–17. Clumps of condylomata acuminata are frequently excised rather than vaporized. The key to laser excision is tissue traction and countertraction.

PREGNANCY

Warts occurring during pregnancy should be treated to safely allow vaginal delivery and to avoid infant contamination. Treatment is best done during the second trimester and never beyond 34 weeks. Extensive cervical vaporization should be avoided. All warts occurring in pregnancy have large vessels and may bleed profusely, therefore treatment should utilize large spots and no more than 15 W of power.

COMPLICATIONS

The majority of complications relating to vaporization of condylomata acuminata occur because of improper patient selection, improper selection of anesthesia, and improper spot size and power settings.

As noted above, condylomata acuminata may present as an extensive disease involving multiple sites especially in immunologically compromised women. To attempt a 2 to 3 hour vaporization late in pregnancy may subject the fetus and mother to risk, e.g., premature labor or hemorrhage. When pregnancy is far advanced and wart disease is extensive, demonstrating rectal, vaginal, or cervical involvement, I believe it is wise to delay treatment of the warts and deliver by cesarean section.

Bleeding is the principal complication associated with extensive vaporization of mucosa and skin surface. Severe bleeding will occur if the operator chooses to perform surgery utilizing high power densities, particularly when combined with the transverse electromagnetic (TEM_{00}) mode; small spots are prone to this problem. When bleeding occurs, especially of an arterial nature, laser coagulation with CO_2 lasers is often futile and simply leads to extensive tissue damage. Excision of stalks of condylomata acuminata with a small tightly focused beam is analogous to cutting with a knife.

No patient with extensive warts or for that matter wide geographic spread of warts should have laser surgery performed under local anesthesia with the idea of vaporizing all visible disease at one sitting. Long treatment sessions are intolerable for the patient and require too much local anesthesia; fatigued patients are more prone to accentuate discomfort and pull away with the possibility of a laser accident.

When extensive loss of skin occurs, patients will experience immediate discomfort. This is best relieved with analgesics and sitz baths. Commonly, delayed pain begins 7 days after vaporization. Interestingly, even extensive *vaginal* vaporization rarely results in pain.

BRUSHING

The technique of *brushing* or lightly blanching the stratified squamous epithelium with a defocused laser beam was described by Baggish. When properly performed this technique results in destruction of the epidermis with little or no damage to the underlying dermis. Virtually no postoperative discomfort has been noted even after extensive brushing. Healing, likewise, is very rapid. The principal benefit of brushing is the destruction of skin surfaces neighboring overt warts and

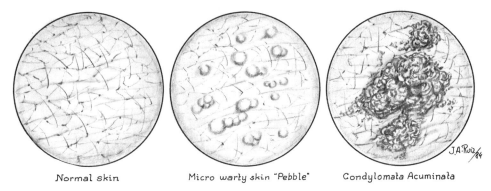

Normal skin   Micro warty skin "Pebble"   Condylomata Acuminata

Figure 15–18. Drawing showing normal skin, micro-warty (pebbly skin), and frank condylomata acuminata.

epithelial surfaces showing pebble-like patterns, i.e., warty change without overt condylomata (Fig. 15–18). Brushing significantly improves the cure rates and is best performed with a large spot, i.e., 2 mm or greater at power settings of 10 watts or less. Condylomata acuminata proliferating in the prickle or basal layers are thus destroyed (Fig. 15–19).

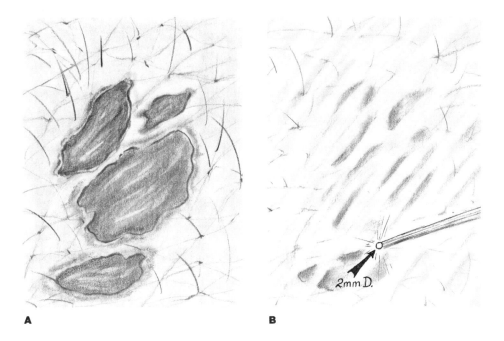

A   **B**

Figure 15–19A. Laser vaporization of C. acuminata. Gross warts are vaporized to the level of the surrounding normal skin surface. **B.** The "brushing" technique blanches skin showing pebbly change or skin in proximity to confluences of condylomata acuminata. The brush technique merely destroys the epidermis, while sparing the underlying dermis.

POSTOPERATIVE CARE

Oral contraceptives have been shown to alter immunity, therefore, it is worthwhile to discontinue these drugs and supply the patient with an alternative method of contraception. We believe this will improve *the primary cure rate.*

When anal warts have been vaporized, stool softeners, e.g., dioctyl sodium sulfosuccinate (Peri-Colace) or mineral oil should be prescribed. Patients are taught to cleanse the anal verge with cotton balls doused in 2.5 percent acetic acid.

As detailed in the chapter on vulvar carcinoma in situ, all patients receive sea water (instant ocean) sitz baths four times daily.[10] These ocean water baths promote healing, diminish infection, and add to the patients' comfort. All patients

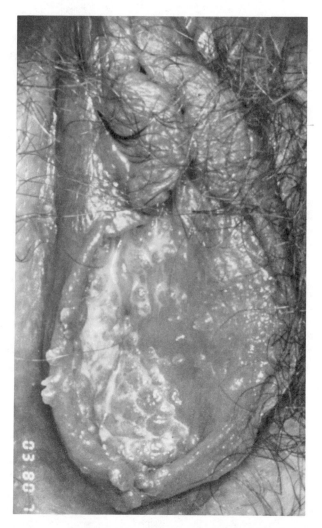

Figure 15–20. Frequently patients with genital wart disease have an associated milky discharge and "wet" perineum.

are instructed to squirt a 1:4 diluted solution of Betadine onto the perineum after urination or defecation. After sitz baths, Betadine squirts, and showers, the operative site is blow dried with an electric hair dryer under "air cycle" or "low heat." We prefer this method rather than towel drying since it preserves the young, thin layers of new squamous cells and promotes rapid healing.

A common characteristic of the perineum afflicted with condylomata acuminata is its wetness (Fig. 15–20). This is usually associated with a heavy vaginal and cervical discharge. We have found it advantageous to get rid of perineal wetness by prescribing daily vaginal douches utilizing a dilute acetic acid solution made-up by adding 1 tablespoon of vinegar to 1 quart of water.

RESULTS

A total of 575 women with genital warts have undergone treatment with the CO_2 laser and have been reported in the gynecology literature.

In 1980, this author reported laser vaporization treatment in 110 women with condylomata acuminata.[8] The overall cure rate in this series was 90 percent and no vulvar, vaginal, anal, or cervical scar formation was observed. Sixty-three patients in this study had abnormal cervical cytology and over 90 percent had a past history of failed podophyllin, 5-FU, cryosurgery, or excisional treatments. Fifteen women were treated during pregnancy. The following year, Hahn published data on 49 women whom he had treated with the laser.[11] Eighty-two percent of his cases had previous nonlaser therapy and had either persistence or recurrence of disease. Calkins et al.[12] reported a 91 percent success rate in 90 women undergoing laser vaporization and Baggish reported a second series of 228 cases with an overall cure rate of 92 percent.[13] Laser surgery in the earlier (1980) group was performed under local anesthesia and approximately 50 percent of the later (1982) series was performed under local anesthesia. In this author's patients, 150 out of 228 women were cured after a single laser exposure (65.8 percent); 184 (80 percent) with 2 treatments; 202 (89 percent) in 3 treatments; 211 (92.5 percent) with 4 treatments. Seventy percent of the women were discovered to have warts in the anal canal and 82 percent of resistant cases had male partners who demonstrated penile warts. Virtually all failures were among immunosuppressed patients. Ferenczy has extensive experience with laser treatment of genital warts; he reported 43 pregnant women who underwent laser vaporization for condylomata acuminata with an overall failure rate of 5 percent. Ferenczy warned that 40 percent of infants and children developing laryngeal warts were delivered from mothers who had genital condylomata.[14,15]

SUMMARY

The CO_2 laser is currently the best method for eliminating genital warts. Not only is the method highly efficacious (90 percent cure) but it provides the means for treating lesions in virtually any location. Additionally, the operator can assure himself or herself that the lesion is physically removed. Finally the laser provides the means for eliminating the causative virus in neighboring epithelia which may not even show overt wart disease.

Several key measures must be followed to insure favorable results. These include:

1. Exploration and elimination of all sites of wart infestation, i.e., cervix, vagina, vulva, anus, urethra, mouth, nose, external skin surfaces (Fig. 15–21, see Color Plate IV).
2. Evaluation and treatment of the male partners.
3. Elimination of immunosuppressive drugs, e.g., oral contraceptives, corticosteriods, if possible.
4. Liberal use of the brushing technique.
5. Frequent, careful follow-up examinations utilizing colposcopy and prompt retreatment when required.

REFERENCES

1. Oriel D: Genital Warts in Sexually Transmitted Diseases. Caterall RD, Nicol CS (eds): London, Academic, 1967, p 186
2. Monif GRG: Viral Infections of The Human Fetus. London, Macmillan, 1969, pp 45, 61
3. Halverstadt DB: Venereal warts. Medical Aspects Human Sexuality. 12, 1972 (June)
4. Reid R, Laverty CR, Coppleson M, et al: Noncondylomatous cervical wart virus infection. Obstet Gynecol 55:476, 1980
5. Reid R, Stanhope R, Herschman BR, et al: Genital warts and cervical cancer. Cancer 50:377, 1982
6. Quick CA, Krzyzek RA, Watts SL, Faras AJ: Relationship between condylomata and laryngeal papillomatia. Ann Otol 89:467, 1980
7. Fearon B, MacRae D: Laryngeal papillomatosis in children. J Otolaryngol 5:493, 1976
8. Baggish MS: Carbon dioxide laser treatment for condylomata acuminata venereal infections. Obstet Gynecol 55:711, 1980
9. Laverty C: Noncondylomatous wart virus infection of the cervix: Cytologic, histologic and electron microscopic features. Obstet Gynecol Surv 34:820, 1979
10. Baggish MS, Dorsey JH: CO_2 laser for the treatment of vulvar carcinoma in situ. Obstet Gynecol 57:371, 1981
11. Hahn GA: Carbon dioxide laser surgery in treatment of condyloma. Am J Obstet Gynecol 141:1000, 1981
12. Calkins JW, Masterson BJ, Magrina JF, Capen CV: Management of condylomata acuminata with the carbon dioxide laser. Obstet Gynecol 59:105, 1982
13. Baggish MS: Treating viral venereal infections with the CO_2 laser. J Reprod Med 27:737, 1982
14. Ferenczy A: Using the laser to treat vulvar condylomata acuminata and intraepidermal neoplasia. Canad Med Assoc J 128:135, 1983
15. Ferenczy A: Treating genital condyloma during pregnancy with the carbon dioxide laser. Am J Obstet Gynecol 148:9, 1984

16

Prevention of Complications in Gynecologic Laser Surgery

Vernon W. Jobson

INTRODUCTION

Serious complications are infrequent after gynecologic laser surgery. Disregard for safety standards and inappropriate clinical judgment create untoward results and their consequent liability. Good clinical judgment is paramount in the prevention of complications. Errors in clinical judgment can occur at several times during the patient's care—preoperatively, intraoperatively, and postoperatively. Each of these time periods has unique characteristics that allow the prudent laser surgeon to successfully plan for, carry out the procedure, and provide follow-up care with a minimal chance of complications.

PREOPERATIVE EVALUATION

In the preoperative period, proper attention to accurate histologic diagnosis will reduce the chance for bad results. A patient with an abnormal cervical Papanicolaou (Pap) smear should have adequate colposcopy. Multiple colposcopically directed biopsies should be taken and, if the proximal edge of the transformation zone is not seen, an endocervical curettage should be performed. Only after this thorough evaluation documents the absence of invasive cancer is the patient a candidate for laser ablative conization. An incomplete preoperative evaluation with omission of vital steps may easily result in the misapplication of ablative therapy to a patient with an obvious or occult invasive cervical cancer. Hemorrhage will be likely during the procedure and the neophyte laser surgeon stands a good chance to become involved in litigation shortly thereafter. Adequate histologic diagnosis is a safeguard to prevent inadvertent treatment of invasive disease with therapies currently acceptable only for preinvasive lesions.

Patients presenting with lesions of the vulva or vagina also require careful and complete histologic sampling prior to selection of laser as the treatment modality. If there is any doubt as to whether a lesion is microinvasive or frankly invasive, an excisional operation (laser or knife) should be planned. Also important in the preoperative period is an assessment of the patient's level of understanding of her disease, general personality, and ability to cooperate and participate in her operative and postoperative care. An ill-informed, immature, and unreliable patient is not a suitable candidate for laser therapy. Although most patients tolerate ambulatory procedures quite well without anesthesia or with local anesthesia, unsophisticated and younger patients are more likely to tolerate this approach poorly. Good rapport should be built prior to the operative procedure. Adequate time on the part of the physician spent toward education of the patient and planning with the anesthesiologist to be involved with the care of the patient is critical to successfully avoid intraoperative complications due to patient noncompliance. Adequate visual aids and patient education performed by your nursing staff will also reinforce your patient's knowledge and build her confidence.

OPERATIVE CARE

During performance of the operative procedure itself, specific steps may be taken to avoid complications. The laser has specific limitations due to the physical characteristics of the energy being delivered. Many of the details relative to free hand or microscopic application are described elsewhere in this book and will not be repeated here. Suffice it to say that inappropriate transection of large vessels with the laser will result in significant intraoperative hemorrhage. Absolute purism and a nonflexible approach to using the laser for control of all bleeding will only result in increased blood loss for the patient. It is important to utilize other adjuncts including topical hemostatic astrigents such as ferric subsulfate, electrocoagulation, and, where need be, sutures to control bleeding.[1,2]

Another iatrogenic complication is circumferential excision and/or ablation around orifices with subsequent scarring and stenosis. This is particularly problematic when treating vulvar or vulvovaginal lesions which result in removal of tissue in a circumferential fashion around the introitus (Fig. 16–1, see Color Plate IV*).

Introital stenosis can be avoided by staging these operations into two separate surgical sessions, treating first one side and later the other. Anal stenosis can occur following circumferential ablation. The scarring which will result in the patient shown (Fig. 16–2, see Color Plate IV) could have been avoided by properly staging this procedure for treatment of perianal carcinoma in situ into two or three treatment sessions. Instead the surgeon treated the entire area in a single operation. Additionally the lesion was ablated deeper than necessary. These factors combined resulted in her referral for management to a medical center.

Depth of penetration beam must also be carefully monitored, when working in the vagina because the inherent risk of penetration to an adjacent viscus and cre-

---

*Color Plate IV appears following p. 177.

**TABLE 16–1. FREQUENCY OF
COMPLICATIONS FOLLOWING
GYNECOLOGIC LASER SURGERY**

Type of Complication	Frequency (%)
Minor bleeding	9.0
Major bleeding	1.0
Cervical pain	2.0
Vulvar pain	27.0
Infection	0
Introital stenosis	<0.5
Cervical stenosis	0
Labial agglutination	<0.5

(Adapted from Baggish, M.[1])

ation of a fistula. A final aspect of operative care to emphasize is that of the intraabdominal application of carbon dioxide laser energy. It is critical to recognize that the laser is nonselective and will vaporize any tissue within the focal length of its beam. Neglect in properly packing away other viscera, such as small or large bowel, or protecting the bladder adequately with wet drapes can result in delayed fistulas from these organs into the intraperitoneal cavity postoperatively. When ablating such intraabdominal lesions as endometriosis, careful attention to operative detail can prevent these late complications. Intraoperative pain control can be achieved by local anesthesia in most cases. Extensive procedures or excision of tissue however requires general anesthesia.

The spectrum of complications includes bleeding, pain, stenosis, scarring, etc. The relative frequency of these are summarized in Table 16–1.

POSTOPERATIVE CARE

The third time frame and most critical one in the prevention of late complications is during the postoperative period. Even before operation, the patient's education with respect to her own self-care should be started. Postoperatively, further instructions, both by the nursing staff and by the medical staff taking care of the patient, will result in an increase in her educational level. Postoperative attention to care of operative sites of excision/vaporization will facilitate healing of what are really mixed second and third degree burns. For vaginal ablative surgery, topical use of estrogen creams is useful. Following vulvar surgery, Silvadene burn cream is a useful adjunct. Prevention of labial agglutination is shown in Figure 16–3 (see Color Plate IV).

Postoperative cervical ablative cases are best handled with an acidifying agent such as Trimosan or Aci-Jel which can be applied starting 5 to 7 days postoperatively (Table 16–2). Restoration of normal acidity helps promote nonbacterial population and therefore aids in healing. When overgrowth of a single organism is prevented, healing can progress nicely. The acid environment also promotes

TABLE 16–2. SUMMARY OF USEFUL POSTOPERATIVE MEDICATIONS AFTER
LOWER GENITAL TRACT LASER SURGERY

Operative Site	Medication	Timing
Cervix	Trimosan or Aci-Jel	Begin 1 week postoperatively
Vagina	Premarin	Begin immediately postoperatively
Vulva	Silvadene	Begin immediately postoperatively

metaplastic changes in the exposed original columnar epithelium. An example of a well-healed cervix is shown in Figure 16–4 (see Color Plate IV).

Proper instruction of patients regarding sexual activity is vital from two standpoints. First, avoidance of sexual activity in the immediate postoperative period will reduce the incidence of infection, pain, and hemorrhage. It is important, however, for patients to resume sexual activity as soon as reepithelialization has occurred. This is particularly true for patients following vaginal and vulvar surgery.

For intraabdominal applications of laser, the postoperative period is one during which the patient must be carefully observed. This is particularly important if the operative procedure was done in a closed fashion, i.e., carbon dioxide (CO_2) laser laparoscopy. Laser laparoscopy is still investigational in the United States. Until more experience is gained, close observation of these patients in hospital would seem advisable to avoid complication rates like those seen in the early 1970s after introduction of standard laparoscopy with electrocoagulation units.

SUMMARY

Severe complications from laser surgery for gynecologic lesions should be infrequently encountered even by beginning laser surgeons. Careful attention to safety factors as well as thoughtful attention to preoperative selection, careful operative application, and meticulous postoperative care will reduce the chance for bad results. This will lead to satisfied patients, more widespread application of the technique, and avoidance of unnecessary litigation.

REFERENCES

1. Baggish M: Complications associated with carbon dioxide laser surgery in gynecology. Am J Obstet Gynecol 139:568, 1981
2. Jobson V: Serious complications following carbon dioxide laser surgery in gynecology. Unpublished manuscript

17

Infertility Amenable to Laser Surgery

Augusto P. Chong

INTRODUCTION

The surgical approach to disease of the pelvic organs is a technologic advance that is capable of producing anatomic or physiologic alterations of the reproductive process which remarkably enhances the chances for successful pregnancy outcome.

Surgical intervention in the management of the infertile female is an art which requires expertise, experience, patience, and the continuous exercise of good judgment. Surgeons who embark on this odyssey must remember that in their hands is the reproductive future of that patient who has invested her total confidence and trust in them. Often it is this first surgical intervention which will determine the future reproductive performance of this patient.

A conservative estimate of the incidence of conditions conducive to infertility in the female's upper reproductive tract requiring surgical intervention is approximately 50 percent. Tubal disease, uterine abnormalities, pelvic adhesions, pelvic endometriosis, and ovarian lesions are by far the most common causes of infertility in the female. Appropriate management of any one of these conditions with the appropriate surgical technique yields highly rewarding success.

In the last decade, the use of fine, atraumatic instruments, nonreactive or slightly reactive sutures, magnifying instruments (double-headed operating microscopes), gentle handling of tissues, and maintenance of tissue moisture during a procedure have all significantly improved surgical techniques, with the inevitable corollary of improving pregnancy success rates. In the last few years, medicine and surgery have acquired their share of high technology by incorporating the use of the laser, which provides another excellent surgical tool in the vast armamentarium of new instruments for reconstructive surgery of the female pelvis.

The use of the carbon dioxide (CO_2) laser to treat disorders in gynecology has steadily increased,[1,2] the major applications being laser vaporization and excision to treat early neoplasms of the vulva, vagina, and cervix.[2,3]

Recently, laser surgery has proven to be of substantial benefit in the treatment of certain epidemic venereal diseases.[4] However, its use intraabdominally has been infrequent, and only a few people have published their experiences with the CO_2 laser in the last 5 years. These publications have shown certain advantages and favorable results for animal tubal anastomosis, as well as for repair of occluded human fallopian tubes.[5-8]

This chapter is devoted to the use of the CO_2 laser for several conditions in the female pelvis which lead to infertility and require surgical intervention to enhance chances for successful pregnancy.

LASER SURGERY OF THE FALLOPIAN TUBES

The tubal factor is responsible for 25 to 30 percent of infertility. Infections are, by far, the most frequent cause of tubal occlusion, but the high incidence of permanent separations and divorce in our society, as well as regretted past decisions to be permanently sterilized,[9-11] lead to increasing requests for tubal reversal, suggesting that the above cited figure may be even higher.

It must be strongly emphasized that tubal surgery should only be performed after the couple has completed an infertility work-up with tests, such as endometrial biopsy to assess adequate ovulation, semen analysis and postcoital tests to rule out male factor involvement, and hysterosalpingogram to determine the area of obstruction and the severity of the lesion.

Technique

Before performing tubal microsurgery on human subjects, experiments were carried out on virginal rabbits. They were sterilized by three methods: (1) Pomeroy ligation, (2) bipolar coagulation, or (3) silicone elastic bands. After 6 to 8 weeks, the animals underwent a second laparotomy, and the obstructed tubal segments were excised with the laser beam. Two methods for approximation of the segments were used: (1) "welding" by numerous intermittent bursts at 0.1 to 0.2 second intervals with 600 to 700 W/cm^2 power density, using a single suture at 6 and 12 o'clock through muscularis and serosa, at the mesosalpingeal and antimesosalpingeal margin, respectively, and (2) conventional suturing after removal of the obstructed segment. Observations from this experimental study showed by standard error of the mean (SEM) that the minimal extent of damage resulting from laser section of the human tube was within an area of 500 to 1000 μm,[7] suggesting that the placement of sutures be 1.0 to 1.5 mm distal to the cut edge of the oviduct. Similarly, these studies refuted the theoretic basis for the laser welding technique. As the weakest portion of the anastomosis, i.e., impact to 500 μm, is the site of welding, it should be no surprise that the "welded" tissue undergoes dehiscence due to normal peristalsis of the bowel and possibly the tube itself, prior to the adequate healing time. These observations indicate that laser welding had little value for the anastomosis of the human fallopian tubes. For details of the technique and results, the interested reader is referred to the article published elsewhere.[7]

The technique used by this author is dependent upon the site of tubal obstruction. When the patient is under general anesthesia, an HUI uterine injector (Unimar, Canoga Park, Calif.) is placed into the uterine cavity for transcervical chromopertubation. I find this instrument very helpful to inject methylene blue or indigo carmine at the time when patency of the tube is to be demonstrated before the anastomosis, to test the anastomatic site for leakage, and to fill the distended clubbed tube before the incision.

Mid-Segment Occlusion: Isthmic-Isthmic, Isthmic-Ampullary and Ampullary-Ampullary

At laparotomy, proper exposure using a self-retaining retractor is used. Ringer's lactate with 5000 units of heparin/L is available for constant irrigation of the pelvic organs. The double-headed operating microscope used by the author is a Zeiss Opmi 6SP (Carl Zeiss, Inc., Wellesley, Mass.) with an adjustable accordian appliance which allows the fiber light to be moved around any laser micromanipulator, with 300 mm lenses; however, any double-headed operating microscope with a micromanipulator can be used. Microsurgical instruments constructed with titanium are used (Codman and Shirtliff, Inc., Randolph, Mass.) with the laser. Stay sutures of 5–0 Vicryl with small atraumatic needles are used to stabilize the stump of the fallopian tube, and then high power densities of approximately 15,000 to 22,000 W/cm^2 are used to excise the occluded area. Injection of 1 or 2 ml of a 1:30 diluted solution of vasopressin is instilled into the operative site to obtain vascular spasm and minimal bleeding with a bloodless field. Manipulating and backstop accessories are required when the laser is used intraabdominally. Initially, glass or quartz rods were utilized, but the laser light beam fatigued the glass and led to unpredictable fractures. Currently, we are using light-absorbing titanium rods which absorb stray laser energy as the target tissue is severed. These rods measure 9 inches in length and range from 1 to 4 mm in diameter. Recently we have experimented with titanium spatulas which have irregular surfaces so as to disperse any possible reflected light (Fig. 17–1). For testing before directing the laser beam to the desired target, a wet tongue depressor is used. This allows one to test the power density grossly by looking at the size of the spot diameter and to see if the CO_2 laser coincides with the helium-neon laser.

After the tube has been opened with the laser, the small amount of charred tissue is gently wiped off with a moist cotton swab and anastomosis is accomplished under the microscope. We use 8-0 or 9-0 nylon with tapered, atraumatic needles at 12, 3, 6, and 9 o'clock muscularis to muscularis, and then at the same points serosa to serosa without splints. After the completion of the anastomosis, methylene blue is injected again, using the syringe attached to the HUI uterine injector to test for leaks in the anastomatic area. Additional stitches are placed if there are gross leaks. I do not think it is necessary to have a perfectly watertight anastomosis since this is not a vascular anastomosis. However, it is extremely important to try the best possible approximation for better healing and decrease in the incidence of ectopic pregnancies. The same procedure is performed in the opposite site, in the presence of another existing blocked tube. Several washings of the pelvic cavity with Ringer's solution, containing heparin 5000 U/L, is then performed until the pelvic organs are devoid of any blood or debris. Prior to closing the abdomen, 100 to 200 ml of dextran 32 percent (Hyskon) are left (Pharmacia Laboratories, Piscataway, N.J.) in the pelvis.

Results shown in Table 17–1 are preliminary and perhaps are not comparable with results reported using conventional microsurgical techniques.[17–19] Neverthe-

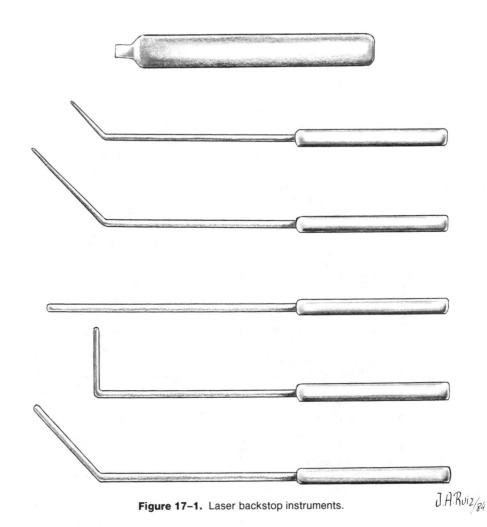

Figure 17–1. Laser backstop instruments.

J.A.Ruiz/84

TABLE 17–1. HUMAN TUBAL SURGERY AND ADHESIOLYSIS UTILIZING THE CO₂ LASER: 90 CASES (DECEMBER 1979 TO MARCH 1983)

Type of Surgery	No. of Patients	(%)	No. Pregnant	(%)
Adhesiolysis only (fimbriolysis)	26	28.9	16	61.5
Salpingoneostomy	24	26.7	8	33.3
Interestitial-isthmic anastomosis	7	7.7	1	14.2
End-to-end anastomosis	33	36.7	17	51.6
Total	90	100.0	42	46.7

less, the follow-up in this series is incomplete, and only time can ascertain the validity of the CO_2 laser for reanastomosis of the fallopian tubes.

Proximal Obstruction of the Fallopian Tube

Interstitial or cornual obstruction is usually due to infections, salpingitis isthmica nodosa, or electrocoagulation for sterilization purposes. Pregnancy success rates are reported to be between 12.5 and 15 percent utilizing the sharp wedge excision technique[12,13] for uterotubal implantation; 14.3 to 64 percent for the reamer technique [12,13]; 50 percent utilizing the open uterine approach[14]; and 64.3 to 71 percent for microsurgical techniques.[13,15]

The use of the laser for tubocornual anastomosis is of little value at the present time according to the preliminary reports presented at the First World Conference on Fallopian Tube in Health and Disease, May, 1983, in West Palm Beach, Florida.[16] Results are shown in Table 17–1. Even though the number of patients is small, it is difficult to argue against the high pregnancy success rate obtained by the conventional microsurgical technique using the "shaving" method for tubocornual anastomosis.

Distal Occlusion of the Fallopian Tubes

Some of the most challenging reconstructive pelvic surgeries for infertility are the cases in which the fallopian tubes have hydrosalpinx and no fimbria. These cases are usually the result of previous pelvic infections due to *Neisseria gonorrhea,* to *Chlamydia trachomatis,* or to ascending infections as a result of the use of intrauterine devices (IUDs). The degree of damage and dilation, the absence of fimbria, or the flattened endosalpingeal cilia do not seem to have a direct relationship with the successful pregnancy rates.

Several techniques have been advocated to reconstruct the obstructed and dilated tubes. Prosthetic devices using the Rock-Mulligan silastic hood in two stages, requiring two laparotomies, showed a conception rate of 22 percent,[20,21] 25 percent,[22] and 37.5 percent.[23] Higher success rates have been accomplished using microscopic techniques.[21,24]

The CO_2 laser can be of excellent aid in performing salpingoneostomies. After lysis of adhesions, using low power densities (Table 17–2) to free the tube, the dimple is identified (Fig. 17–2), stay sutures are placed, and 1 to 2 ml of vasopressin (1:30) is injected (Fig. 17–3). A Y incision is made with high power densities (Fig. 17–4), using the micromanipulator adapted to the Zeiss Opmi 6SP double-headed operating microscope. Further lengthening of the incision is made

TABLE 17–2. SPECIFICATIONS FOR CO₂ LASER TREATMENT IN HUMAN TUBAL SURGERY

Procedure	Power (W)	Spot (mm)	Time (Sec)	Power Density (W/cm²)
Lysis of adhesions	5–15	0.4–1.0	0.1–continuous	480–9000
Tubal excision	20–30	0.3–0.8	Continuous	4800–22,000
Cornual shave	20–40	0.3–0.8	Continuous	7000–22,000

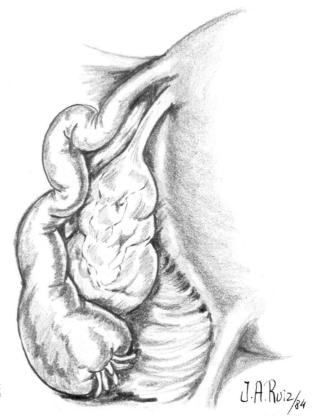

Figure   17–2. Hydrosalpinx: notice the dimple and absence of fimbria.

J.A.Ruiz/84

using the titanium rods to protect the neighboring and underneath structures, with continuous irrigation of Ringer's lactate. The new stoma is maintained by suturing the fimbrial surface to the serosa in a cuff technique fashion (Fig. 17–5), using 8–0 or 9–0 nylon, with atraumatic tapered needle. The operation is bloodless with the use of the CO_2 laser. Since the tube is filled with dye, the target area initially does not need to be protected for fear of going through the fallopian tube. Sometimes the use of the free handpiece of the articulated arm of the CO_2 laser can be used instead of the micromanipulator; this requires experience and expert assistance. On the third or the fourth postoperative day, a hydrotubation is performed, and is subsequently performed once or twice a week for a period of 3 to 4 weeks. The solution used for this purpose is composed of dexamethasone 20 mg and 20 ml of normal saline. If the first two hydrotubations offer no resistance, with little or no backflow, the ensuing hydrotubations are performed using 20 ml of Hyskon.

The question of using hydrotubations is a long-standing, controversial issue. While the work of Grant[25] showed significant pregnancy success rates with fewer ectopic pregnancies in patients on whom hydrotubations were performed, others denied the benefit of this adjunct technique[26]; some others use it, but do not enthusiastically endorse it,[24,27] awaiting further studies. In my experience, hydro-

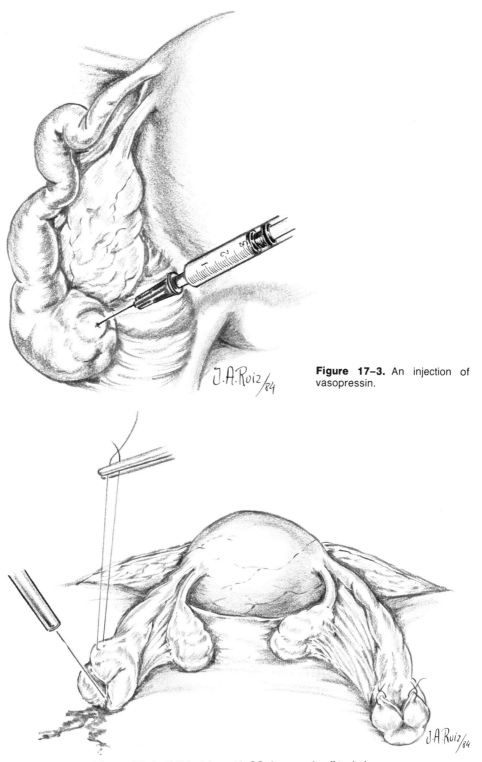

Figure 17–3. An injection of vasopressin.

Figure 17–4. "Y" incision with CO_2 laser and cuff technique.

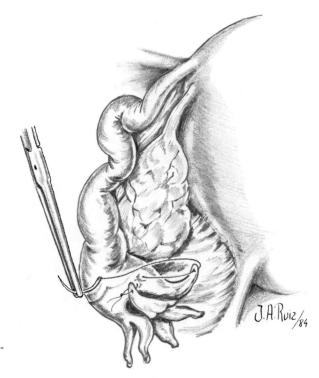

Figure   17–5. Salpingoneostomy: finished cuff technique.

tubations seem to help, however, no randomized studies were conducted to ascertain the validity of this procedure. In the past, I performed hydrotubations using
Elase in lyophilized powder form (bovine fibrinolysin and desorybonuclease combined; Parke-Davis, Division Warner-Lambert Co., Morris Plains, N.J.) in addition to dexamethasone and normal saline. One patient suffered cardiac arrest a
few minutes after the procedure, however, and two others had a severe reaction.
Fortunately, all recovered soon after, without sequelae. Whether or not Elase was
the cause of these unpleasant experiences, the drug was removed from the author's
hydrotubation protocol.

LASER ADHESIOLYSIS FOR INFERTILITY SURGERY

We are more cognizant today of the importance of tubal physiology and know that
tubal patency is not enough to achieve successful intrauterine pregnancy. Tubal
motility and mobility[28] are extremely important mechanisms at the critical time
of ovulation, when synchronicity is the key for blastocyst implantation.

The presence of adhesions in the pelvic reproductive organs, especially around
the fallopian tubes and ovaries, compromise this "pick-up" mechanism leading to
infertility or to ectopic pregnancies. There are three major causes of pelvic adhesions in the female: (1) infection, (2) pelvic endometriosis, and (3) pelvic surgery.

These conditions are frequently encountered, making what is called "peritoneal factor" a relatively common cause of infertility. While in the pelvic cavity, the pelvic surgeon should always have crucial steps in mind, i.e., gentle handling of organs and tissues, constant irrigation with isotonic solutions, and the use of minimal nonreactive sutures. Blunt dissection is not adequate since it leaves raw and oozing areas, which predispose to adhesion reformation. One of the most important uses of the CO_2 laser in infertility surgery is adhesiolysis. It provides an almost ideal technique for separation of adherent tissues by providing clean incision by means of vaporization with minimal necrosis and no bleeding. It allows the surgeon to reach nonvisible, recessed, or poorly accessible areas by utilizing the reflective power of the laser beam from metal or anodized rhodium mirrors (Fig. 17–6).

Before utilizing the CO_2 laser on living tissue, one should calibrate the laser at different power settings on a moist tongue depressor to determine the spot size and the accuracy of aim. The instrument may be attached to a microscope and controlled by a micromanipulator, or it may be operated by means of an articulated arm and free handpiece. To maintain a sterile field, the laser's articulated arm is draped with a double thickness stockinet. Traction and counter traction is of paramount importance when one incises tissue with the laser. Basic backstop instruments are utilized frequently for adhesiolysis (Table 17–3). Titanium rods are extremely useful, either straight or at a 45 or 90 degree angle. The most versatile rod is the 2 mm diameter, 45 degree angle rod since it can obtain access to

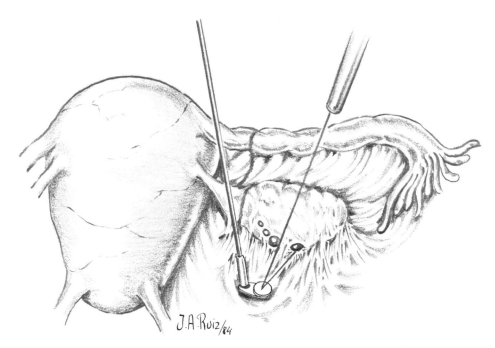

Figure 17–6. Vaporization of endometriosis using the reflecting power of the laser.

TABLE 17–3. REQUIREMENTS OF ACCESSORY INSTRUMENTS

Requirements
Backstop
Absorption of laser light
Minimal reflection
Nonflammability
Nonbreakability
Ease of manipulation
Manipulating rods
Relative Smoothness
Nonreflectiveness (round, irregular surface)
Absorption of heat and light
Nonbreakability
Microsurgery instruments
Light absorption (anodized)

almost any area by placing it behind the target area (Fig. 17–7). Vaporization of veil adhesions is accomplished quickly and completely, and often it is not necessary even to use backstop instruments, but instead to employ low power settings of 5 to 9 W and spot diameters of 0.4 mm or more (Table 17–2). When dense adhesions are excised, the use of backstop instruments are mandatory to protect the vital structures behind the lesions (Fig. 17–7). The major advantage of the laser is the bloodless operative field since small vessels are sealed by the traversing beam, making sutures unnecessary and saving time. Since the heat of the laser

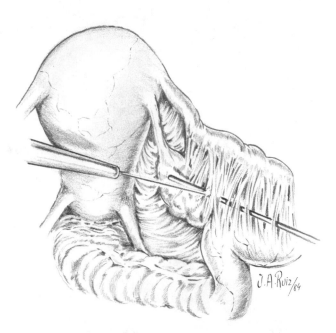

Figure 17–7. A laser adhesiolysis.

TABLE 17–4. FOLLOW-UP STATUS OF WOMEN TREATED BY CO$_2$ FOR TUBAL DISEASE

Length of Follow-Up	No.	Pregnant	(%)	Lost to Follow-Up
36 mo	9	4	44.4	2
24–35 mo	14	7	50.0	1
18–23 mo	15	5	33.3	2
12–17 mo	22	14	63.6	—
6–11 mo	14	6	43.9	1
6 mo	16	4	25.0	—
Total	90	42	46.7	6

beam is so intense, the impact area is sterilized, preventing dissemination of infection. Salpingolysis is an ideal condition for the use of the laser; results reported[28,30] showed pregnancy success rates between 50 and 75 percent, depending on the severity of the adhesive disease. Our preliminary report tallied 61.5 percent (Table 17–1), however, most of the cases had moderate or severe adhesions. In seven patients who had mild to moderate fimbrial adhesions, six became pregnant within 18 months (85.7 percent). If the CO$_2$ laser is not available because of malfunctioning, the author now finds it hard to substitute conventional surgery for adhesiolysis in infertility surgery. The follow-up period is too short at this time to quantitate any significant difference in outcome between this laser-treated series of patients and women treated by conventional surgical methods (Table 17–4).

MYOMECTOMY AND METROPLASTY

When large intramural leiomyomas or subseptate uteri is the only possible cause of infertility, the CO$_2$ laser is of substantial value to excise the myomas or to remove the septum. Prior to the use of the laser, hemostasis is accomplished with vasopressin injection. The site for septum removal is traced with a superficial (low power) laser incision, performed with the handheld piece of the laser instrument. Traction is accomplished with skin hooks, and the septum is excised at high power in a blood-free field. The myometrium is then etched approximately 3 to 4 mm deep to create an edge and to facilitate placement of the first layer of sutures with 3-0 Vicryl gastrointestinal (GI) needle.

Myomectomy is performed in a similar manner, and dissection is performed with the laser with low power densities, traction, and countertraction. This technique provides excellent hemostasis, making these operations less bloody than the usual techniques.

PELVIC ENDOMETRIOSIS

Endometriosis is a poorly understood condition which is characterized by the ectopic growth of endometrial glands and stroma, most frequently on pelvic peritoneal surfaces and adjacent structures in the pelvis, such as ovaries and supporting ligaments of the uterus.

This disorder was thought to afflict predominantly white women of the upper socioeconomic class who attempt childbearing later in their reproductive life cycles rather than women in other classes.[31] This long believed theory has now been discredited. As to the ages of the women suffering pelvic endometriosis, the disorder can occur as early as the teenage years.[32] It is estimated that endometriosis is found in 15 to 25 percent of women undergoing gynecologic laparotomy[33] and in 25 percent of women undergoing laparoscopy for infertility.[34] The actual incidence of pelvic endometriosis among infertile women is difficult to assess, however, a realistic estimate is 25 to 35 percent, a figure which is based on operative statistics from infertility specialists. Although several theories of origin have been postulated over the years, and numerous clinical and experimental models have reportedly demonstrated the plausibility of one theory over all others, the etiology of this disease remains nebulous. An animal model[35,36] has substantiated the classic "retrograde menstruation" theory of Sampson.[37] Endometriosis has been found, however, at sites distant from the pelvic peritoneum, i.e., bronchial tree, nasal mucosa, lacrimal glands, and the theory of retrograde flow cannot explain these occurrences; therefore, vascular or lymphatic transport of endometrial tissue is possible.[38] Moreover, the transformation of coelomic epithelium into endometrial glands and/or stroma as a result of unspecified stimuli[39] might answer the obscure presence of ectopic endometrial tissue outside the abdominal cavity. The principal symptom associated with pelvic endometriosis is pelvic pain, most often intensifying just prior to and during menses. Dyspareunia and infertility often accompany pelvic endometriosis. The latter do not bear any relationship to the degree and quantity of endometriotic implants, there being a common clinical observation of finding an inverse relationship between the severity of dysmenorrhea and the degree of pelvic endometriosis.

Two major therapeutic approaches for the amelioration of endometriosis have evolved over recent years, i.e., medical or surgical treatment. Medical management currently consists of pseudopregnancy produced by continuous oral contraceptive administration and pseudomenopause secondary to danazol treatment. One surgical approach may be radical, i.e., total abdominal hysterectomy (preservation of the ovaries may be associated with the risk of persistence of the disease and of the symptoms). Conservative surgery is the other choice, which preserves the pelvic reproductive viscera while removing all visible foci of endometriosis. This conserving doctrine is usually combined with one or more of the following procedures: adhesiolysis, uterine suspension, and/or presacral neurectomy. Laser surgery utilizing the carbon dioxide laser for the conservative management of pelvic endometriosis is a method which provides the pelvic surgeon with a new, versatile surgical tool.

Technique

Several CO_2 laser machines can be used to vaporize focal endometrial implants, excise endometrial cysts, and lyse pelvic adhesions: the Xanar Articulator (Xanar Surgical Systems, Colorado Springs, Colo.); Biolas Model 405 (Advanced Biomedical Instruments, Woburn, Mass.); Sharplan 733 (Advanced Surgical Technologies, Inc., Schaumburg, Ill.); and other laser machines are suitable for this type of surgery. Each of the lasers is equipped with an articulated arm, to which an autoclavable handpiece can be attached. A coincident helium-neon (He-Ne) laser provides a visible red target, onto which the CO_2 laser beam can be directed. Each laser can be attached to a double-headed operating microscope by means of a micromanipulator. It is recommended that one utilize a mobile light system in order to provide the best illumination of the operative area.

Manipulating and backstop accessories are required when the laser is used intraabdominally (see Fig. 17–1). Initially, glass or quartz rods were utilized, but the laser light beam fatigued the glass, which led to unpredictable fracture. Moistened wooden tongue depressors have served as backstops when adhesions or tubular structures were to be lased. The backstop obviously absorbs stray laser energy as the target tissue is severed. Recently we have experimented with titanium spatulas, the surfaces being irregular so as to disperse any possible reflected light.

The laser's articulated arm is draped with a 6 inch sterile double-thickness stockinet, with a small opening cut into the arm. The microscope to which the laser micromanipulator and articulating arm are attached is covered with a standard plastic drape, open at the bottom to allow the laser light to be fired unimpeded.

For vaporization of implants (Fig. 17–8) power settings ranged from 2 to 5 W, and spot size ranged from 0.4 to 2.0 mm in diameter. Time exposure ranged from 0.1 second to continuous. For lysis of adhesions power settings ranged from 5 to 15 W, with other settings remaining constant. For ovarian excision power was set at 20 to 30 W (Table 17–2).

Fine absorbable sutures (5-0 to 7-0 Vicryl or Dexon) can be used to approximate resected ovaries and to attach free peritoneal grafts when extensive raw surfaces result from adhesion dissection.

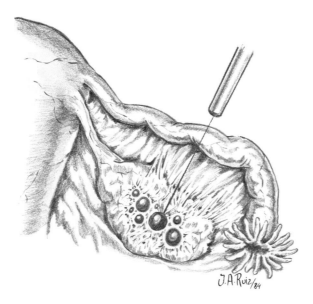

J.A.Ruiz/84

Figure 17–8. Laser photovaporization of endometriotic implants.

Constant irrigation with Ringer's lactate solution, adding 5000 units of heparin/ L, is recommended to maintain tissue moisture and to prevent fibrin deposition. It is recommended that 100 to 200 cc of 32 percent dextran (Hyskon, Pharmacia Laboratories, Piscataway, N.J.) be left in the pelvis prior to closing the abdomen in order to minimize adhesion formation.[40]

The most important single technical aid to laser excisional surgery is careful, constant traction and countertraction at the line of incision. Not only does this allow for more rapid dissection, but it also protects surrounding tissue from heat damage.

The action of laser light on endometrial implants is precise and predictable. The laser spot can be focused to less than 0.5 mm or to more than 2.0 mm, depending on the size of the lesion to be destroyed. For very precise vaporization, we prefer to use power densities of 1000 W/cm^2 or less, at intermittent time exposures of 0.1 to 0.2 second. The initial impact causes brownish fluid to exit the lesion and to vaporize into a mist. When no further fluid is observed and the vaporization has created a shallow crater less than 1 mm deep, laser exposure is discontinued. No sutures are placed in the craters and usually no bleeding is observed (Fig. 17–9). Foci of endometriosis on the posterior aspect of the ovary and deep in the cul-de-sac are vaporized indirectly by reflecting the laser beam from a stainless steel mirror (see Fig. 17–6). Bleeding is virtually absent in every case. Fine adhesions are vaporized under microscopic control, which aids the surgeon in identifying and sighting the direction of tissue planes. In addition, the fine laser spot delivered by intermittent bursts provides easy, precise cutting and complete hemostasis. Whenever possible, a manipulating rod is slipped behind the adhesion for protection of neighboring tissues and for traction on the adhesion (see Fig. 17–7).

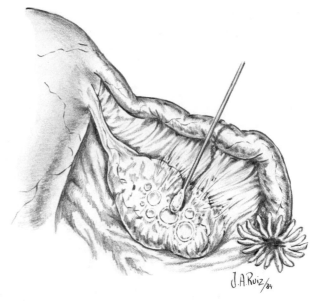

Figure   17–9. After   laser vaporization.

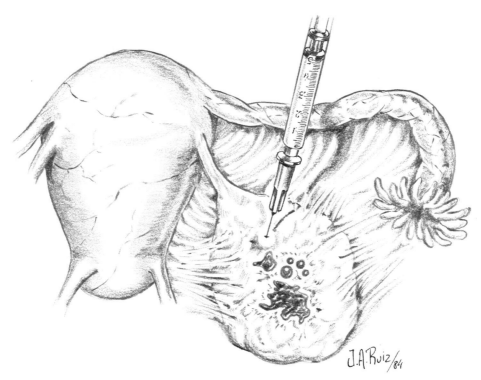

Figure 17–12. Injection of Pitressin.

In addition to hemostasis, the use of the laser to excise or uncap ovarian endometriomata provides a unique advantage (Fig. 17–10, see Color Plate IV*). Whenever the endometrioma occupies a substantial part of the ovary, so that its total removal might result in ovarian failure, the cyst is opened by the laser (Fig. 17–11, see Color Plate IV). Injection of 1 or 2 ml of 1:30 diluted solution of vasopressin is injected into the operative site to obtain vascular spasm to further accomplish minimal bleeding (Fig. 17–12). An elliptic portion of the cyst wall is then excised (Fig. 17–13), and the chocolate fluid contents drained (see Fig. 17–11). The interior of the cyst is next exposed by eversion, and the interior lining is superficially vaporized (Fig. 17–14). The cavity is finally closed by approximating the walls with fine sutures.

Improvement of pelvic pain and visible amelioration of endometriosis can be expected in 40 percent of patients treated with danazol, according to Friedlander.[41] Dmowski and Cohen[42] and Greenblatt and Tzingounis[43] report a 50 percent response rate. Following conservative surgery employing a combination of sharp dissection and needle cautery, regression of disease varies from 30 percent[44] to 94

*Color Plate IV appears following p. 177.

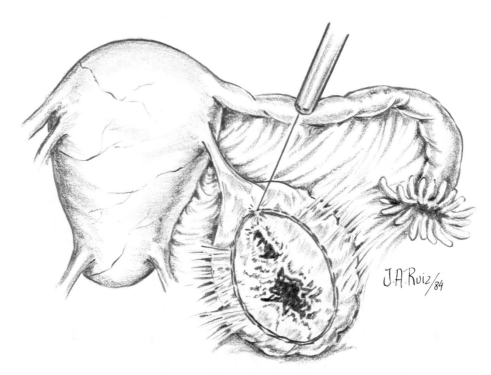

Figure 17–13. Laser wedge resection.

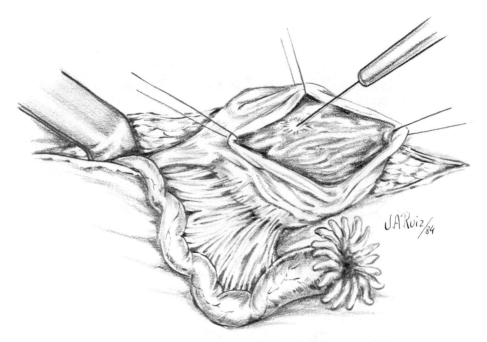

Figure 17–14. Laser photovaporization of endometriotic cystic wall.

TABLE 17–5. SEVERITY OF ENDOMETRIOSIS AND INCIDENCE OF PREGNANCY IN 24 PATIENTS

Stage	No. Trying	Pregnant	(%)
I	—	—	—
II	13	11	84.6
III	8	3	37.5
IV	2	—	—
Total	23	14	60.8[a]

[a]Average.

percent.[45] Buttram[46] has correlated successful surgical treatment with the severity of disease, i.e., 84 percent success with the mild stages, but 75 and 56 percent respectively when faced with moderate or severe endometriosis. In order to better correlate and compare treatment programs, the American Fertility Society has proposed a standardized staging system based on a grade point analysis.[47]

Our preliminary results showed 60.8 percent pregnancy success rate (Table 17–5).[48] In this series, patients with Stage I pelvic endometriosis, as classified by the American Fertility Society,[47] were not treated by the CO_2 laser; therefore, the results are for Stages II, III, and IV (Table 17–6).

Postoperative danazol (Danocrine) has been used with success.[49] Its pre- or postoperative use cannot be recommended at the present time, however, since there are not enough meaningful, available data to support this antigonadotropic agent as adjunctive therapy.

SUMMARY

Technically, the CO_2 laser has some strategic advantages over other operative methods for the conservative management of endometriosis. Hemostasis, predictable precision, and the ability of the laser beam to reach into recessed or otherwise poorly visible areas are benefits representing a technologic advance previously unavailable to the gynecologist.

TABLE 17–6. SEVERITY OF ENDOMETRIOSIS IN 54 PATIENTS TREATED BY CO_2 LASER

Stage	No.	(%)
I	0	0
II	37	67
III	14	27
IV	3	6
Total	54	100

The preliminary reports appearing in the literature on the use of intraabdominal laser surgery, as well as the upcoming, controlled, randomized studies, will allow the gynecologist to find the proper use for the laser so that he or she will be able to apply this modern surgical tool with wisdom, less passion, and more science. I am sure that we should be able to see the light at the end of the tunnel in the near future, hopefully without deleterious reflections.

REFERENCES

1. Stafe A, Wilkinson EJ, Mattingly RF: Laser treatment of cervical and vaginal neoplasia. Am J Obstet Gynecol 128:128, 1977
2. Baggish MS: High power-density carbon dioxide laser therapy for early cervical neoplasia. Am J Obstet Gynecol 136:117, 1980
3. Dorsey JH, Diggs ES: Microsurgical conization of the cervix by carbon dioxide laser. Obstet Gynecol 54:565, 1979
4. Baggish MS: Carbon dioxide laser treatment for condylomata acuminata venereal infections. Obstet Gynecol 55:711, 1980
5. Grosspietzsch R: Microtubular reanastomosis in animal model and early human results. Gynecological Laser Surgery. New York, Plenum, 1981
6. Klink F, Grosspietzsch R, Klitzing L, et al: Animal in vivo studies and in vivo experiments on human tubes for end-to-end anastomotic operation by CO_2 laser technique. Fertil Steril 30:100, 1978
7. Baggish MS, Chong AP: Carbon dioxide laser microsurgery of the uterine tube. Obstet Gynecol 58:111, 1981
8. Bruhat MA, Mage G: Use of CO_2 laser in salpingoneostomy. In Kaplan I (ed): Laser Surgery III, Part 1. Jerusalem, Academic Press, 1979, pp 271–278
9. Norris AS: An examination of the effects of tubal ligation: Their implication for prediction. Am J Obstet Gynecol 90:431, 1964
10. Woodruff JD, Paurstein CJ: The Fallopian Tube, 1st ed. Baltimore, Williams & Wilkins, 1969, p 336
11. Campanella R, Wolff JR: Emotional reaction to sterilization. Obstet Gynecol 45:331, 1975
12. Rock JA, Katayama KP, Martin EJ, et al: Pregnancy outcome following uterotubal implantation: A comparison of the reamer and sharp wedge excision techniques. Fertil Steril 31:634, 1979
13. Diamond E: A comparison of gross and microsurgical techniques for repair of cornual occlusion in infertility: A retrospective study, 1968–1978. Fertil Steril 32:370, 1979
14. Peterson EP, Musich JR, Behrman SJ: Uterotubal implantation and obstetric outcome after previous sterilization. Am J Obstet Gynecol 128:662, 1977
15. Winston RML: Microsurgery of the fallopian tube: From fantasy to reality. Fertil Steril 34:521, 1980
16. Chong AP, Baggish MS: The use of carbon dioxide laser in tubal surgery. Int J Fertil 28:24, 1983
17. Diamond E: Microsurgical reconstruction of the uterine tube in sterilized patients. Fertil Steril 28:1203, 1977
18. Gomel V: Microsurgical reversal of female sterilization: A reappraisal. Fertil Steril 33:587, 1980
19. Jones HW Jr, Rock JA: On the reanastomosis of fallopian tubes after surgical sterilization. Fertil Steril 29:702, 1978

20. Garcia C-R, Aller J: Surgical approach to tubal disease. Clin Obstet Gynecol 17:102, 1974

21. DeCherney AH, Kase N: A comparison of treatment for bilateral fimbrial occlusion. Fertil Steril 35:162, 1981

22. Roland M, Leisten D: Tuboplasty in 130 patients: Improved results due to stents and preoperative endoscopy. Obstet Gynecol 39:57, 1972

23. Young PE, Egan JE, Barlow JJ, Mulligan WJ: Reconstructive surgery for infertility at the Boston Hospital for Women. Am J Obstet Gynecol 108:1092, 1970

24. Gomel V: Salpingostomy by microsurgery. Fertil Steril 29:380, 1978

25. Grant A: Infertility surgery of the oviduct. Fertil Steril 22:496, 1971

26. Verhoeven HC, Berry H, Frantzen C, Schlösser H-W: Surgical treatment for distal tubal occlusion: A review of 167 cases. J Reprod Med 28:293, 1983

27. Rock JA, Katayama KP, Martin EJ, et al: Factors influencing the success of salpingostomy techniques for distal fimbrial obstruction. Obstet Gynecol 52:591, 1978

28. Spadoni LR: Tubal and peritubal surgery without magnification: An analysis. Am J Obstet Gynecol 137:189, 1980

29. Bronson RA, Wallach EE: Lysis of periadnexal adhesions for correction of infertility. Fertil Steril 28:613, 1977

30. Diamond E: Lysis of postoperative pelvic adhesions in infertility. Fertil Steril 31:287, 1979

31. Goutschis JG, Vorys N, Neri AS: Endometriosis. In Gold JJ (ed): Gynecologic Endocrinology, ed 2. Hagerstown, Maryland, Harper & Row, 1975, p 245

32. Schrifrin BX, Erez S, Moore JG: Teen-age endometriosis. Am J Obstet Gynecol 116:973, 1973

33. Kistner RW: Endometriosis. In Sciarra J (ed): Gynecology and Obstetrics, Vol 1. Hagerstown, Maryland, Harper & Row, 1977

34. Dmowski, WP, Cohen MR, Wilhelm JL: Endometriosis and ovulatory failure: Does it occur? Should ovulation stimulating agents be used? In Greenblatt RB (ed): Recent Advances in Endometriosis. Proceedings of a Symposium, March, 1975. Amsterdam, Holland, Excerpta Medica, 1976, p 129

35. Scott RB, TeLinde RW, Wharton LR Jr: Further studies on experimental endometriosis. Am J Obstet Gynecol 66:1082, 1953

36. Dizerega GS, Barber DL, Hodgen GD: Endometriosis: Role of ovarian steroids in initiation, maintenance and suppression. Fertil Steril 33:649, 1980

37. Sampson JA: Peritoneal endometriosis due to the menstrual dissemination of endometrial tissue into the peritoneal cavity. Am J Obstet Gynecol 14:422, 1927

38. Oliker AJ, Harris AE: Endometriosis of the bladder in a male patient. J Urol 106:858, 1971

39. Merrill JA: Endometrial induction of endometriosis across millipore filters. Am J Obstet Gynecol 94:780, 1966

40. DiZerega G, Utian W: Efficacy of 32% dextran-70 in the utility of second-look laparoscopy in infertility surgery (abstract). Fertil Steril 37:291, 1982

41. Friedlander RL: The treatment of endometriosis with danazol. J Reprod Med 10:197, 1973

42. Dmowski WP, Cohen ME: Treatment of endometriosis with an antigonadotropin, danazol: A laparoscopic and histologic evaluation. Obstet Gynecol 46:147, 1975

43. Greenblatt RD, Tzingounis V: Danazol treatment of endometriosis: Long-term follow up. Fertil Steril 32:518, 1979

44. Spangler DB, Jones GS, Jones HW Jr: Infertility due to endometriosis. Am J Obstet Gynecol 109:850,1971

45. McCoy JB, Bradford WZ: Surgical treatment of endometriosis with conservation of reproductive potential. Am J Obstet Gynecol 87:394, 1963

46. Buttram VC Jr: Surgical treatment of endometriosis in the infertile female: A modified approach. Fertil Steril 32:635, 1979

47. The American Fertility Society: Classification of endometriosis. Fertil Steril 32:633, 1979

48. Chong AP, Baggish MS: Management of pelvic endometriosis by means of intraabdominal carbon dioxide laser. Fertil Steril (abstract) [Supp] 39:429, 1983. Fertil Steril (in press)

49. Wheeler JM, Malinak LR: Postoperative danazol therapy in infertility patients with severe endometriosis. Fertil Steril 37:291, 1982

18

Laser Microsurgery of the Oviducts

G. Mage
J. L. Pouly
M. A. Bruhat

INTRODUCTION

Microsurgical treatment of tuboperitoneal infertility experienced great progress in the 1970s. Prior to that time, the results of tubal surgery were often inconsistent and unsuccessful, and only a few pioneers such as Palmer in France were interested in it. Today, microsurgery is practiced by many medical teams and has given rise to numerous publications. Carefully controlled animal studies, especially those involving microsurgical anastomosis, have provided a better understanding of the functions of the different tubal segments. The nomenclature adopted in Madrid in July 1980 represents the beginning of a classification system that will permit better comparisons of results to be made. Recently, many surgical improvements have been proposed, among them the use of the carbon dioxide (CO_2) laser.[1-5,8]

The CO_2 laser beam is a particularly useful tool in tubal microsurgery because it can section with concomitant hemostasis and minimal tissue damage. It represents a new and easy surgical procedure. In tubal microsurgery, regardless of which method is used, sectioning procedures are followed by those of reconstruction. The use of a microscope improves the success of these operating methods, especially reconstruction. Conventional dissection is accomplished either by means of a unipolar microelectrode in adhesiolysis or neosalpingostomy with immediate hemostasis, or by means of the "cold knife" method in tubal section prior to anastomosis. In this case, hemostasis is achieved secondarily by means of unipolar or bipolar microelectrode coagulation.

The CO_2 laser represents an alternative to these conventional techniques. Quality tissue dissection is obtained along with immediate hemostasis for the small blood vessels (in theory, up to 0.5 mm in diameter), and a minimal tissue damage (<100 μm with correct use). So the CO_2 laser can be used to perform all sectioning procedures, including complete section of the tube before anastomosis, without having to obtain complementary hemostasis. This results not only in improving the surgical procedure but also in reducing the operating time. The small amount of tissue damage produced by CO_2 laser section does not diminish the success rate.

PATIENT SELECTION

The purpose of tubal surgery is to restore as faithfully as possible, tuboovarian anatomy. Anatomic repair, however, is not synonymous with functional recuperation and, even under the best conditions, does not guarantee the occurrence of an intrauterine pregnancy.

For a given degree of tubal damage, there is a maximal probability of success. The purpose of tubal surgery is to approach this maximum. It is too much to hope that any new surgical procedure can provide a large increase of the success of infertility surgery.

Consequently, patient selection involves:

1. Estimation of the maximal chance of success for each case. It is based on a detailed medical evaluation and the experience of the surgeon.
2. Definition of the lowest probability of success which still represents a reasonable indication of tubal surgery. The views of the patient should be carefully considered in the decision-making process. The following medical, psychologic, and economic factors must also be considered:
   a. Medical: May the surgeon refuse to operate if he considers the chances of success to be very low?
   b. Psychologic: Should the surgeon operate and thus provide some hope for a patient whose chance of success are virtually nonexistent, or should the surgeon refuse to operate on such patients and thus deprive them of all hope?
   c. Economic: The money needed for a single tubal microsurgical operation (if it were known in advance to be useless) could be used instead to vaccinate, for example, 10,000 third-world children against rubeola.

Improvement and wide-spread use of the in vitro fertilization technique will dramatically influence the decision as well.

Patient selection depends on estimating the maximal probability of success on the basis of three factors: (1) association with other factors of infertility, (2) the severity of tubal and peritoneal involvement, and (3) the risk of persistent inflammatory disease or recurrence of adhesions.

Evaluation of Other Parameters of Sterility

Minimal examinations are required: spermogram, spermoculture, postcoital testing, detection of ovulation based on basal body temperature, and evaluation of the corpus luteum.

Classic contraindications include age over 40, a medical risk for pregnancy, tubal tuberculosis, azoospermia, and sperm-smear incompatibility confirmed by two cross-over tests.

The following are not definitive contraindications: anovulation, dysovulation, and hyperprolactinemia responding to bromocriptine treatment.

Masculine hypofertility represents a great dilemma. Both masculine hypofertility and tubal involvement must be considered in determining the appropriateness of surgery. We think that microsurgery is contraindicated when the spermogram consistently shows less than 5×10^6 normal and mobile spermatozoids per milliliter in 4 hours. In cases of infected sperm, intervention must be delayed until a complete and permanent cure has been obtained.

Evaluation of Tubal Lesions

Preoperative evaluation of tubal damage comprises hysterosalpingography and laparoscopy. These are not mutually exclusive but complementary.[6] Failure to do one or the other will result in error of judgment. Sometimes discordance between them obliges one to repeat one of the procedures (especially hysterosalpingography) for a perfect evaluation.

This tubal check-up permits the surgeon to evaluate:

1. The location and extent of tubal obstruction
2. The condition of the tubal wall
3. The involvement of the tubal epithelium
4. The size and degree of adhesions
5. The probable etiology of the lesions
6. The stability of the lesions
7. Diagnosis of certain specific lesions.

Location and Extent of Obstruction
Tubal obstruction can occur in four principal locations for which prognosis and surgical procedures are different:

1. Terminal obstruction is the most common and is corrected by salpingostomy. Conditions of the tubal wall and endosalpinx determine, to a large extent, the success of surgery. In cases, of incomplete obstruction, the chances of success with fimbrioplasty, which faithfully restores the fimbria, are greater than those of salpingostomy.
2. Isthmic or isthmointerstitial obstruction requires anastomosis. This procedure produces excellent results if the lesion is isolated, as after tubal sterilization.
3,4. The other tubal obstruction sites are infrequent and the results of therapy often are poor. These include a complete interstitial obstruction requiring tubal reimplantation, or a medioampullary obstruction requiring either ampulloampullary anastomosis or medioampullary salpingostomy. In these two types of obstructions, surgical intervention is performed only when the other tubal conditions are satisfactory. The association of several obstructions on the same tube lowers the chances of successful treatment. Bifocal obstruction (distal and proximal) represents an extensive infection of the tube and the prognosis is poor.

Condition of the Tubal Wall

Persistent inflammatory disease of the tube is associated with histologic sequelae. The involvement of the muscle layer of the tube is characterized by fibrosis which interferes with transport function. At an advanced stage such tubes can be permeable but not functional.

Numerous degrees of damage exist which are not well classified. This evaluation is often subjective. Hysterosalpingography may show a frozen tube from one film to the next in cases of parietal sclerosis.

Laparoscopy provides more information especially when blue dye testing permits through transparency determination of the thickness of the tubal wall.

In cases of a hydrosalpinx, which is moderately dilated and whose wall is fine and flexible, there is good chance of success. A distended hydrosalpinx with a fine wall means a partial destruction of the tubal musculature which lowers the chance of success. Distal obstruction without dilation, but involving a thick and sclerotic wall is a contraindication for surgery.

Epithelial Involvement

The tubal mucosa plays a major role in the physiology of the tube. The best evaluation is histologic. Unfortunately, tubal biopsy during laparoscopy remains an unresolved problem. Hysterosalpingography is the most simple evaluation technique.

The prognosis is poor for patients with an absence of ampullary mucosal folds or with the presence of irregular and reticular images of the ampulla which indicates the presence of intraampullary adhesions (honeycomb). On the other hand, the prognosis is good if there are mucosal folds even when the obstruction is complete.

Adhesions

Peritubal ovarian adhesions are one of the main factors of surgical failure, for tuboperitoneal infertility. Three parameters appear to be important: (1) the type of adhesion, (2) the number of organs involved, and (3) the degree of involvement in each organ.

Three types of adhesions are generally recognized: (1) type A—fine and avascular adhesion, (2) type B—thick and poorly vascularized adhesions; and (3) type C—thick and vascularized adhesions (Fig. 18–1).

Adhesion type A or B are easily removed during laparoscopy or laparotomy. Adhesion type C requires laparotomy and peritonization. Risks of recurrence are important for adhesions type C and minimal for adhesions type A.

Organs involved include all parts of the tube but especially the ampulla, the ovary, the uterus, the pouch of Douglas, and the gastrointestinal tract.

One expresses involvement as a function of the extent of adhesion formation for each organ ($\frac{1}{3}$, $\frac{2}{3}$, $\frac{3}{3}$, or $\frac{1}{4}$, $\frac{1}{2}$, $\frac{3}{4}$ or $\frac{4}{4}$). The problem is that this is a subjective evaluation. Generally the greater the extent of the adhesions, the greater is the risk of recurrence.

Adhesion involvement is thus polymorphic and the prognosis differs widely, as, for example, between type A adhesions, partially involving some pelvic organs, and type C adhesions, encompassing the ovaries.

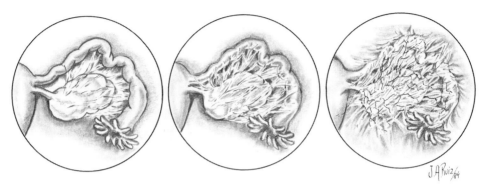

Figure 18–1. Three types of adhesions are illustrated: fine, filmy adhesions; moderately thick adhesions; thick, vascularized adhesions.

Objective determination of the chance of successful adhesiolysis is therefore, difficult, especially since the status is rarely equal for both adnexa. The experience of the laparoscopist is very important in estimating the chances for success. For a more objective approach, we use a numerical scoring system which takes into account the type of adhesion and its extension to each organ (Table 18–1). Currently, the new scoring, which is done for each adnexa, does not enable us to make definitive conclusions. But it seems that a score of 25 or more on the most favorable adnexa represents a contraindication.

Etiology of the Lesions

Patient history, hysterosalpingography, and laparoscopy permit us to specify the etiology of tubal sterility and dramatically influence the prognosis of tubal surgery. The five main causes are (1) salpingitis, (2) ectopic pregnancy, (3) genital tuberculosis, (4) endometriosis, and (5) nongynecologic pelvic infection, e.g., peritonitis, appendicitis, and infectious sequelae of abdominal or pelvic surgery.

Sequelae of nongynecologic pelvic infection represent the best indication since, in general, there is little involvement of the tubal wall. Endometriosis constitutes a specific problem for which the results are often satisfactory. On the other hand, tubal surgery is not successful in the case of genital tuberculosis. Intermediate success is achieved in treatment of sequelae of salpingitis or ectopic pregnancy where an overall evaluation of the lesion, especially tubal wall involvement, plays a significant role.

Stability of the Lesions

Any surgeon has been surprised at least once to discover, upon tubal microsurgery, more extensive lesions than those indicated during preoperative laparoscopy. There is hardly a worse situation imaginable, than that of discovering, upon intervention, that the tissues are still inflammatory. The persistence of inflammation can be evocated on the basis of important discrepancies between the hysterosalpingographic findings and those of laparoscopy, usually obtained several weeks

TABLE 18–1. PRE- AND POSTOPERATIVE TUBAL EVALUATION AND SCORING

Evaluation

Adhesions						Tube	
Ovary						Permeability	
	No	**1/4**	**2/4**	**3/4**	**4/4**	Normal	0
						Proximal obstruction	5
A	0	1	1	1	1	Distal partial obstruction	2
B	0	2	4	6	10	Distal total obstruction	5
C	0	5	10	15	20		
Proximal part of the tube						Tubal wall	
	No	**1/3**	**2/3**	**3/3**			
A	0	1	1	1		Normal	0
B	0	2	4	6		Thin or thick	5
C	0	3	5	10		Sclerosis	10
Distal part of the tube						Tubal mucosa	
	No	**1/3**	**2/3**	**3/3**			
A	0	1	1	1		Normal folds	0
B	0	2	4	6		Decreased folds	5
C	0	5	10	15		No folds or honey comb	10

Scoring[a]

	Left	Right
Adhesions (before lysis)	☐	☐
Tube	☐	☐
Total	☐	☐
Adhesions (after lysis)	☐	☐

[a]Tubal damage: Mild <5, moderate 5 to 10, severe >10, adhesions: mild ≤5, moderate 6 to 19, severe > 20.

later. The laparoscopic profile includes an inflammatory aspect and, especially, a tendency for hemorrhage upon adhesiolysis, as well as false peritoneal cysts.

Conclusive signs are rare: blood count and sedimentation rate that are generally normal; bacteria in the cul-de-sac liquid and in the tubal fluid are seen only occasionally. Blood cultures for *Chlamydia,* if positive, have diagnostic value. In practice, however, the best criterion is histopathologic confirmation. Since biopsy of the tube is very traumatic, we prefer biopsy of the adhesions. If it confirms a persistent inflammation, a long-term antibiotic and corticoid treatment is indicated prior to surgery. A second preoperative laparoscopic evaluation is advised.

Particular Lesions

It is not well known today whether interstitial polyps can cause sterility. In the absence of successful treatment of other suspected causes of infertility, surgical treatment may be proposed. Laparoscopy indicates whether the lesion is associated with an isthmic nodosis salpingitis or other peritoneal lesions.

The pathogenicity and nature of isthmic nodosis salpingitis is poorly known.

Diagnosis is made with the laparoscopy with enlargement of the juxtauterine isthmic portion. Surgery is difficult to justify if there is a satisfactory tubal permeability. If permeability is unsatisfactory or if there is a hysterosalpingographic image of tubal endometriosis, surgery may be indicated.

Synthesis

The decision to operate is based on a number of factors and in particular the condition of the most favorable adnexa.

Reversal of Sterilization

Factors to consider include:

1. Sterilization method: results are usually excellent with Hulka clips or Yoon bands, but are disappointing with electrocoagulation.
2. If the time between tubal sterilization and surgery is greater than 5 years, the chances of success are decreased.
3. The length of the remaining tube.
4. The type of anastomosis: an isthmoisthmic or isthmointerstitial anastomosis is prefered. Tubal reimplantation has only a fair prognosis.

Postinfection Isthmointerstitial Obstruction

Isolated: Prognosis is good if the condition of the tubal wall and epithelium is satisfactory. The chances of success depend on the length of the obstruction; too large a resection has deleterious consequences.

The combination with other lesions is unfavorable. The three types of other lesions that may be associated are terminal obstruction, thick tubal wall, and extensive pelvic adhesions.

The combination of one of these three conditions with postinfection isthmointerstitial obstruction is not a contraindication but the chances of success are dramatically reduced. The combination of two of these lesions is an absolute contraindication.

Distal Obstruction

1. Isolated: their prognosis is rather favorable if the tubal wall and epithelium are not too involved.
2. Their combination with another lesion worsens the prognosis and one can consider these as contraindications. Presence of intraampullary adhesions (honeycomb) involving nearly all the ampulla, a very thick and sclerotic tubal wall, and perituboovarian adhesions of the C type are contraindications.
3. Intermediate involvement includes absence or reduction of the mucosal folds, thin tubal walls, and extensive adhesions of the B type.

Combination with one of these does not constitute a contraindication. When two are associated with a distal obstruction, however, operative indications should be rejected.

Adhesiolysis

In our mind, laparotomy for adhesiolysis in patients with healthy tubes should be infrequent. Indeed, results following laparoscopic removal are good (generally over 50 percent of intrauterine pregnancies). Moreover, when adhesiolysis by laparoscopy (extensive type C adhesions) is impossible, the prognosis is poor even with laparotomy. This is true only for medical teams trained in performing operative laparoscopies.

Scoring System

To reduce the subjective nature of the indications for microsurgery and to better specify the chances of success as a function of the combination of lesions, we use a prospective overall scoring system that takes into account for each adnexa both the condition of the tube and the degree of involvement of the adhesions (see Table 18–1).

The lack of sufficient data does not permit us to make generalizations regarding the value of this system, but it seems that a score of more than 25 for adhesions, a score of more than 15 for tubes, or a general score over 30 indicates a very poor prognosis (<5 percent—for the most favorable adnexa).

INTERVENTION

Time of Intervention

It seems desirable to perform the operation some time after laparoscopy for the following reasons:

1. The decision to undergo surgery rests with the patient; it is preferable to obtain the patient's agreement after she is made aware of the results of laparoscopy.
2. If material is obtained during laparoscopy for tubal biopsy, endometrial biopsy, and culture of Chlamydia, it is only logical to await the results of these tests.
3. Sometimes it is necessary, in order to evaluate the tubes correctly by means of laparoscopy, to remove the adhesions. In this case, it is preferable to await healing and operate after the adhesiolysis.
4. In case of tubal lesions that are still inflammatory, antibiotic treatment is recommended prior to surgery.
5. The organization of the operating theater makes it difficult to schedule laparotomies whose performance depends on the findings of laparoscopy.

The best time for the operation is the preovulatory period of the menstrual cycle when ovarian manipulation does not run the risk of causing hemorrhage due to a corpus luteum.

Installation

Position of the Patient
The surgeon must be able to operate in a comfortable position. It is best to use a moving operating table to eliminate the inconvenience of the central pedestal. An extension of 60 cm attached to the end of a standard operating table can be used (Winston).

Exposure of the Lesions
It is imperative in microsurgery that the lesions be correctly exposed. A wide Pfannenstiel incision with careful hemostasis of the wall is sufficient, and it is unnecessary to section the large abdominal muscles. A Kirschner frame is especially useful to take full advantage of the parietal incision. Douglas packing raises the adnexa* which are placed on a Silastic sheet.

Hydrotubation
A solution of methylene blue (0.02 or 0.04 percent) must be injected either by median transfundic puncture (a clamp being placed in the cervical region) or by a No. 10 Foley catheter placed, via the transcervical route, into the uterus and inflated to 2 cc. We prefer the intrauterine catheter because it is not always easy to identify the uterine cavity with transfundic puncture.

Microscope
We have no preference for any particular microscope from among the many on the market. We use a Zeiss (Opmi 6) two-way stereo microscope which permits the surgeon and his assistant to see the identical image. In the beginning, a single operating microscope is perfectly satisfactory. The microscope should not get in the way during surgery and should provide a clear bright field of vision. An imperfect image could be the result of one of the following which should be checked preoperatively: the ocular is inadequately set into the binocular heads, the ocular is not properly adjusted to correct for the surgeon's vision, and the distance between both oculars is not correctly adjusted.

The microscope should be handled in a sterile fashion—plastic drapes to enclose the microscope or autoclavable plastic caps placed over the controls are two of the simpler techniques.

Instrumentation
Special instruments are required for microsurgery but simplicity does not exclude efficacy. Basic microsurgical instruments include fine tissue forceps (straight and angled), needle holder and scissors, glass rods, and catheters. The fine sutures used vary from 6.0 to 8.0; nonresorbable thread is preferred; polyglycolic can be used, but catgut is never used. There is no need for sophisticated equipment for constant irrigation. Simple irrigation is done by means of 50 cc syringe containing

---

*It is sometimes necessary to perform adhesiolysis before placing Douglas packing (see section on Adhesiolysis).

physiologic saline. Special equipment to ensure safety from laser refractions will probably be available and useful in the near future (see Chap. 5).[7]

CO_2 Laser

Apparatus
There do not seem to be fundamental differences between the various models currently available. A CO_2 laser delivering 10 W of power is sufficient for tubal microsurgery. The laser may be connected either to a microscope or to a handpiece. The connection to a handpiece is preferred for the following reasons:

1. The focal length of the handpiece (50 to 120 mm) which is less than that of a microscope (250 mm), provides a smaller impact diameter useful in microsurgery.
2. The better ease of handling the handpiece always permits one to obtain a perpendicular tissue section, something not always possible with a connection on the microscope.
3. The handpiece permits one to obtain either a focalized or defocalized shot.
4. The main advantage of the connection to the microscope is the precision of the impact, thanks to a micromanipulator placed on the microscope.

Power Density†
Proper use of the CO_2 laser is required in microtubal surgery.[3] The main advantage of the CO_2 laser is the quality of tissue sectioning it provides. It combines immediate hemostasis with minimal tissue damage. Tissue damage, however, depends very much on the power density used for sectioning,[11] as the following results of a study show:[3]

- On day 0 the uterus of a rabbit was sectioned longitudinally, with the CO_2 laser, for 2 cm using an impact diameter of 0.3 mm delivered by a handpiece of 120 mm focal length. The time required for sectioning was recorded for progressively high power densities.
- On day 1 hysterectomy was performed to determine the tissue damage caused by the sectioning. Figure 18–2 clearly shows that it is necessary to use sufficiently high power density which, by lowering tissue exposure time to the CO_2 laser, diminishes tissue damage.

In practice, proper use consists of a connection to the handpiece of a 100 to 120 mm focal length lens which delivers an impact diameter of 0.2 to 0.3 mm at the focal point. This is accomplished with 10 W of power which is necessary and sufficient to guarantee both the least possible tissue damage and an acceptable sectioning rate.

---

†Abbreviations used are: HPD (high power density $\simeq$ 20,000 W/cm^2); LPD (low power density $\simeq$ 1000 W/cm^2).

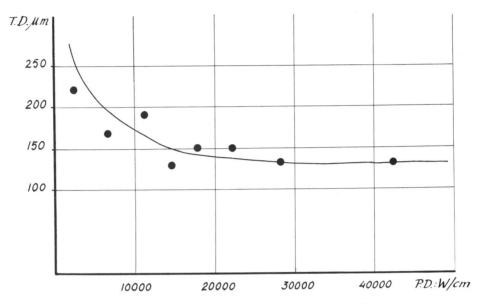

Figure 18–2. Relationship of power density and thermal injury.

Used improperly (i.e., low power density), the CO_2 laser can cause considerable tissue damage, which would diminish its value in microsurgery. This finding was confirmed by a recent study.[8]

Experimental Studies
From the many experimental studies done with the CO_2 laser in tubal microsurgery, it is possible to extract the following two essential points:

1. The CO_2 laser seems to have greater value than the unipolar microelectrode in adhesiolysis.[9,10] Although it is always difficult to extrapolate experimental results to the clinic, this finding suggests that one use of the CO_2 laser instead of a unipolar microelectrode to remove perituboovarian adhesions whose recurrence is one major cause of failure in salpingostomy. Use of the CO_2 laser, however, does not prevent the recurrence of adhesions, i.e., it should be accompanied by other methods designed to prevent such a recurrence.
2. The sectioning of a tube by CO_2 laser does not decrease the quality of subsequent anastomosis.[3] In a comparative study of isthmoisthmic anastomosis in the rabbit, either after CO_2 laser sectioning or after scissor sectioning and hemostasis by bipolar coagulation, we found no statistically significant difference in permeability levels and nidation index between the two techniques, although the results were slightly better after CO_2 laser sectioning (Table 18–2). The main advantage of the CO_2 laser is hemostasis provided concomitantly with sectioning, which shortens the

TABLE 18-2. RESULTS OF EXPERIMENTAL REANASTOMOSIS

Procedure	No. Animals	Tubal Permeability (%)	Nidation Index (%)	Adhesions (%)
Conventional	10	75	59.2	50
Laser CO_2	19	85	64.8	35

operating time and decreases postoperative adhesions. Similar results have been found after anastomosis on the uterine horn of the rabbit.[11]

It appears that one can use the CO_2 laser for all tubal sectioning. Tissue damage is compatible with correct healing and does not interfere with tubal function even after an anastomosis or neosalpingostomy. The immediate hemostasis achieved with the CO_2 laser makes it a technique which is advantageous over all other conventional methods.[12] It also appears that for adhesiolysis and prevention of the recurrence of adhesions, the CO_2 laser is better than a microelectrode.

Principles of Microsurgery

Respect for the principles of microsurgery is at least as important if not more so than the actual use of an operating microscope.[13] It results in surgery with the least amount of trauma. Use of the microscope makes the surgeon realize the need for light-handed surgery, respecting as much as possible the integrity of structures, particularly the peritoneal serosa.[14]

Hemostasis
Although the role of bleeding in the formation of adhesions is not clear, it is evident that careful hemostasis is necessary in microsurgery. It is also evident that it must cause the least possible tissue damage. Use of the CO_2 laser for tissue sectioning (tubal wall or adhesions) often provides simultaneous hemostasis. It is sometimes necessary, however, to perform coagulation of a vessel whose diameter exceeds the hemostatic capacity of the CO_2 laser. For that, one can use either a unipolar microelectrode or a bipolar coagulation. Irrigation of the hemorrhagic area with physiologic saline permits one to accurately localize the responsible vessel and perform timely hemostasis. Immediately after hemostasis is obtained, one should perform peritoneal cavity lavage. The great value of the CO_2 laser is that it assures coagulation of all the small capillaries, whose hemostasis is not otherwise always accomplished spontaneously and which causes tissue damage.

Avoidance of Peritoneal Trauma
The least trauma of the peritoneal serosa may be the focus for prevention of adhesion formation. The following measures are recommended to avoid adhesion formation:

1. Use polished glass rods to manipulate organs.
2. Eliminate talc from gloves by washing before opening the peritoneum.

3. Constantly irrigate the surgical field with physiologic saline.
4. Carefully suture all wounds of the peritonea serosa after dissection.
5. Position peritoneal grafts on large denuded areas. These peritoneal patches may be obtained from the vesicouterine cul-de-sac where the peritoneum is easy to dissect. The size of the peritoneal patch is determined grossly. The patch is carefully separated from the underlying fatty tissue, placed on the deperitonized area, and sutured at the free border of the peritoneum. Cicatrization is most often excellent. On the ovary, it is impossible to use the peritoneal patch, which could hinder follicular rupture. It is possible to suture all the wounds of the ovarian cortex.
6. Avoid complementary procedures such as ovarian suspension with catgut or shortening of the round ligaments as well as resection of the omentum.
7. Carefully suture the parietal peritoneum with polyglycolic thread.

Surgical Technique

There are three main types—terminal plasty, tubotubal anastomosis, and tubouterine anastomosis.

Terminal plasty consists of restoring the normal anatomy of the entire ovary-fimbria. Usually, the lesions occur after an attack of salpingitis, but they can also occur after surgery on the pelvis or after endometriosis. Great care must be taken to ensure that the postinfection lesions are not still developing. Surgical intervention of inflammatory lesions is bound to result in failure.[15,16]

Adhesiolysis

Special attention must be given to performing adhesiolysis. It is the first order of affairs prior to so-called tubal operations and should not be considered secondary or of minor importance. It would be regrettable indeed to have done excellent plastic surgery of the tube only to learn that the operation was unsuccessful due to a recurrence of adhesions.

Adhesiolysis is somewhat tedious but requires considerable meticulousness. An operating microscope is only necessary for perifimbrial adhesions, and the beginning of adhesiolysis can generally be done with magnification.

Adhesions must be delicately raised by means of a special laser rod and sectioned at their extremities by a focused CO_2 laser beam with HPD. Adhesiolysis is usually performed adnexa by adnexa from inside out. It is possible that some thick adhesions cannot be revealed by a glass rod in which case it is necessary to dissect them by excising between the two fixed organs with a small scissors. Hemostasis is then accomplished on demand by bipolar coagulation, since the CO_2 laser is of little value in this case. After freeing the uterus and then the adnexa, the latter are placed in Douglas packing covered by a white plastic platform. The operating microscope can then be installed for microscopic control. It is then necessary to carefully dissect all adhesions between the fimbria and the ovaries in such a way as to restore normal mobility between these two structures. Fine adhesions which can be revealed on a glass rod pose no dissection difficulties. On the other hand, it is often the case that the ampulla and the fimbria are attached to the ovary by a thick adhesion. Dissection then must be done with a microsurgical scissors, cutting from the ampulla toward the fimbria, while trying to remain in the excision field between the ovarian capsule and tubal serosa. This is sometimes difficult because neovascularization may be present; hemostasis in this event should be preventive and wherever possible done with bipolar coagulation. The CO_2 laser is not easy to use in this type of dissection. It is suitable to free the fimbria of the ovarian capsule so as to create normal mobility and enable it to cover nearly the entire surface of the ovary. Dissection must be continued until the vascular pedicle of the fimbria is revealed but not compromised. In some cases, there are thick adhesions on the surface of the ovary which make excision difficult. It is possible to vaporize these adhesions directly with a defocused beam with LPD without injuring the fragile ovarian cortex. All areas of dissection or CO_2 laser vaporization must be carefully washed and wiped with cotton swabs soaked in physiologic saline in order to remove carbonized debris (Figs. 18–3, 18–4).

At the end of adhesiolysis, the surgeon should look for (through the microscope) defects in the peritoneal serosa or ovarian cortex and suture them with nonresorbable 8.0 suture. Large deperitonealized areas, especially subovarian regions, should be covered with a patch of free peritoneum or with a peritoneal rotation flap from the Douglas cul-de-sac and sutured with 6.0 thread.

Numerous publications exist on the subject of adjuvant treatment for prevention of recurrence of adhesions. Steroid therapy is a useful one in adhesiolysis as has been well shown. As with the CO_2 laser, however, one should not expect mir-

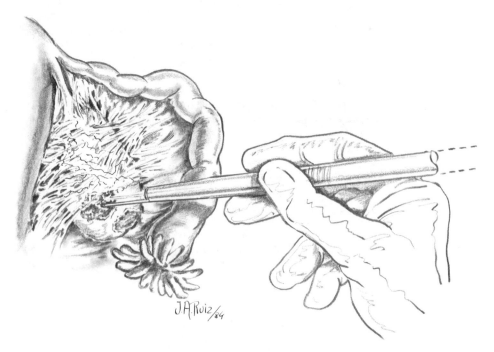

Figure 18–3. Investment adhesions virtually encase the ovary. The laser, utilizing low power densities can vaporize these adhesions bloodlessly even when they are crisscrossed with numerous parasitic vessels.

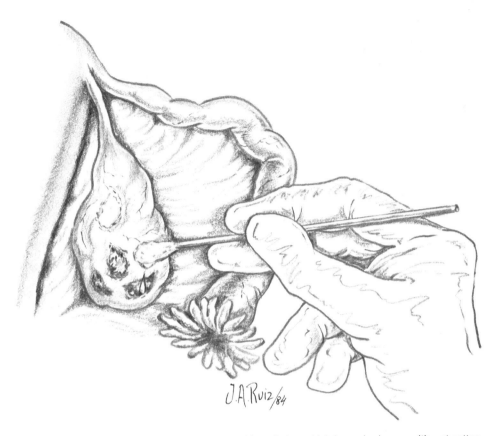

Figure 18–4. Vaporized tissue may leave a residue of char which is washed away with wet cotton swabs.

acles. We administer steroid therapy for 6 days beginning the day before surgery as is done by many other teams (Table 18–3). It is definitely effective if the peritoneal serosa is not severely damaged and if the areas devoid of peritoneum have been sutured. Hydroflotation is also a reasonable adjuvant treatment. The best fluid to use is probably a solution containing 32 percent dextran; 100 to 200 ml are poured into the peritoneal cavity prior to parietal suturing at the end of surgery.

TABLE 18–3. PREOPERATIVE STEROID THERAPY (DECADRON)

	J − 1	J 0	J 1	J 2	J 3	J 4	J 5
AM		20 mg IM	8 mg IM	20 mg	10 mg IM	5 mg	5 mg
PM	8 mg IM	8 mg IM	8 mg IM	20 mg IM (orally)	10 mg (orally)	5 mg (orally)	

Salpingostomy

Salpingostomy consists of creating a new tubal ostium either at the terminal portion of the ampulla (terminal salpingostomy), or after resection of the terminal portion (medioampullar salpingostomy), or after resection of the entire ampulla (isthmic salpingostomy).

The result on fertility is inversely proportional to the extent of ampullary resection so that, in practice, terminal salpingostomy is the method of choice. Isthmic salpingostomy is rarely performed at present.

Salpingostomy is performed in three steps: restoration of ampulla-ovary mobility; opening of the ampulla; and eversion.

1. *Restoration of ampulla–ovary mobility.* It is very important to restore good mobility of the tubal ampulla whose neoostium should "sweep across" the surface of ovary (see section on Adhesiolysis). It is sometimes useful to inject methylene blue before dissecting. Tubal distention facilitates dissection of the terminal portion of the ampulla in cases of adhesion to the ovarian cortex.
2. *Opening of the ampulla* (Fig. 18–5). The tube is gently distended with methylene blue. Under the microscope, it is generally easy to identify the original site of the ostium by a star-shaped scar. Great care must be taken

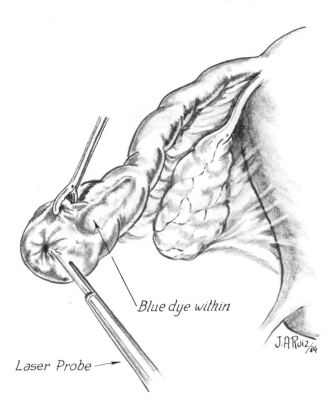

Blue dye within

Laser Probe →

J.A Ruiz/84

Figure 18–5. The hand held laser is employed in order to create the smallest spot and the highest power density, a hole is drilled into the dimple of the hydrosalpinx.

to identify the precise point of opening. It is likely that most of the occlusions following salpingostomy are due to choosing the wrong site for the neostomy. On the clinical setting, linear ampullary salpingostomy for tubal pregnancy has resulted in excellent healing. Only a salpingostomy done at the original site of the ostium has any chance of remaining permeable. A focused CO_2 laser beam with HPD opens the hydrosalpinx at the central point of the ostium. The injected dye prevents damage to the opposite mucosa. It is necessary to make several incisions radiating from 5 to 10 mm along the mucosal folds. The site of these incisions is generally visible under the microscope. Thse incisions are made with a HPD CO_2 laser beam focused on a laser rod introduced via the ostium. Care must be taken not to damage the vascularization of the fimbria. Considerable experience is required in order to know when the ampulla is sufficiently open; one must not make too large or too small an incision, but just enough to permit good eversion of the free folds. When the pavilion is open, one can look for possible intrapavilion adhesions, which are then sectioned on a laser rod by a focused laser beam (Fig. 18–6).

3. *Eversion.* If the tubal wall is supple, eversion can be accomplished by a defocused CO_2 laser with LPD to the serosa of the free folds. There is a retraction of the peritoneal serosa which results in spontaneous eversion. Our experience with second-look laparoscopy has been that this eversion is permanent and that the technique is of value (Fig. 18–7). When the tubal wall does not allow this method, eversion must be maintained by a series of nonresorbable mucoserosal 8.0 sutures. Sometimes two to three are sufficient; at other times a series of points along the entire everted fimbria are necessary.

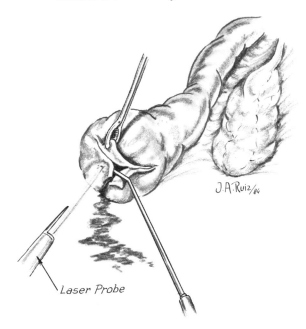

J.A.Ruiz/84

Laser Probe

Figure 18–6. A rod is inserted into the opening created in Figure 18–5. Flaps are cut with the finely focused laser beam. Four cuts are made through the full thickness of the tube.

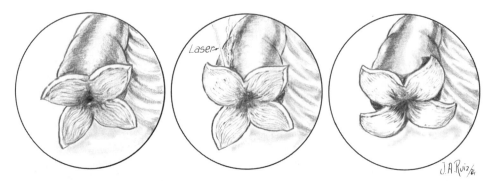

Figure 18–7. A defocused laser beam (low power density) is "played" over the serosal aspect of the flaps to produce flower-like eversion of the endosalpinx.

Particular attention should be given to the following points:

- Opening at the exact site of the former ostium
- Parallel incisions at the mucosal folds in order not to damage the vascularization
- Searching for and freeing of all intraampullary adhesions
- Reestablishing, if possible, the fringe connecting the fimbria to the ovary
- Not everting the ampulla too much like "turning a sock inside out"
- Always being economical with tubal tissue and not performing terminal resection except in the rare case where exploration of the fimbria indicates a mucosa that appears more satisfactory farther from the ostium
- Restoring good tuboovary mobility
- Suturing all defects of the serosa of the tubal ampulla and of the ovarian cortex to avoid adhesions
- Injecting dye at the end of salpingostomy and assuring the absence of dilation upstream from the line of everting sutures

Postoperative Management

It does not appear useful to perform postoperative hydrotubation whose effectiveness remains to be demonstrated. Steroid therapy, along with antibiotic therapy (ampicillin or doxycycline), is advised to help prevent postoperative adhesions (see section on Adhesiolysis).

In the case of difficult operations, a combination of antibiotics and corticosteroids can be prescribed for 2 to 3 weeks.

Tubal Reanastomosis

This is without doubt the technique which benefits most from microsurgery (Fig. 18–8). Overall, the success rate of reversal of sterilization has doubled with microsurgical procedures. The CO_2 laser is especially useful since it generally permits resection of the block before anastomosis without hemostasis, which results in considerable time saving. Tubal block can result from sterilization or from a pathologic condition—infection, endometriosis, or polyp. The technique which does

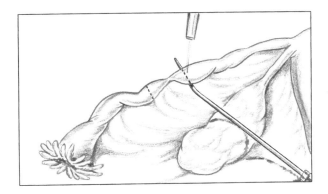

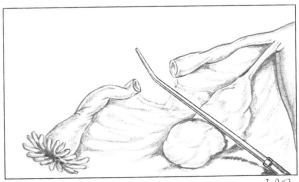

Figure 18–8. An obstructed segment of oviduct is cut away using a backstop rod (beneath to absorb the remaining laser energy).

J. A. Ruiz/84

not differ according to the cause involves two steps—resection of the block and anastomosis.

Resection of the Block. This is accomplished with a focused CO_2 laser beam with HPD in order to minimize tissue damage during tubal sectioning. Our experience suggests that it is possible to section the mucosa with HPD CO_2 laser beam. If the subtubal vessels are not compromised, the sectioning is bloodless, which is advantageous especially if one performs several sectionings before locating the healthy region. The sectioning should be perpendicular to the longitudinal axis of the tube. Organs situated behind the tube should be protected from the laser beam, either by a laser rod or by a very moist compress. The following three points should be emphasized, regardless of the site of anastomosis:

1. Tubal resection on the uterine side should be done until the injection of blue dye in the uterus is accompanied by a definite jet from the section.
2. Placing an intratubal catheter is not necessary, and moreover, it is important to prevent introducing foreign matter into the tube. For the novice or in difficult cases, however, a catheter facilitates anastomosis. If the surgeon is satisfied with the operation, the catheter can be removed imme-

diately, otherwise it can be left in place for several days. It is better to remove the catheter by the abdominal wall rather than via the uterus.

3. Anastomosis after laser sectioning does not differ from classic techniques and involves two series of suture points with 8.0 thread. The first is a series of separate extramucosal points and the second involves the serosa, either in separate points or in two whip stitches. In all cases, a first point is made with 6.0 thread at the mesosalpinx connecting the two regions to be anastomosed so that the suture is made without tension. This is a major factor in the success of microsurgical anastomosis. After the anastomosis is completed, blue dye is injected to ensure that it is permeable and does not leak. Depending on the site of anastomosis one can perform the following:

Tubotubal Anastomosis

1. Isthmoisthmic: This is the easiest to perform with two suture levels. The extramucosal level involves four to five points beginning with the most difficult, i.e., the point near the mesosalpinx.
2. Ampulloampullary: The larger the diameter of the tubal lumen, the greater the number of points required. The thinness of the muscle layer sometimes warrants only a single extramucosal suture.
3. Isthmoampullary: This type poses a problem in incongruence between the two lumens to be anastomosed—those of the isthmus and the ampulla. Of the methods proposed, we use that of Winston which consists of gently inserting a 1 mm diameter grooved probe into the blind end of the ampulla. A laser beam opens the tip of the tube on a few millimeters, and the end of the probe is inserted through this opening. The two lumens are sutured having basically the same size; a plastic splint can be placed in the groove to catheterize the ampulla.

Tubouterine Anastomosis: Isthmointerstitial Anastomosis. This type is always preferred over reimplantation if the intramural portion is permeable over several millimeters (Fig. 18–9). It is also, without doubt, the most difficult type of anastomosis to perform because the suture points on the uterine side are not easy to make. Three points merit attention:

1. The two lumens should be approximated by a 6.0 suture between mesosalpinx and uterus in order to avoid tension.
2. A splint should be used in the slightest case of difficulty to facilitate the anastomosis. Take care to carry out a perfect peritonization.
3. The laser is useful in these anastomoses because the successive sections that are sometimes required to locate the permeable portion generally do not hemorrhage. It is wise to use several slightly defocused laser beams to fashion the tubal extremity in order to facilitate placing the suture points and obtain perfect congruence.

Tubal Reimplantation. This technique is rarely performed because it is generally possible to locate a permeable intramural portion and perform isthmointerstitial anastomosis, and the results of this technique are always less favorable than those of anastomosis (Fig. 18–10).

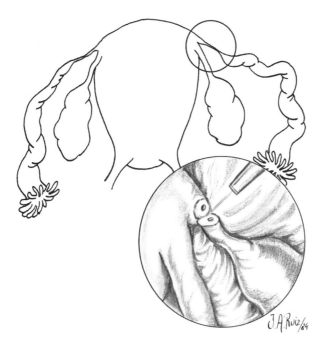

Figure 18–9. The laser may substitute for a knife to "shave" the interstitial (intramural) portion of the oviduct until patency is demonstrated. This direct anastomotic technique is preferred to reimplantation whenever possible.

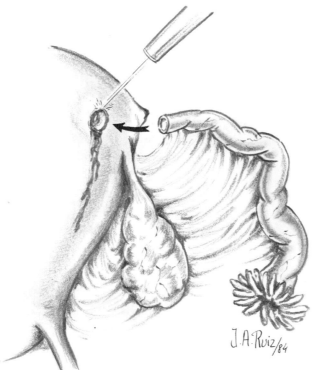

Figure 18–10. When tubal implantation is necessary. High power settings and a 1.5 to 2.0 mm spot allow for a clean hole to be drilled into the posterior aspect of the uterus.

The CO_2 laser is useful here because it permits one to excavate to the desired extent the orifice in the uterine horn. This neoorifice can be created by a focused laser beam cutting the periphery of the opening. Injection of diluted vasopressin is useful since hemostasis with the CO_2 laser is not always complete in the uterine horn. The tubal extremity is cut and bivalved. Each bivalve is connected by a 6.0 or 7.0 polyglycolic thread, each end of which is passed through the new orifice and then through the uterine muscle. The two ends of each thread are then sutured together.

Postoperative Surveillance

Three points merit special attention in the postoperative period. The first is to treat other possible causes of infertility, such as dysovulation, in order that the patient is in the best condition to become pregnant.

The second is to inform the patient of the risk of ectopic pregnancy following plastic surgery of the terminal point of the tube and the importance of quickly notifying the physician in the event of any delay in the menstrual period. Detection of pregnancy by basal body temperature (BBT) is, of course, preferred but not always possible to perform on all patients.

The third is to check tubal permeability postoperatively. If an intrauterine pregnancy does not soon occur, it is wise to ensure tubal permeability. Hysterography is sufficient in cases of anastomosis and we perform it during the third postoperative month. In the case of salpingostomy, we prefer to perform laparoscopy 6 to 8 weeks after surgery. This permits one to check not only the plastic result but to remove any adhesions that may have reformed. This procedure is not followed by all and some perform second-look laparoscopy only in the absence of intrauterine pregnancy after 12 to 18 months.

Evaluation of the Results

Evaluation of the results of tubal surgery is confounded by several factors.

The first is the need for a long-term assessment of the value of any technique, which is particularly true for the CO_2 laser which was installed in our clinic only in the beginning of 1979. The CO_2 laser has been used by numerous surgical teams but there are still insufficient data to permit definitive assessment of the results.

The second factor is the evaluation of the results of salpingostomy. The lack of an internationally adopted classification of the lesion, i.e., the severity of tubal involvement, makes comparison of the results of different studies difficult. Prognosis depends heavily on the extent of tubal involvement and patient selection greatly influences the results.

The third factor concerns the manner of evaluating the results which may easily introduce bias. For example, discounting patients lost to follow-up or those having presented with a postoperative pelvic inflammatory disease, artificially increases the success rate. In addition, in the case of asymmetric intervention, as for example, on one side adhesiolysis and salpingostomy on the other, the patient should be classified in the framework of the more successful intervention and not the opposite. Some investigations lump all forms of fecundation including intrauterine pregnancies, miscarriages, and extrauterine pregnancies.

TABLE 18–4. RESULTS OF MICROSURGERY USING CO$_2$ LASER

Procedure	No. Patients	Minimal Follow-up (mo)	Post-operative Permeability	Intra-uterine Pregnancy (3 mo)	Sponta-neous Abortion	Ectopic Preg-nancy
Salpingostomy	38	18	91%[a]	9 (23.7%)	4 (10.4%)	3(8%)
Reversal of sterilization	15	3	100%[b]	8 (53.3%)	1 (6.8%)	0

[a]On 34 patients.
[b]On 14 patients.

This habit should cease with a classification system to separate ectopic pregnancy, miscarriage, and term pregnancy. The only pregnancy of value to the patient is, of course, the latter.

Naturally, the results should be evaluated in patients having undergone any surgical intervention. Because of the recent use of the CO$_2$ laser in tubal microsurgery, there are no current valid statistics in the literature.

We report below our results in terms of two types of intervention: those involving either pathologic fallopian tubes (salpingostomy) or healthy ones (reversal of sterilization).

Of the 38 patients who underwent, with an 18-month minimal followup, terminal bilateral or unilateral salpingostomy, 9 (23.7 percent) achieved a term pregnancy, 4 (10.4 percent) had a miscarriage, and 3 (8 percent) had an ectopic pregnancy.

The postoperative permeability, evaluated in 34 patients by control postoperative laparoscopy, was 91 percent (Table 18–4).

On the 15 patients who underwent reversal of sterilization with a 3-month minimal follow-up, 8 (53.3 percent) have achieved a term pregnancy or are pregnant for more than 3 months, 1 (6.2 percent) had a miscarriage. None of these patients had an extrauterine pregnancy. The postoperative permeability evaluated in 14 patients (1 patient lost in follow-up) and involving 24 tubes was 100 percent. The short follow-up of some patients permits us to hope for an increased success rate (Table 18–4).

These percentages are similar to those reported in the literature for conventional surgical procedures, which is promising, considering the newness of using the CO$_2$ laser and the future technologic progress designed to decrease the diameter of laser beam impact and improve ease of handling.

REFERENCES

1. Baggish MS, Chong, AP: Carbon dioxide laser microsurgery of the uterine tube. Obstet Gynecol 58:111, 1981
2. Bellina JH: Microsurgery of the fallopian tube with CO$_2$ laser—82 cases with follow-up. Laser Surg Med 36:129, 1982
3. Bruhat MA, Mage G: Progress in CO$_2$ laser tubal microsurgery. Presented at the 4th Congress of International Society of Laser Surgery Tokyo, 1981 (unpublished data)
4. Bruhat MA, Mage G: Use of CO$_2$ laser in Salpingotomy. In Kaplan I (ed): Laser Surgery III, Part One. Jerusalem, Jerusalem Academic Press, 1979, p 271

5. Mage G, Bruhat MA: Pregnancy following salpingostomy. Comparison between CO_2 laser and electrosurgery procedure. Fertil Steril (in press)
6. Bruhat MA, Mage G, Manhes H, et al: Place de la coelioscopie dans le bilan de la stérilité féminine. J Fr Gynecol Obstet Biol Reprod 9:337, 1980
7. McLaughlin DS: Advanced surgical instrumentation needed for intra-abdominal application of the carbon dioxide laser in reproductive biology. Lasers Surg Med 2:241, 1983
8. Fayez JA, Jobson VW, Lentz SS, et al: Tubal microsurgery with the carbon dioxide laser. Am J Obstet Gynecol 146:371, 1983
9. Schiedel P, Walleizener G, Hepp H: CO_2 laser in treatment of pelvic adhesions: Experimental results. In Kaplan I (ed): Laser Surgery III, Part One. Jerusalem, Jerusalem Academic Press, 1980, p 269
10. Tadir Y, Ovadia J, Margara R, Winston RHL: Intraperitoneal adhesiolysis by CO_2 laser. In Atsumi, K, Nimsakul N (eds): Microsurgery in Laser. 4th Congress of the I.S.L.S., Tokyo 13:27, 1981
11. Choe JK, Dawood MY, Andrews AH: Conventional versus laser reanastomosis of rabbit ligated uterine horns. Obstet Gynecol 61:689, 1982
12. Verschueren R: In Van Gorgum (ed): The CO_2 Laser in Tumor Surgery. Amsterdam, Assem, 1976
13. Chamberlain G, Winston R (eds): Tubal Infertility. London, Blackwell, 1982
14. Gomel V (ed): Micro-Surgical Techniques in Infertility. Clin Obstet Gynecol. Hagerstown, Harper and Row, 1980
15. Oviducte et Fertility. (Proceeding of Société Nationale pour l'Etude de la Stérilité et de la Fécondité). Paris, Masson, 1979
16. Cornier E (coordinateur): Techniques Microchirurgicales de la Sterilite. Paris, Masson, 1982

19

Laser Surgery for Adhesions

Robert W. Kelly

INTRODUCTION

"Pelvic adhesions from one source or another represent the greatest single cause of failure in modern reproductive surgery. If adhesions are not present prior to surgery, it is probable they will be present after surgery." Engrossed as we are in the technologic revolution of the 1980s, we can still imagine these statements being made by a prominent reproductive surgeon in 1954. Little would he know his statements would remain applicable for at least three decades. Even though our knowledge of the healing process has increased tremendously in the last 30 years, adhesions still remain a major problem. A multitude of surgical techniques and adjuncts have come and gone over the years in the search for an answer to this dilemma. One of the most important advances, however, has been the introduction of the operating microscope and "microsurgical tissue handling" techniques. This trend, which was largely propagated by the work of Swolin, began in 1967[1] and has continued to grow. Magnification, delicate instruments, fine suture, reduced tissue handling, removal of lint and talc, and less traumatic methods of dissection have probably all contributed to the reduction in postoperative adhesion formation, but have not totally prevented it. There seems to be no common denominator in the process of postoperative scarring. It remains a complicated physiologic and anatomic process, the course of which remains unpredictable and difficult to alter.

PELVIC ADHESIONS

The literature is replete with articles dealing with the surgical management of patients with pelvic adhesions as a cause of infertility. Pregnancy rates have varied widely from study to study. Valid comparison of the reported pregnancy rates has been extremely difficult because of the lack of institution of a uniform system of classification for adhesions. Varying degrees of ovarian and tubal involvement with adhesions, the rarity of adhesions as an isolated problem, and associated infertility factors, e.g., anovulation, make the situation very complex. For example, it would take the average practitioner many years to collect 30 or more patients with essentially the same degree of pelvic adhesions of the same etiology with no fimbrial damage and no other infertility factors. Clinical studies are subsequently observational and involve patient groups that are heterogeneous with regard to the extent of adhesions, the presence of associated tubal obstruction in varying locations along the tube, associated infertility factors such as anovulation, and the etiology of the adhesions. It is possible for instance that adhesions which have been caused by previous surgery are more prone to give a poor surgical outcome than are adhesions which have resulted from endometriosis or infection. This is of course speculation, but it emphasizes the multitude of variables which may exist and which ultimately must be addressed in a comprehensive system of adhesion classification. Hulka and colleagues[2] published a classification system in 1978 which divided adhesions into two major groups depending on whether they were thin, filmy, and avascular or thick, fibrous, and vascular. They further subdivided each of these two groups according to the amount of ovarian surface that was visible, i.e., I—100 percent, II—>50 percent, III—<50 percent, and IV—not visible. Their system did not have a mechanism for dealing with peritubal adhesions which did not involve the ovary, i.e., tube adherent to bowel or omentum. They did not have sufficient data to give pregnancy rates for each of the eight groups possible. Unfortunately, this system was not widely adopted by tubal surgeons even though it represented a reproducible mechanism by which surgical techniques might be evaluated. Thus, we continue to determine the efficacy of various surgical techniques and adjuvants in a time-consuming and inconsistent fashion, extrapolating from apples to oranges.

ADJUVANTS FOR PREVENTION OF ADHESIONS

No discusson of surgery for pelvic adhesions would be complete without at least brief mention of the numerous adjuvants that are currently in vogue. One of the most basic concepts is that of preoperative removal of the powder from surgical gloves. This is best done with careful rinsing of the gloves using a continuous flow of solution or at least two washes in separate basins. The importance of lint, talc, and corn starch granulomas as a cause of adhesions is clearly demonstrated by the works of Diamond[3] and Yaffe et al.[4] Another commonly used adjuvant is that of 32 percent dextran 70 which received strong support by Di Zerega and Hodgen in 1980[5] in their study in monkeys where they compared 32 percent dextran 70, 10 percent dextran 40, and the combination of dexamethasone, promethazine, and ampicillin. They found only the 32 percent dextran 70 to be effective in preventing adhesions in monkeys, but emphasized the need for controlled, objective studies in women to determine its usefulness in humans. Early second-look laparoscopy has been suggested by many authors. The importance of this technique has been reaffirmed more recently by Surrey and Friedman[6], and also by Raj and Hulka.[7]

Again, further controlled studies will be needed before the efficacy of early second look can be clearly determined. Other adjuvants including frequent irrigation, heparinized irrigation, and nonsteroidal anti-inflammatory agents are also embroiled in the controversy that still remains to be settled.

ACCESSORY INSTRUMENTS

There are many available accessory instruments for use in laser surgery for treatment of adhesions. Undoubtedly, the most useful instruments are the quartz and the Pyrex rods. These materials absorb the laser energy and dissipate the heat generated. They are primarily used as backstops during dissection. While the quartz rods are probably superior in terms of durability, they are far more expensive. In 1983, a 1-year supply of 6 mm Pyrex could be purchased for about the same cost as one quartz rod.

The Pyrex rod is available through scientific product suppliers in 3-foot lengths. It can be pulled and fire polished with the use of an inexpensive propane torch to the desired length and configuration. Its surface is smooth and it will not abrade tissue. The 6 mm rods are thick enough so that they can be used as gentle tissue retractors with safety in the abdomen. Smaller diameter rods should probably be avoided because of the danger of breakage. The Pyrex rod will get subsurface fractures from laser impact at high power densities. When a significant number of these fracture lines appear, the rod should be discarded, i.e., usually after 2 to 3 cases. The most common configuration for the rod is a 15 to 18 cm length with a 2 to 2.5 cm right angle at one end, but any shape or length the surgeon finds useful is acceptable.

A useful alternative to the rods is wet Telfa. This material holds water well, making it virtually impenetrable by the laser as long as it is kept wet. It can be cut to any shape or size; it is inexpensive, readily available, nonabrasive and disposable.

The physical properties of the laser allow it to be reflected off mirrored surfaces. This can be both advantageous and hazardous. The hazard comes if the laser is reflected off a polished instrument such as a retractor and damages surrounding structures. Fortunately, however, this has not often been reported as a complication of laser usage. The advantage of this ability to be reflected is that it allows access to otherwise inaccessible areas of the pelvis. Either a stainless steel mirror or a silver-fronted dental mirror can be used for this purpose. The laser is focused on the image in the mirror and the surgeon operates on the image. There is no necessity for mentally reversing the image. If the surgeon makes the mistake of focusing on the mirror instead of the image, the mirror will likely be damaged. A brief amount of practice time with the mirror will usually be sufficient for mastery of the technique and procedures will become substantially easier.

Without a doubt the surgeon's best ally for intraabdominal laser surgery is irrigation. Since the laser energy is entirely absorbed by 1 mm or less of water, flooding those areas surrounding the operative site offers total protection from damage to underlying or surrounding structures. It is important, however, that the tissue which is the subject of dissection not be covered with solution. Laser impact on even small pools or irrigation causes the solution to boil and results in thermal damage to underlying tissue. Tissues are kept moist by frequent irrigation, but excesses are removed from the area of dissection by suction prior to laser impact.

CO_2 LASER FOR LYSIS OF ADHESIONS

The specifications necessary for a laser unit to be acceptable for use in the abdomen have been addressed elsewhere in this book. The problem then is to decide how one desires to use the TEM_{00} mode CO_2 laser, i.e., either with the hand scalpel or the micromanipulator. Many laser surgeons desire to use the hand scalpel while viewing with optical loops or with the operating microscope much as one would do when using the microcautery with standard microsurgery. Proponents of this technique feel that the smaller spot size (125 μm) allows higher power densities and decreases thermal damage. This is true, but the depth of focus for this system is limited and this factor may well offset the proposed advantage. The focal length for the hand scalpel is only 125 mm. If one is out of the focal plane by only 5 mm, the power density is decreased by 83 percent leaving only 17 percent of the calculated power density. On the other hand, the ability to defocus the handheld system at will during the procedure is a distinct advantage. By simply moving the laser scalpel back from the tissue, the beam is defocused and the power density is reduced. This is very useful when working with adhesions. Working deep in the cul-de-sac, however, is cumbersome with the hand scalpel and the focal distance again becomes a problem. In contrast to the hand scalpel is the micromanipulator attached to the microscope. This system can have a focal length of 250 to 400 mm, but can still give a spot size of 200 μm. A 300 mm system gives adequate working room under the microscope and offers a comfortable position for the surgeon. With the greater focal length, the depth of focus is greater. Being out of focus 5 mm reduces power density of a 250 mm focal length system by only 47 percent as compared to 83 percent for the 125 mm handheld system. To defocus this system, however, requires manipulation of the adapter lens. This is generally easily done in a matter of 2 to 3 seconds, but still does not allow the very large spot size that can be attained by defocusing with the hand scalpel. Another major advantage to the micromanipulator is the precision of control it offers over the hand scalpel. A 7 mm movement of the micromanipulator "joystick" moves the beam only 1 mm in the operative field.

Few animal studies have been done comparing the degree of adhesion formation after laser microsurgery to that after standard microsurgery. Choe et al.[8] looked at the effect of the CO_2 laser on adhesion formation after microsurgical reanastomosis of the ligated uterine horn in the rabbit and compared their results to a control group done with standard microsurgery. Fourteen rabbits had ligation and division of both uterine horns. Four weeks later, seven rabbits had conventional microsurgical resection of the ligated stumps and reanastomosis. The other seven rabbits had laser resection of the ligated stumps followed by reanastomosis. They used a laser with a TEM_{01} mode and a spot size of 2 mm with power densities ranging from 637 to 796 W/cm^2. These power densities are considerably lower than the power densities currently used by most laser microsurgeons. These authors showed a significant reduction (P < .001) in adhesion formation in the laser group.

Martin et al[9] performed tubal incision and anastomosis in 18 virgin Sprague Dawley rats at the time of a single laparotomy. They used three different incisional modes: 1000 W/cm^2, 12,000 W/cm^2, and sharp incision. They noted no difference in the percentage of animals forming adhesions or in the severity of adhesions among the three groups of animals.

Clinical application of the CO_2 laser to adhesion removal is done in many different ways. In general, as a surgeon becomes more proficient with the laser, he will use higher power densities and move away from the interrupted modes of application (single or repeat pulse). These changes allow dissection to proceed more rapidly with less thermal damage to tissue. As a rule of thumb, the surgeon should operate with the highest power density he can comfortably and safely control in a given situation to get the desired result.

Filmy adhesions are excised by holding them with a forceps and vaporizing both ends. The 6 mm Pyrex rod is invaluable for this type of dissection. It is also wise to flood the pelvis with irrigation for this process. Multiple rods can be used to place the adhesions under gentle traction. While cutting over the rod, however, one should hold the rod slightly away from the tissue to be lased if possible. This prevents transmission of heat from the Pyrex to the tissue. This transmission is easily detected when the rod is in contact with the tissue because the tissue will be noted to fuse to the rod. If this occurs, irrigation and gentle traction are generally sufficient to separate the surfaces. Adhesions are transected immediately adjacent to the serosal surface of the involved organ. If this is carried out properly, there should be no blanching or other detectable change of the organ surface. Power densities in the range of 3000 to 5000 W/cm^2 are usually adequate for this type of dissection, although higher power densities are appropriate. A small spot size is preferable here, usually 200 to 800 μm in diameter. Thick, fibrous adhesions between surfaces require more tedious dessection, but can frequently result in a good outcome. If the beam can be applied parallel to the axis of the adhesive plane, a small spot size with high power density seems to work best, e.g., ovary adherent to the uterine corpus. If the beam must be applied tangentially, it is sometimes necessary to use a larger spot size (1 to 2 mm) with lower power density, e.g., tube adherent to ovary. This allows separation of the surfaces with gentle traction and avoids actual incision of the serosal surface or ovarian capsule. The beam is applied at the leading edge of the adherent surface in a sweeping motion allowing vaporization of the adhesive fibers. Traction facilitates removal of the underlying normal tissue from the path of the beam and keeps a fresh supply of adhesive fibers exposed. Traction is best applied with opposing finger pressure or pressure from the Pyrex rods. Clamps and pick-ups should be avoided if possible and used only on tissue that is to be excised. The surgeon soon becomes comfortable operating with the laser beam close to the gloved fingers or other vital structures as he appreciates the precise way in which the laser can be applied. In situations where structures are poorly accessible by direct line of vision, mirrored surfaces become essential to the laser surgeon. This author prefers a silver fronted dental mirror that is at a 45 degree angle to the handle. The handle should be smooth and of an appropriate length for optimal control. The mirror is heated to body temperature by warm irrigating solution prior to use. Rewarming is generally necessary at frequent intervals. The surface of the mirror must be dried before laser impact lest one boil the water on the mirror surface. If the mirror surface becomes coated with liquid, dried blood, or debris, it will rapidly become pitted and unsuitable for further use. Since the laser plume is primarily water vapor, it must be suctioned off before it coats the mirror. Usually placement of the suction tip immediately adjacent to the mirror is sufficient to accomplish this purpose.

Frequently one encounters relatively large surface areas on the ovary or uterus that are covered with adhesions that are not amenable to excision. These areas can be vaporized using a spot size of 2 mm or more with power densities in the range of 500 to 1000 W/cm^2. A gentle sweeping motion to vaporize the involved areas works well and avoids capsular or serosal disruption although slight serosal blanching may occur. Raw surfaces can be treated in a similar fashion to prevent capillary oozing. Many feel this maneuver decreases the likelihood of postoperative adherence of neighboring structures, but this effect remains to be proved. After surface adhesions are vaporized, there can be a significant amount of carbonized debris present on the surface. Some feel this should be removed by debriding with wet cotton swabs. The author feels this type of removal is traumatic, often leading to bleeding, and prefers copious irrigation of the surfaces instead. All of the carbonized debris may not be removed by irrigation, but at second-look laparoscopy there is usually little or no carbon visible,[10] having been removed by the normal activity of peritoneal macrophages.

The technical advantages of the laser as an adjunct to microsurgery readily become apparent as one uses it. These advantages have been almost universally acknowledged by those microsurgeons using the laser. They include shortened operating time, improved hemostasis, increased precision of application, and decreased tissue damage. The laser's ability to be reflected off mirrored surfaces improves access to difficult areas. The construction of the micromanipulator decreases the significance of intention tremors or other extraneous movements by the surgeon. Densely adherent surfaces are more easily separated and the resulting surfaces are more likely to be intact.

The impact of the CO_2 laser on pregnancy rates in patients having microsurgery for pelvic adhesions is unknown as of this writing. To date, the only published series dealing with adhesiolysis that has classified adhesions such that other investigators might reproduce the study is that of Kelly and Roberts.[10] The overall study included 69 patients in three groups. There were 28 patients with hydrosalpinges, 27 of whom had associated adhesions. Current data on those patients show a 21.4 percent term pregnancy rate and a 7 percent ectopic rate. Eighty-three percent of those patients had demonstrated patency of at least one tube or their only remaining tube from 3 to 12 months postoperatively. In their adhesiolysis group there were an additional 21 patients who were staged according to Hulka and colleagues' 1978 classification. There were insufficient numbers for calculation of pregnancy rates in each of the adhesion subgroups, but the overall term pregnancy rate was 29 percent with one ectopic reported. As these authors expand their series over time and as other series are reported, the effect of the CO_2 laser on the outcome of infertility surgery for adhesions can be determined.

SUMMARY

The use of the CO_2 laser as an adjunctive tool in the treatment of pelvic adhesions as a cause of infertility appears to be promising. Its ability to make fine hemostatic incisions with great precision and minimal trauma to surrounding structures is a very positive feature. Technically, it is superior to cautery for this type of surgery. We must remember, however, that as of this writing, the laser has not been clearly shown to improve pregnancy rates in patients having infertility surgery for pelvic adhesions. The laser does not compensate poor surgical technique or poor patient selection. The surgeon must educate himself thoroughly in the physics and use of the laser lest it become his enemy.

REFERENCES

1. Swolin K: Fifty fertility operations: Literature and methods. Acta Obstet Gynecol Scand 46:234, 1967
2. Hulka JF, Omran K, Berger GS: Classificaiton of adnexal adhesions: A proposal and evaluation of its prognostic value. Fertil Steril 30:661, 1978
3. Diamond E: Lysis of postoperative pelvic adhesions in infertility. Fertil Steril 31:287, 1979
4. Yaffe H, Beyth Y, Reinhartz T, Levij I: Foreign body granulomas in peritubal and periovarian adhesions: A possible cause for unsuccessful reconstructive surgery in fertility. Fertil Steril 33:283, 1980
5. Di Zerega GS, Hodgen GD: Prevention of postoperative tubal adhesions: Comparative study of commonly used agents. Am J Obstet Gynecol 136:173, 1980
6. Surrey MW, Friedman S: Second look laparoscopy after reconstructive pelvic surgery for infertility. J Reprod Med 27:658, 1982
7. Raj SG, Hulka JF: Second look laparoscopy in infertility surgery: Therapeutic and prognostic value. Fertil Steril 38:325, 1982
8. Choe JK, Dawood MY, Andrews AH: Conventional versus laser reanastomosis of rabbit ligated uterine horns. Obstet Gynecol 61:689, 1983
9. Martin DC, McCoy TD, Poston WM: Comparative study of reanastomosis following laser incision and sharp incision of the rat uterine horn. Presented at the First World Conference: Fallopian Tube in Health and Disease, Palm Beach, Florida, May, 1983
10. Kelly RW, Roberts DK: Experience with the CO_2 laser in gynecologic microsurgery. Am J Obstet Gynecol 146:285–588, 1983 (updated by personal communication)

20

Laser Techniques for Pelvic Adhesions

Daniel C. Martin

Pelvic adhesions causing infertility and pelvic pain can be the result of gynecologic operations, pelvic inflammatory disease, or endometriosis. One of the first steps in the use and knowledge of laser surgery for adhesions is to attempt to prevent their occurrence. Meticulous care at ovarian cystectomies, prompt treatment of pelvic inflammatory disease, and early recognition and therapy for endometriosis can decrease adhesion formation and can help the patient avoid the need for therapy.

PRINCIPLES

The laser is a surgical unit that can aid in reconstructive pelvic surgery. The laser is not a replacement for gentle, precise, and hemostatic surgery. If the laser is used as if it creates its own magic, the laser can do more damage than good. With ongoing experience, the surgeon can anticipate an increased ease in difficult dissections, decreased operating time, decreased blood loss, and increased extent of surgery performed through the laparoscope.[1]

GENERAL

David[2] has adequately covered the general considerations prior to any surgical therapy for pelvic adhesions or distal tubal disease. The controversies regarding these considerations are well recognized. He has included:

1. Preoperative medications which may include steroids, antihistamines, and antibiotics
2. Hemostatic incision into the abdomen
3. Washing powder from the surgical gloves
4. Packing the intestines with moist pads which can be wrapped with Silastic
5. Using microsurgical equipment and suture
6. Using either Ringer's solution with heparin or Macrodex
7. Adhering to general microsurgical principles.

To these are added:

1. Using a wound protector to decrease oozing into the abdomen
2. Using a Kirschner retractor or equivalent to avoid damage to the lateral nerves.

EDUCATION

As laser surgery will be a new concept to most surgeons, operating without touching the tissue and cutting without resistance will require the development of new skills. This will require education available in microsurgery courses, intraabdominal laser courses, intraabdominal laser preceptorships, and practice on surgical specimens or other objects in the operating room. Empiricism with laser techniques should be in the laboratory or in the operating room with surgical specimens, steak, grapefruits, or other objects. Do not expect that a few courses or a few months of work will create competence with the laser. If an orientation towards preoperative preparation is not followed, preventable damage can occur.

LASER TECHNIQUE OF INCISION

The laser incises by vaporization. The laser destroys or removes tissues by use of three techniques: coagulation, excision, or ablation. Coagulation denatures the protein and results in subsequent necrosis. Excision of tissue can be performed by undermining a lesion by vaporizing the tissue beneath the lesion. Ablation converts the tissue into a carbon plume.

The Nd:YAG laser predominantly causes coagulation. The argon laser acts by a combination of coagulation and ablation. The CO_2 laser is most useful for ablation and excision. The action of a laser at this level is one of flash vaporization in a controlled vaporization width which is usually from 0.2 to 1.0 mm. Tissue in the immediate zone surrounding this receives superficial thermal damage and heals well. The thermal damage is predominately a function of exposure to heat from the target tissue. Although this is generally limited by the 100°C vaporization point of water, temperatures in excess of 200°C can be created by burning fat. Tissue can be welded to quartz rods at temperatures in excess of 1665°C.

CLINICAL STUDIES

Many studies suggest that laparoscopic laser, microscopic laser, and contemporary surgical techniques are equally efficacious.[1,3,4,5,6,7,8–10] These studies have been reviewed and summarized by Daniell.[11] In the largest series, 230 patients were followed for 2 years. In this study, 3 of 8 (38 percent) of patients with bipolar disease, 37 of 114 (32 percent) patients with previous reconstructive surgery, and 44 of 102 (43 percent) patients with no previous surgery conceived.[3] In a multicenter study of 106 patients, at second-look laparoscopy, adhesions were decreased at pelvic sites. Nonlaser surgery appeared to have an equal efficacy for prevention of some adhesion reformation.[12] Similar results were noted following ovarian resections in 25 patients.[8]

Adhesion formation appears to be related to the presence of previous adhesions, foreign bodies, infections, and ischemia. Ischemia appears to be the most important of these. Large spot sizes and low power densities increase the time of exposure and thus increase stomal necrosis and ischemia. This should be expected to cause increased fibrosis and stenosis.[13] Small spot sizes and high energy densities decrease the time of exposure and thermal necrosis with a slight decrease in hemostasis.[14] Pulse modes also decrease thermal necrosis.

MODES OF DELIVERY

Handheld Lysis

The handheld unit most resembles the scalpel and is initially the easiest to use. It also has the greatest range of motion. This range, however, gives it the greatest chance of being reflected from other instruments or aimed at unintended targets. The exact impact area of the beam should be observed at all times. The hand held unit also has the greatest range of power densities and can produce spot sizes of from 0.2 mm to greater than 10.0 mm for incision, ablating, and coagulating with much ease. This range of spot sizes results from the short focal length and short depth of field. The short depth of field requires either a depth gauge or much practice to keep the instrument in focus for cutting. The depth gauge has the disadvantage of interfering with motion and of being disconcerting as it is 2 to 3 mm lateral to the laser beam. Often the depth gauge will result in the operator pulling the instrument back out of focus 5 to 15 mm in an attempt to keep the depth gauge from pulling across tissue. Moving back from the focal spot decreases the power density significantly. The hand held unit at 1 cm out of focus has been measured as losing 93 percent of the power density when compared to tight focus. (Table 20–1). As the power density decreases, the time of incision increases. This increases tissue necrosis, ischemia, and fibrosis.[13]

The hand held unit is most useful for lysis of midline adhesions and distal tubal occlusions. A barrier must be placed behind the adhesions to stop the penetration of the laser beam as cutting past the target tissue and damaging other organs is a significant possibility. The barrier can be soaked sponges, solutions, rods, adhesions, the tissue itself, or peritoneal sidewall. The rods can be made of Pyrex,

TABLE 20–1. POWER DENSITY IN THE DEFOCUSED AREA[a]

Distance from Focal Length	125 mm Handheld		250 mm Microscope	
	Microns	*W/cm²*	*Microns*	*W/cm²*
0 mm	220	26,000	450	6500
5 mm	530	4400	600	3500
10 mm	840	1800	750	2200

[a]Power = 10 W, port beam = 8 mm.

quartz, or etched metals. The water, Pyrex, quartz, adhesions, and peritoneum will all absorb the beam. Wet solutions will boil off at 100°C as they absorb the beam. Quartz and Pyrex rods will be etched and have been shattered. Glass rods and rods of less than 3 mm in diameter should be avoided as the heat distribution from these exceeds 1200°C and can shatter the rods rapidly. Under experimental conditions glass, quartz, and Pyrex rods have been shattered in the lab. Etched metal rods scatter the beam sufficiently so that damage is unlikely except in the immediate perimeter.

With the backstop in place, adhesions with small vessels can be lysed in a hemostatic fashion. With larger arterioles and small veins, bleeding can occur which will have to be controlled with either coagulation or free ties. When bleeding occurs in spite of the laser, attempts at coagulating this with a defocused laser are generally unsuccessful and result in much tissue destruction. More thermal necrosis occurs the longer this is attempted. It is easier, quicker, and less traumatic to use coagulation or free ties for this type of bleeding.

Microscopic Lysis

The microscope gives the best recognition of cutting depth. The magnification allows recognition of dissection planes once the initial blanching has resolved. Although the spot size of the microscope (0.4 to 0.8 mm) is larger than that of the hand held attachment (0.2 mm), the power density is still sufficient for incision. Furthermore, the increased depth of field of the microscope produces a more uniform incision (Table 20–1). With severe adhesions, the magnification can cause disorientation and has resulted in transection of the tube with both microsurgical technique and laser microsurgical technique.

If it is necessary to change the focus, when shifting powers of magnification, the microscope is not parfocal. This can result in an unintended defocused beam. To avoid this problem, it is necessary that the microscope be parfocused so that the focal plane is constant at all powers. Parfocus is accomplished by setting the microscope distance at the highest power and then setting the eye pieces at the lowest power. With the microscope set in this fashion, the powers should interchange without affecting the focus.

The main advantage to the microscopic laser appears to be in minimizing retraction and tissue handling. The laser will reach difficult sites in the pelvis much easier than other contemporary techniques. It is also possible to place a mirror beneath the ovary and dissect subovarian adhesions with minimal retraction as the beam is aimed down into the pelvis at the mirror and reflected upward at the adhesions (Fig. 20–1). The beam is easily aimed at the target by viewing the mirror. This requires careful observation as misdirected reflections of the beam off the mirror or metal instruments may injure the patient or operating room personnel. The same mirror reflection techniques can be attempted with the handheld attachment but are very awkward. In addition, the handheld attachment generates much higher power densities which can easily vaporize the face of the rhodium front surfaced mirror.

When working with mirrors it is necessary to remember that these must be front surfaced. The most common used is a #5 dental rhodium mirror which can be obtained from any dental supply house. If the mirrors are back surfaced, the laser

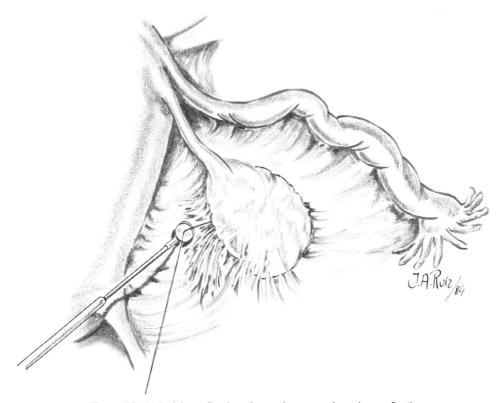

Figure 20–1. Incising adhesions beneath ovary using mirror reflection.

will destroy the glass on the front surface without reaching the mirrored surface. With high power densities, even the rhodium front surface mirrors can be vaporized. Because of this potential, rhodium mirrors will probably be replaced by gold and stainless steel mirrors as these become available.

The microscopic laser has been the major source of damage to operators' hands. Surgeons have moved their fingers through the microscopic field and into the beam of the laser causing superficial incisions and coagulation. These have healed well and resulted in no permanent damage. Permanent damage could occur with a deep cut. Just as surgeon's hands in the fields have been cut, patient organs such as the bowel can easily move into the path as the laser is aimed at distant targets. As with handheld attachments, extreme care must be utilized to be certain that unintended targets such as bowel are not allowed in the beam's path.

Laparoscopic Lysis

Laparoscopic lysis of adhesions should not be attempted until mastering intraabdominal use of the laser at laparotomy. This should include a working knowledge of handheld techniques and of microscopic techniques. Laparoscopic techniques should start with nodular endometriosis on the uterosacral ligaments and should progress slowly over 10 to 250 cases before attempting difficult adhesions. If adequate laboratory exposure is not present, 100 or more cases may be needed before attempting these techniques. Dense and vascular adhesions on the underside of the ovaries should be lysed with the laparoscope only in those patients who have agreed to elective laparatomy. Lysis of dense and vascular adhesions is not commonly of benefit to the patient unless endometriosis is found in these areas.

The laparoscope provides magnification and adequate assessment of the incisional depth. This magnification allows identification of intraluminal folds at salpingostomy. Field width is compromised in using this magnification. This compromise of the field width requires an adequate knowledge of the location of surrounding organs so as to prevent damage to them.

Single puncture and second puncture equipment is available. The single puncture equipment is most useful for angles which cannot be appropriately obtained with a double puncture as well as for adhesions and endometriosis on the posterior aspect of the uterus. The second puncture trocar should be placed so that it is high enough on the abdomen to maintain an angle into the pelvis, but low enough so that it does not interfere with the laparoscope. If the second puncture trocar is placed close to the pubis, the angle can result in aiming the laser into the upper abdomen and exposing bowel to this technique. Superficial burns of the ascending colon have occurred in this situation. A simple technique for determining the appropriate placement site is to place pressure on the abdomen with a finger while viewing the depression through the laparoscope. Pressure applied directly above the symphysis will push the peritoneal wall against the uterine fundus (Fig. 20–2). The finger is progressively moved up the abdomen until the depressed area is noted to be far enough away from the symphysis to be above the target site (Fig. 20–3). This helps avoid aiming the laser into the upper abdomen.

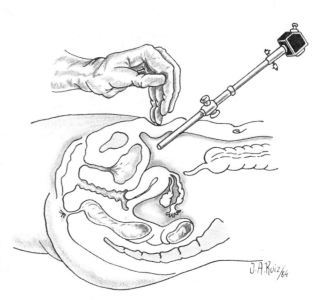

Figure 20–2. Depression of abdominal wall to determine placement of second puncture (location too low).

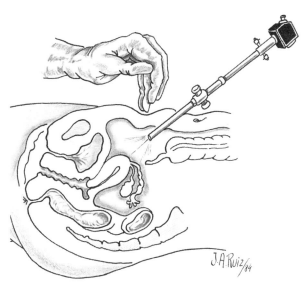

Figure 20–3. Depression of abdominal wall to determine proper placement of second puncture (correct location).

Backstops for the laparoscopic laser include fluid solutions, etched metal rods, Pyrex rods, quartz rods, adhesions, lateral sidewall, the target itself, and a backstop probe. Fluid solutions can be placed in the pelvis and the adhesions stretched over this area so that the beam aims into the solution after cutting the adhesions. The rods are the same as previously mentioned. When quartz or Pyrex rods are used, these are not used for retraction. The trocar used with these rods has either no valve or a smooth ball valve. Trumpet style valves can crush the rod.

Adhesions and lateral peritoneum are used when other backstops are not adequate and only after much work with other backstops. When using the adhesions or the lateral peritoneum as a backstop, surface damage to the peritoneum has been tolerated in the initial series of patients. The ureter and lateral vessels are identified and avoided as the potential for damage to these is significant.

A hydrosalpinx wall can be used as its own backstop and the laser targeted tangentially into the wall. This results in an incision which is limited by the beginning of the next incisional point. Tension is maintained to speed the incision and decrease the time of thermal damage.

The backstop probe is a modification of the basic laparoscopic probe. The basic probe is an open-ended second puncture probe very similar to a handheld attachment. The backstop probe is built so that the beam is aimed onto a platform which is part of the probe itself (Fig. 20–4). This platform permits the penetration of the laser. The probe can occasionally be awkward to utilize, but in most instances gives much peace of mind regarding the penetration of the laser. The backstop area can either be the same size as the range of the laser or smaller. When it is the same size as the range of the width of laser motion, the laser will not go past the edge of the backstop. This provides a greater margin of safety, but limits overall capabilities. When the backstop allows the laser to be moved off of the edge of the backstop, the laser can also be used as a straightahead instrument to vaporize

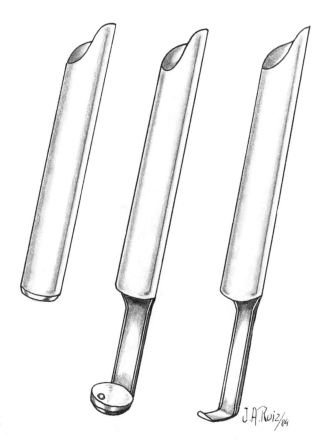

Figure 20–4. Probe types:
open (*left*), full backstop (*center*), partial backstop (*right*).

peritoneal lesions such as endometriosis. If the backstop covers the full range of
motion and a peritoneal lesion is to be vaporized, the backstop probe must then
be exchanged for the open-ended probe (Fig. 20-5).

   With the backstop probe, the manipulator at the top of the instrument is used
to align the beam of the backstop. This beam can be aligned at any edge or point
on the backstop. The point of alignment is based on the orientation needed. When
adhesions are to be cut on the upper side, the beam is moved to the upper side
(Fig. 20–6).

   There can be times that a high angle is needed to get behind the uterus and
single puncture equipment is not available. In these situations, an accessory puncture can be placed lateral to the umbilicus. This will produce approximately the
same angle as the laparoscope when aimed at the target area.

   Bipolar coagulation should be available for bleeding from vessels too large for
control by the laser. If the surgeon persists in trying to coagulate bleeding in laparoscopic situations, a carbon build-up occurs. As the carbon is vaporized, temperatures in excess of 1200°C are created which can melt the solder of certain parts

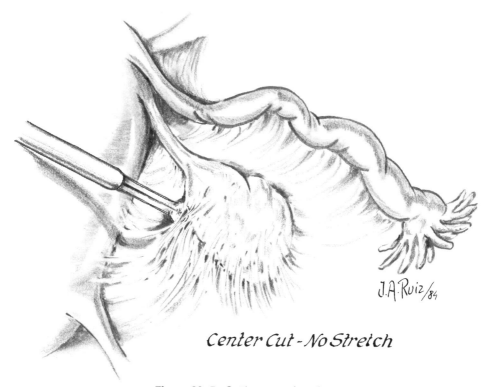

Center Cut - No Stretch

Figure 20–5. Cutting on probe edge.

of the equipment. Equipment which was previously soldered is now being put together with screws due to this potential. Preoperatively, the patient must understand the possibility of laparotomy to control bleeding of this nature. Laparotomy was necessary once in the first 800 patients, due to bleeding from the uterosacral ligament and an inability to maintain the pneumoperitoneum.

INTRAPERITONEAL SOLUTIONS

Various intraperitoneal solutions have been suggested by different authors for wetting tissue, peritoneal lavage, and tubal flotation. These include Hyskon, Macrodex, saline solutions, Ringer's solution, heparin solution, and steroid solutions. Copious lavage with any of these solutions is used to remove carbonized debris. There is concern that this carbonized debris can be a focus for long-term inflammatory reaction or for infection. This possibility also exists for bipolar and unipolar coagulation. These solutions are left for flotation at the end of the procedure.

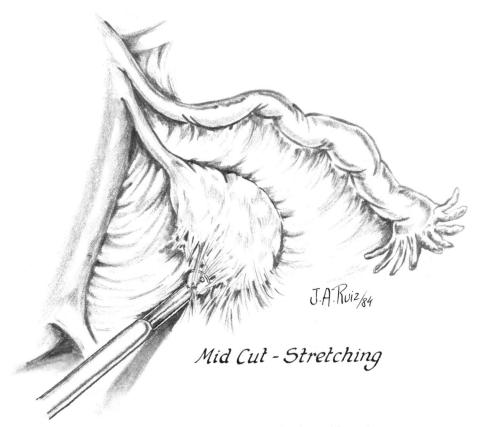

J.A.Ruiz/84

Mid Cut - Stretching

Figure 20–6. Probe used to stretch adhesions while cutting.

CONCLUSIONS

Current data suggest that the laser has the same efficacy as micropoint cautery. It has the advantages of decreasing operating time, increasing the ease of difficult dissections, decreasing blood loss, and increasing the extent of surgery which can be performed through a laparoscope. The main disadvantage is the cost and time of training for both the surgeon and operating room personnel. The potential danger of this high power equipment has been controlled by careful precaution and preparation on the part of the surgeons and operating room personnel.

REFERENCES

1. Baggish MS: Status of the carbon dioxide laser for infertility surgery. Fertil Steril 40:442, 1983
2. David SS: Microsurgical management of distal tube disease. In Reyniak JV, Lauersen

NH (eds); Principles of Microsurgical Techniques in Infertility. New York, Plenum, 1982, pp 161–183

3. Bellina JH: Microsurgery of the fallopian tube with the carbon dioxide laser: Analysis of 230 cases with a two-year follow-up. Lasers Surgery Med 3:255, 1983
4. Daniell JF, Herbert CM: Laparoscopic salpingostomy utilizing the CO_2 laser. Fertil Steril 41:558, 1984
5. Daniell JF, Pittaway DE: Use of the CO_2 laser in laparoscopic surgery: Initial experience with the second puncture technique. Infertility 5:15, 1982
6. Grosspietzsch R, et al: Experiments on operative treatment of tubal sterility by CO_2 laser technique. In Kaplan I (ed): Proceedings of the Third International Congress for Laser Surgery. Tel-Aviv, OT-PAZ, 1979, pp 256–262
7. Kelly RW, Roberts DK: Experience with the carbon dioxide laser gynecologic microsurgery. Am J Obstet Gynecol 146:585, 1983
8. Mage G, Bruhat MA: Pregnancy following salpingostomy: Comparison between laser and electrosurgery procedures. Fertil Steril 40:472, 1983
9. Pittaway DE, Maxon W, Daniell JF: A comparison of the CO_2 laser and electrocautery on postoperative intraperitoneal adhesion formation in rabbits. Fertil Steril 39:402, 1983
10. Tadir Y, et al: Intraperitoneal adhesiolysis by CO_2 laser microsurgery. In Atsumi K, Nimsakul N (eds): Laser-Tokyo '81. Tokyo, Japanese Society for Laser Medicine, 1981, pp 27–28
11. Daniell JF: The role of lasers in infertility surgery. Fertil Steril 42:815, 1984
12. Diamond NP, et al: Tubal patency in pelvic adhesions at early second look laparoscopy following intraabdominal use of the carbon dioxide laser: Initial report of the intraabdominal laser study group. Fertil Steril 42:717, 1984
13. McCoy TD, Martin DC, Poston W: Reanastomosis of rat uterine horn following laser and sharp incisions. Fertil Steril 41:805, 1984
14. McLaughlin DS: Evaluation of adhesion reformation by early second look laparoscopy following microlaser ovarian wedge resection. Fertil Steril 42:531, 1984

21

Laser Laparoscopy

James F. Daniell

INTRODUCTION

The medical use of a laser through an endoscope is already well established in gastroenterology and otolaryngology, and new endoscopic applications for the laser are currently being investigated in orthopedics, urology, and gynecology. This chapter reviews the North American development of laparoscopic attachments which facilitate intraperitoneal use of the carbon dioxide (CO_2) and the argon laser in gynecology.

DEVELOPMENT OF INSTRUMENTATION

The initial development of instruments for directing the CO_2 laser through a laparoscope and early investigations of their clinical utilization began independently on three continents in the late 1970s with reports by Bruhat et al. in France,[1] Tadir et al. in Israel,[2] and Daniell and colleagues in North America.[3,4] Initial animal studies and clinical trials were not begun in America until 1980 when a prototype laparoscope was designed jointly by Eder Instrument Company, Chicago, Illinois and Advanced Surgical Technologies, Incorporated. This prototype allowed articulation of a laser beam focusing lens to the surgical arm of a Sharplan 733, CO_2 laser. Aiming and firing the focused CO_2 beam was then feasible through the 5 mm operating channel of the laparoscope.

With initial evaluation in animals, this prototype laser laparoscope was found to be impractical and difficult to use because of poor optics and the operator's inability to keep the CO_2 beam from reflecting off the inner walls of the operative channel of the laparoscope.

An initial prototype for a second puncture laparoscopic probe allowing use of the CO_2 laser beam intraperitoneally was developed in an attempt to improve the system. Using the second puncture instrument to introduce the laser beam into the pelvis allowed utilization of a standard laparoscope and solved the problem of inadequate visibility. The problem of poor beam alignment, however, was not corrected and loss of pneumoperitoneum due to the lack of air-tight articulations continued to be a problem. The reduced visibility due to intraperitoneal smoke with firing also was bothersome. The introduction of the CO_2 laser beam through an accessory trochar site made the procedure more cumbersome as the intraperitoneal ends collided during the manipulations necessary to align the laparoscope, the laser probe, and accessory instruments that are needed for traction, suction of smoke, or for use as a backstop for the beam. Often when attempting use of the CO_2 laser intraperitoneally, one found that four or five instruments were needed simultaneously. Thus the system was unwieldy and clinically difficult to master.

With subsequent evolution of instrumentation allowing more efficient and practical use of the CO_2 laser via laparoscopy, the majority of technical problems have now been overcome. This was only accomplished by constant communication between the manufacturers of both the laparoscope and laser, and the investigators carefully evaluating each new modification in animal models and patients.

PRESENT SYSTEMS FOR USE OF THE CO_2 LASER VIA LAPAROSCOPY

Although modifications of the CO_2 laser laparoscope continue, at the present time two systems for use of the CO_2 laser with the laparoscope are available and these are suitable for clinical application by the laparoscopist, who is both experienced with operative laparoscopy and familiar with the intraabdominal use of the CO_2 laser.

Operative Channel Use of the CO_2 Laser

The present operative laparoscope for use with the CO_2 laser is a 12.7 mm diameter instrument with refined optics and a 5 mm operating channel (Fig. 21–1). This instrument can be used as a regular operating laparoscope with 5 mm accessory forceps. When the decision to use the laser through the laparoscope is made, the operator simply attaches the articulated arm of the laser with its special micromanipulator mirror and focusing lens to the operating channel. The lens and mirror allow final focusing and correct alignment of the laser beam which subsequently passes through the operating channel of the laparoscope. The CO_2 insufflation tubing is then attached to allow flow of carbon dioxide down the beam channel. By flowing the CO_2 from the insufflator down this shaft, warm intraperitoneal CO_2 does not fog the mirror or focusing lens in the housing. The flow of CO_2 also keeps intraperitoneal smoke, which can reduce the power of the beam, out of the laser channel.

Prior to use, the laparoscope is fired at a moist tongue blade to check the alignment of the helium-neon (He-Ne) optical aiming beam, and to center the beam down the operating channel of the scope with the alignment mirror. The laparoscope is then reintroduced into the abdomen, and the orange optical aiming beam is correctly positioned before firing. It is necessary to pass a second instrument into the pelvis to vent off the smoke of vaporization that occurs. The operator must keep the suction probe close to the impact site of the laser beam and immediately start to vent off the smoke as it occurs. if this smoke diffuses throughout

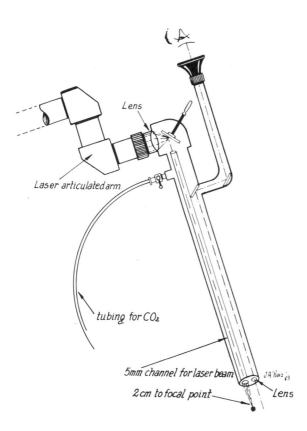

Figure 21–1. This drawing illustrates how the present laser laparoscope uses a micromanipulator mirror to direct the focused CO_2 laser beam down the operating channel of the scope. The CO_2 flow leads to the pneumoperitoneum source and keeps smoke and moisture out of the mirror and lens housing. This system is very functional with good optics and a beam that can be kept easily centered on the target.

the peritoneal cavity, one has the unpleasant sensation of trying to operate through a dense fog. If this happens, the laparoscope should be removed and entire pneumoperitoneum replaced with fresh CO_2 from the insufflator.

Laparoscopic Use of the CO_2 Laser through an Accessory Trocar

The present second puncture probe for using the CO_2 laser with the laparoscope is a double ring probe 7 mm in external diameter. This probe attaches to the same lens and mirror coupler that is used with the operating laparoscope. The CO_2 insufflation tubing is attached to the probe at its proximal end. The smoke of vaporization is drawn out the outer ring channel of the probe and is controlled by a separate valve that allows controlled suctioning of the intraperitoneal smoke. A second double-barrelled probe, which has a specially designed backstop, is also available for use when one is vaporizing adhesions. Both of these special probes are shown in Figure 21–2. The probe with the fixed backstop eliminates the risk of accidental injury to intraperitoneal structures as the beam passes through tissue and impacts on underlying structures.

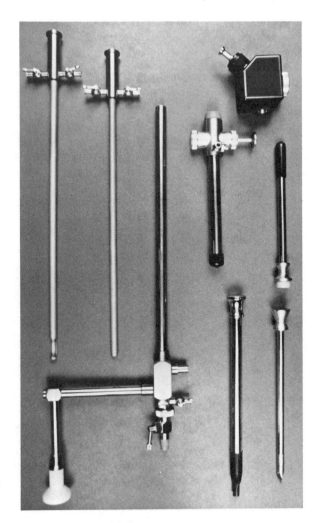

Figure 21–2A. A complete set of laser laparoscopic equipment for both single and double puncture techniques.

ALTERNATE LENSES FOR LASER LAPAROSCOPY

The standard focusing lens for the laser laparoscope is 350 mm with the focal point 2 cm from the end of either the operating scope or the second puncture probe. This long focal length produces a spot that is 2 mm in diameter. This relatively large diameter limits the power density that is obtainable. This long focal length lens makes it difficult to defocus the laser as done at open handheld CO_2 laser surgery by pulling the scope back from the tissue since one must move back several centimeters from the area of planned impact to significantly increase the spot diameter. The long focal length of the second puncture system also results in

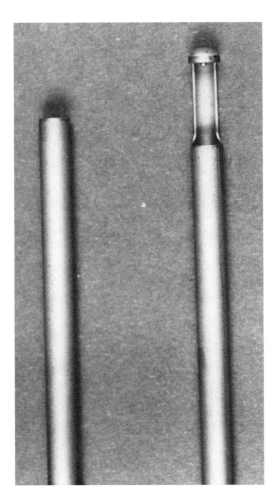

Figure 21–2B. The two second puncture probes for using the CO_2 laser laparoscope are pictured here with the double puncture scope. A backstop for safe vaporization of adhesions can be seen on the end of the instrument on the right.

an instrument that is longer than optimal for comfortable use with multiple puncture techniques in thin patients.

Because of these problems, a lens and mirror attachment has been designed that contains two focal lengths, a 250 and a 350 mm lens. This feature gives the system greater flexibility. Use of the 250 mm lens with a shorter second puncture probe (230 mm) results in an instrument that is less cumbersome. This also allows higher power densities to be obtained due to the smaller diameter of the focused beam spot. Similarly, the 250 mm lens when aimed and fired through the 330 mm long operating channel of the laser scope results in a significant defocused beam and less power density. Variable power densities are necessary to perform vaporizations and for making incisions with the laser beam. These differences become clear when one understands the operative procedures now possible with the CO_2 laser laparoscope.

**TABLE 21–1. CLINICAL USES FOR THE
CO₂ LASER LAPAROSCOPE**

Terminal salpingostomy
Ablation of endometriosis
Uterosacral ligament transection
Pelvic adhesiolysis
Vaporization of small uterine fibroids
Ovarian cystotomy
Destruction of hydatid cysts

CLINICAL APPLICATIONS FOR THE CO₂ LASER LAPAROSCOPY

To date, several operations have been successfully carried out with the CO_2 laser laparoscope (Table 21–1).

The true efficacy of the CO_2 laser for these procedures is still uncertain because of limited clinical experience presently confined to a small number of investigators. Preliminary data, however, suggest that the CO_2 laser laparoscope may provide distinct advantages for the treatment of some types of pelvic pathology.

CO₂ Laser Laparoscopy for Terminal Salpingostomy

The results of primary salpingostomy/fimbrioplasty for the treatment of hydrosalpinges are uniformly poor, with most series reporting no better than a 20 to 30 percent term pregnancy rate.[5] Many women who undergo distal salpingostomy or fimbrioplasty for hydrosalpinges develop a recurrent obstruction. These patients are poor candidates for a repeat tuboplasty because of the dismal results from a second procedure or their lack of desire for a second major operation. Nevertheless, Gomel reported a technique of laparoscopic salpingostomy[6] which resulted in the successful achievement of pregnancy in a small number of cases. Because of the limitations of conventional unipolar cautery utilized in his procedure, the technique of laparoscopic CO_2 laser salpingostomy seemed to offer a reasonable alternative in selected patients who desired pregnancy but did not want a laparotomy for repair of distal tubal disease. Because of Vanderbilt University's early activity in the area of in vitro fertilization, many patients with a recurrent hydrosalpinx were inquiring about their acceptability for that clinical program in 1981–82. This led us to begin selective recruitment of patients who, on review of their medical record, were thought at that time to be probable candidates for laser laparoscopic neosalpingostomy.[4] These patients were thought to need screening laparoscopy for acceptance into Vanderbilt University's in vitro fertilization program. They were asked to give consent for an attempt at CO_2 laser laparoscopic salpingostomy at the time of this screening laparoscopy.

At laparoscopy, the tubes and ovaries were inspected for adhesions or other significant pathology. The tubes were distended with indigo carmine dye transcervically. If the distal tube was mobile and distended well with dye, and if the CO_2 laser beam could be aimed at right angles to the end of the hydrosalpinx through the second puncture laser probe, an attempt was made to perform the operation. A linear incision was then made with the finely focused beam with the carbon dioxide laser set at 35 W (Fig. 21–3). Then as blue dye began to spill through the opened tube, the incised ends of the tube were carefully grasped with accessory forceps (Fig. 21–4). Two grasping forceps were used. A 3 mm forceps was passed through the channel of the laparoscope and a 5 mm alligator forceps was passed through a third puncture for traction on the incised edges of the tube. A second incision in the end of the hydrosalpinx was then made with the high power density laser beam at a 90 degree angle to the first linear incision. After making these radial incisions in the hydrosalpinx, the laser power was reduced to 5 W and the beam was defocused by pulling the probe back from the area of planned impact 4 to 5 cm. The target was the lateral peritoneum of the hydrosalpinx a few millimeters back from the incised edges (Fig. 21–5). As this lower power density beam hit the tissue, the tubal serosal peritoneum would constrict slowly, everting the edges of the hydrosalpinx. This newly constructed "fimbria" would then flower back opening up the ampullary portion of the tube. Copious irrigation with heparinized Ringer's solution and vigorous chromopertubation was then carried out. The accumulated cul-de-sac fluid was suctioned from the pelvic cavity and 200 ml of 32 percent dextran-70 instilled intraperitoneally before terminating the laparoscopy.

This procedure, although technically cumbersome, can be performed with most thin-walled, mobile hydrosalpinges. In our initial series of 20 patients with only 6 months' follow-up, we had a postoperative patency rate of 80 percent and a pregnancy rate of 15 percent which is almost compatible to conventional open microsurgery (Table 21–2). This is significantly better than the results obtained by

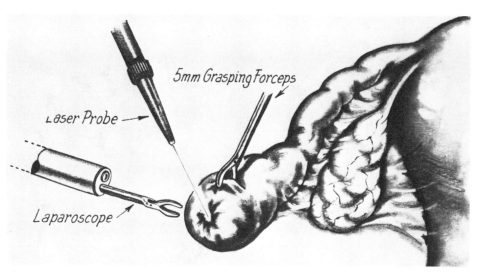

Figure 21–3. The end of the hydrosalpinx is incised at its thinnest area using the CO_2 laser beam with the tube distended with dye.

350

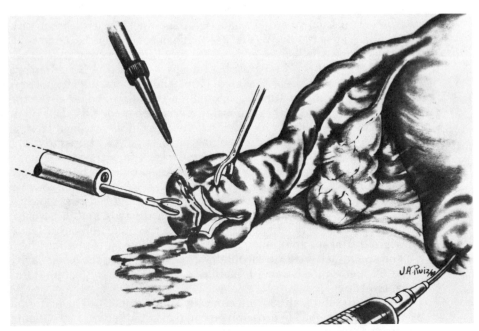

Figure 21–4. As dye begins to spill through the incised tube, the two grasping forceps are used for traction while the incisions in the end of the hydrosalpinx are completed.

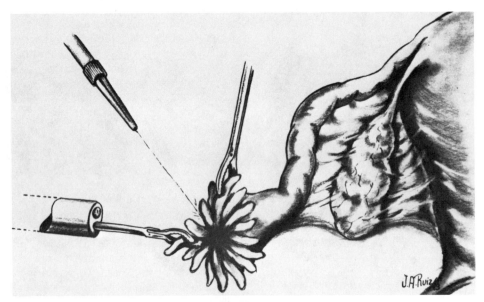

Figure 21–5. After the radial incisions in the hydrosalpinx are completed, the CO_2 laser beam is used at a lower power density to constrict the peritoneal surfaces of the tube. This causes the new "fimbria" to evert outward like a flower.

TABLE 21–2. RESULTS OF CO₂ LASER LAPAROSCOPIC SALPINGOSTOMY

Total Patients	Patency at HSG (6 wk Postop)	Follow-Up at 6 Mo	
		IUP	*Ectopic*
20	16 (80%)	3 (15%)	1 (5%)

Fayez for laparoscopic salpingostomy without the laser.[7] In 19 patients he reported only a 31 percent patency rate at follow-up hysterosalpingography. Only 2 of his 19 patients conceived and both of these were ectopic gestations.

All these patients undergoing laparoscopic laser salpingostomy were discharged by 24 hours postoperatively. There were no complications in this series. The savings to patients in hospitalization, expense, lost time from work or routine activities, and discomfort were significant. Although further clinical evaluation is needed before any conclusions concerning the efficacy of this operative procedure can be made, it appears that this laparoscopic technique of salpingostomy may be of benefit to selected patients. In addition, it is a technically difficult multipuncture technique of advanced laparoscopy.

Laser Laparoscopy for Endometriosis

The CO_2 laser is an ideal method for vaporizing implants of endometriosis. The beam produces instant vaporization of the lesion as it impacts on the tissue. There is no injury beyond the visible tissue destruction and the depth of the vaporization is limited to 1 to 2 mm and easy to control with proper application of the beam. Any lesion that can be visually identified by the laparoscopist becomes an easy target for the CO_2 laser beam (Fig. 21–6). The risks associated with cautery are eliminated and one can safely vaporize implants on the bladder, the tube, and over the uterus with ease.

Either delivery technique for directing the laser beam intraperitoneally may be used for patients with endometriosis, but firing the beam through the operating channel of the laparoscope is usually easier and less cumbersome.

Once preliminary inspection of the pelvis is completed, the laser arm is attached to the operating channel of the laparoscope. A second puncture instrument is needed for traction and repositioning of the pelvic structures such as rolling the ovaries upward to allowing firing at the posterior ovarian surface where implants are commonly encountered. A 5 mm round suction probe is ideal for use as the second puncture instrument, because it permits simultaneous suction of the smoke of vaporization and retraction.

Each lesion is then vaporized with the laser set at 20 W power and the beam somewhat defocused to give a spot diameter large enough to rapidly cover the lesion's surface. By using this slightly defocused beam and rapidly moving the laser over the surface of each lesion, the depth of penetration is minimal and easily controlled. The laparoscope can be periodically moved in close proximity to the lesion to judge the depth of vaporization obtained with the laser. The clinical decision regarding "optimal" depth is difficult. Usually, adequate vaporization

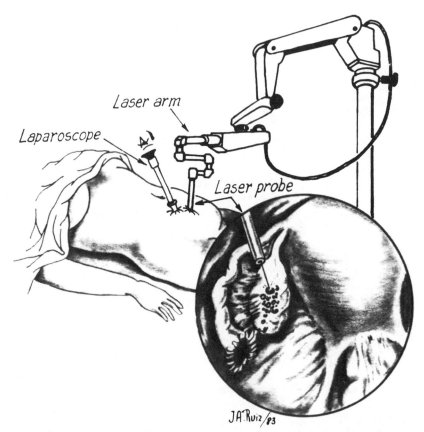

Figure 21–6. Using a regular laparoscope and the second puncture CO_2 laser probe, the beam can be used to vaporize pelvic endometriosis. This drawing shows the set up as used clinically and the view through the laparoscope.

requires a depth of 2 to 3 mm with elimination of the visible boundaries of the lesion and visualization of a clean impact surface lined with retroperitoneal adipose tissue.

Intermittent lavage of each impact site with heparinized lactated Ringer's solution (5000 units of heparin in 1000 cc) through the second puncture instrument cleanses the area to allow easy assessment of the effects of vaporization. If any excess fluid is not first suctioned off the planned impact site, excess smoking occurs with firing of the beam. This occurs because the beam must first boil off all the fluid in its path before it can impact directly on the tissues.

Early clinical results of use of the CO_2 laser for mild or moderate endometriosis have been encouraging. There have been no complications in any cases to date. Table 21–3 shows that in the first 20 patients treated at Vanderbilt Unversity with this technique the relief of symptoms and early pregnancy rates have been rea-

TABLE 21-3. EARLY RESULTS OF LASER LAPAROSCOPY FOR PELVIC ENDOMETRIOSIS

	Stage of Disease	Primary Presenting Symptoms		6 Mo Follow-Up Results	
		Pain	*Infertility*	*Pain Resolved*	*Pregnant*
Mild	12	2	10	2	5
Moderate	8	2	6	2	2
Total	20	4	16	4 (100%)	7 (47%)

sonable with 6 months' follow-up. Multicenter larger clinical trials are now in progress to further evaluate this new treatment for endometriosis.

Uterosacral Ligament CO_2 Laser Ablation

Although uterosacral ligament divison by laparoscopic cautery and scissors has been reported to be modestly successful in transecting the nerves passing into the cervix, the conventional technique is considered risky and ineffective by many laparoscopists. Criticism of laparoscopic division of the uterosacral ligaments has primarily focused on the difficulty in completely burning the ligaments and in cutting the associated nerve fibers and on the fear of bleeding from adjacent vessels or damage to the ureter.

With the CO_2 laser beam, the uterosacral ligament can be vaporized safely without bleeding or lateral damage to adjacent tissue. In patients with dysmenorrhea, either with or without visible endometriosis, the uterosacral ligaments can be easily transected at the time of a diagnostic laparoscopy using the CO_2 laser. The technique is simple and merely involves vaporizing a 2 cm section of the ligament just where it enters the posterior cervix. This is done to a depth of 1 cm in the center of the vaporized area, producing a shallow rectangular bilaterally (Fig. 21-7).

The clinical results of any therapy for dysmenorrhea are difficult to evaluate objectively, but the initial subjective patient response has been good in the few patients treated to date. Further investigations of this operative procedure seem indicated.

Laparoscopic Adhesiolysis with the CO_2 Laser

Since the tissue vaporized with the CO_2 laser "goes up in smoke," this mode of destruction of pelvic adhesions seems ideal. The undesired tissue can be bloodlessly destroyed and the adjacent normal tissue is totally unaffected. Other forms of laparoscopic adhesiolysis do not allow such precise removal of the transected scar tissue. Unipolar cautery may be associated with the risk of burns to skin, bowel, and other tissues and may cause thermal damage to a wider area than

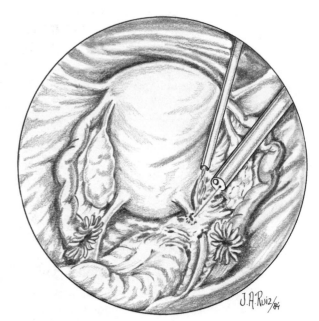

Figure 21–7. The uterosacral ligaments can be selectively vaporized as illustrated. A 5 mm suction probe is being used through a third puncture placed suprapubically to suction off the smoke as it occurs.

desired. Likewise, trying to laparoscopically carefully remove all adhesions is tedious and difficult.

To use the laser for this procedure requires some sort of backstop for the beam. As the laser passes through thin adhesive bands, it passes in a straight line until it is absorbed by some tissue or fluid in its path. This can lead to inadvertent injury to pelvic vital structures.

The special second puncture probe with built-in backstop is suitable for most adhesions if it can be hooked around the tissue. At other times one may elect to use another puncture site to pass a laser rod to use as the backstop. Occasionally, the pelvic side wall, ovary, or uterus itself may serve as an intentional backstop. Cul-de-sac fluid also can serve as a safe site for final beam absorption when working down deep in the pelvis.

When performing adhesiolysis with the laser, we usually use a setting of 10 W and keep the probe or laparoscope close to the tissue to minimize the risk of a loop of bowel suddenly dropping down into the line of fire. We have encountered no complications yet with judicious use of the laser for laparoscopic adhesiolysis. To avoid accidental injury to adjacent tissues, it is absolutely essential to always trace mentally the path of the beam before stepping on the trigger to actually fire the laser.

Miscellaneous Use for the CO_2 Laser Laparoscope

Besides the clinical uses for the laser laparoscope previously discussed, there are other occasional uses for the discrete destruction of tissue that are possible with the properly focused CO_2 laser beam. Small uterine fibroids and ovarian fibromas can be easily ablated with a moderately defocused beam. These lesions can be completely destroyed without injury to adjacent underlying healthy tissue. Hydatid cysts can be likewise vaporized without difficulty when seen. The laser can also perform bloodless drainage of small benign ovarian cysts without difficulty. The laser can be used to drain the small multiple follicles seen in polycystic ovaries near the ovarian surface. This might temporarily relieve the block to anovulation in these patients in a fashion analogous to ovarian wedge resection.

PRESENT DISADVANTAGES OF THE CO_2 LASER LAPAROSCOPIC SYSTEM

In spite of the continuing development of instruments for use of the carbon dioxide laser via laparoscopy, there are still problems with the system. The expense of the surgical laser is significant ($50,000 and up) and still questionably cost effective for hospitals, physicians, and patients. Its use requires specialized equipment that needs constant biomedical maintenance and diligent operating room technical care. The surgical procedures described above are cumbersome, with multiple punctures usually necessary. In addition, there are often technical problems with intraperitoneal smoke accumulation, loss of pneumoperitoneum from gas leakage, maintenance of proper beam alignment, and fogging of the laser lens or mirror. The major theoretic intraoperative risk of the laparoscopic laser is accidental injury to vital tissues. Only strict adherence to the principles of laser surgery will minimize these risks.

ADVANTAGES OF THE CO_2 LASER LAPAROSCOPE

In spite of the problems mentioned with this method of application of the CO_2 laser beam to intraperitoneal pelvic pathology, this technique offers a number of potential advantages. The system allows precise, bloodless destruction of endometriosis, selected pelvic adhesions, small fibroids, and for uterosacral ligament transection. Successful correction of distal tubal obstruction is possible in some cases without laparotomy.

Finally, in the hands of careful, experienced laparoscopists who are familiar with the biophysics of the CO_2 laser and its tissue interactions intraperitoneally, this technique appears safe and effective in early clinical trials.

THE ARGON LASER USED LAPAROSCOPICALLY

The CO_2 laser cannot yet successfully be passed through fibers for clinical use. Other types of laser beams, however, are capable of being passed through flexible fibers. The argon laser is being investigated by Keye et al.[8] to photocoagulate endometrial implants by passing a fiberoptic probe under laparoscopic direction and touching the target. The laser is then activated and the lesion absorbs the laser energy with resultant tissue necrosis to variable depths without surface vaporization. This system seems promising, but does have certain limitations. The biophysics of the argon beam are such that it is only absorbed by tissue with a purplish color since the beam effect is color dependent. The depth of penetration is variable and cannot be accurately controlled at the time of use. It is similar to a cautery wound in that the depth of tissue damage is not always obvious. In addition, it is impossible to make usable incisions or vaporize surfaces with the argon laser.

In spite of these characteristics of the argon laser, cautious further investigations of this new technique are encouraged to determine if there may be benefits to patients that are not obtainable with present forms of operative laparoscopy.

SUMMARY

Although not for the timid, use of the CO_2 or argon laser through the laparoscope offers potential benefits in the correction of certain pelvic abnormalities that were previously untreatable by laparoscopy. It appears that the systems presently available can be used with safety. The judicious use of these new laparoscopic techniques and carefully planned further investigations by adequately trained experienced laparoscopists combined with continuing improvements in the delivery systems will hopefully soon answer the question of the efficacy of laser laparoscopy.

REFERENCES

1. Bruhat M, Mage G, Manhes M: In Kaplan I (ed): Laser Surgery III. Proceedings of the 3rd International Society for Laser Surgery. Tel Aviv, 1979, pp 235–238
2. Tadir Y, Ovadia J, Zuckerman Z, Kaplan I: In Atsumi K, Nimsakul N (eds): The 4th Congress of International Society for Laser Surgery. Tokyo, 1981, pp 25–26
3. Daniell JF, Brown DH: Carbon dioxide laser laparoscopy: Initial experience in experimental animal and humans. Obstet Gynecol 59:761, 1982
4. Daniell JF, Pittaway DE: Use of the CO_2 laser in laparoscopic surgery: Initial experience with the second puncture technique. Infertility 5:15, 1982
5. Harris WT, Daniell JF: Use of corticosteroids as an adjuvant in terminal salpingostomies. Fertil Steril (in press)
6. Gomel V: Salpingostomy by laparoscopy. J Reprod Med 18:265, 1977
7. Fayez JA: An assessment of the role of operative laparoscopy in tuboplasty. Fertil Steril 39:476, 1983
8. Keye WR, Matson GA, Dixon J: The use of the argon laser in the treatment of experimental endometriosis. Fertil Steril 39:26, 1983

22

Hysteroscopic Laser Surgery

Milton H. Goldrath

INTRODUCTION

Over the past 15 years, the hysteroscope has very slowly stimulated the interest of gynecologists towards increasing their diagnostic acumen. It was only a matter of time until therapeutic modalities could be developed. At the present time, hysteroscopic scissors, hysteroscopic biopsy forceps, and hysteroscopic coagulators can be used inside the uterus with direct visualization.

The Sinai Hospital of Detroit has long had a deep institutional interest in the uses of lasers in medicine. The development of optical fibers, that could transmit laser energy, led to the use of lasers endoscopically and more particulary hysteroscopically. In 1979, the first hysteroscopic use of the laser was performed at Sinai Hospital of Detroit.[1] We used the neodymium:yttrium-aluminum-garnet (Nd:YAG) laser to photocoagulate and photovaporize the endometrium in patients suffering from severe menorrhagia. This has been the main thrust of our hysteroscopic laser surgery and will be further discussed later in this chapter.

Since that time we have utilized the Nd:YAG laser to divide uterine septa. This was a natural outgrowth of our laser photocoagulation and photovaporization of the endometrium as we soon saw septa in several of these patients and the great ease with which they could be divided utilizing this laser. The inability of carbon dioxide laser energy to be transmitted via a fiberoptic has, up to now, made its hysteroscopic use quite difficult.

THE HYSTEROSCOPIC LASER TREATMENT OF MENORRHAGIA

Hysterectomy is the most common major operation performed in the United States.[2] While hysterectomies are performed for many indications, i.e., malignancy of the uterus and its adnexa, large benign tumors of the uterus, uterine prolapse, and precursors to uterine and cervical malignancy, the most common presenting symptom in cases where a normal or near normal uterus has been removed was dysfunctional uterine bleeding.[2-6] It is obvious to all practicing gynecologists that many of their patients are greatly distressed by excessive menstrual bleeding and are consulting their gynecologists for relief. The standard management of abnormal uterine bleeding consists first of diagnostic procedures such as hysteroscopy and curettage. Following appropriate diagnostic procedures, hormones, ergot derivatives, and/or antifibrinolytic agents have been used.[7] Oral contraceptives are probably most efficacious in the treatment of these patients. Many patients, however, are fearful of using oral contraceptives or, for various reasons, their use is contraindicated or undesirable. Curettage without removal of an offending lesion, such as a submucous myoma or endometrial polyp, is usually unsuccessful in the management of severe menorrhagia. When these methods fail, cause undesirable side effects, or are contraindicated, the gynecologist usually resorts to either performing a hysterectomy or allowing the patient to endure her heavy vaginal bleeding. Iron is used to prevent or treat anemia.

Many patients will endure profuse menses, which are incapacitating and produce profound anemia, rather than subject themselves to a major operative procedure. Other patients will not even tolerate moderately heavy periods or what many might consider normal periods. In addition, there are patients with various blood dyscrasias and medical illnesses that make major abdominal surgery relatively contraindicated. It is with these thoughts in mind that we devised a new surgical procedure for the treatment of menorrhagia.

In 1948, Asherman described a syndrome that now bears his name.[8] Intrauterine synechiae usually produce amenorrhea or hypomenorrhea and infertility. The common denominator in all of Asherman's cases was a postpartum or postabortal curettage or other intrauterine operative procedure. Asherman's syndrome is rare following a diagnostic curettage in the nonpuerperal uterus.[9] The susceptibility of the postpartum or the postabortal uterus to synechiae formation is well known but poorly understood. The softness of the myometrium, which often comes off in strips, has been implicated as has subclinical infection.[10] It is also known that in the postabortal and postpartum state estrogen levels are low. Perhaps this hinders endometrial regeneration.

Asherman's syndrome, in the rare case that conceives, often results in habitual abortion, premature delivery, and placenta accreta. These sequelae are not pertinent to our discussion unless one of our patients should subsequently conceive. It did lead to some concern regarding tubal sterilization in those patients who had not been previously sterilized. For reasons to be explained further on in this discussion, we no longer do tubal sterilizations as we are convinced that these patients are sterile following laser photovaporization and photocoagulation of the endometrium.

Although Asherman spent a large part of his career trying to help the unfortunate victims of Asherman's syndrome regain their menstrual function and fertility, others soon came to the conclusion that reproducing Asherman's syndrome would be of benefit to a large number of women who were suffering from excessive uterine bleeding or excessive fertility. Many physical and chemical methods were used for this purpose. They include substances such as quinacrine, methylcyanoacrylate, oxalic acid, paraformaldehyde, and silicone rubber.[11] Physical methods used were intracavitary radium,[12,13] superheated steam,[14] and cryocoagulation.[11,15,16] More recently DeCherney and Polan[17] described the use of the resectoscope in the management of intractable uterine bleeding. All of these substances and agents except for intracavitary radium, cryocoagulation, and electrosurgical resection have been abandoned because they were unsuccessful. Radium is no longer used. Droegemueller and colleagues[15,16] devised some ingenious cryocoagulation applications which were successful in a few patients. The procedure, however, is basically blind and areas of endometrium were often spared. They were only able to completely destroy the endometrium in a few patients. Fundal and cornual endometrium was often viable and functioning. This did produce painful hematometra in some patients if the isthmus was obliterated by the cryocoagulation. Droegemueller et al. have subsequently abandoned their procedure. Burke et al. reported a case of uterine abscess formation following cryosurgery of the endometrium.[18] This was most likely due to excessive necrosis of the uterine wall. Again, cryosurgery is a blind procedure and the amount of destruction is not readily ascertainable.

The regenerative capacity of the endometrium is well known to gynecologists. In the normal menstrual cycle, the endometrium sloughs down to the basalis and regenerates in a matter of a few days. Attempts to remove or destroy the tissue in animal models has been largely unsuccessful. Shenker and Polishuk applied various agents to the rabbit endometrium.[19] The following chemical agents were instilled: 10 percent formalin, 2 percent formalin in ethanol, $CuSO_4$ pentahydrate pellets, talc suspension, sodium lauryl sulfate, and quinacrine; 10 percent formalin was the only agent that prevented endometrial regeneration and caused complete occlusion of the uterine cavity by fibrous tissue. We know of no attempts to use this agent in the human nor would we advise such use. The same authors were able to produce intrauterine adhesions in the rabbit with autologous fibroblast implants.[20,21] In 1975, Polishuk[22] described the use of homologous fibroblasts in the rat. In the same publication, he described the successful use of autologous fibroblast implants in a few patients. We know of no further animal or human studies.

Preliminary Studies

We proposed to destroy the entire endometrium under hysteroscopic vision using the Nd:YAG laser. The thick myometrium, usually greater than 2 cm, and relatively thin endometrium, usually less than 1 mm in thickness, makes the human uterus an ideal organ for this modality. It is only necessary to destroy approximately 5 percent of the uterine thickness in order to destroy the endometrium. This provides a great safety factor.

We attempted to approach the hormonal status of the postabortal or puerperal uterus by placing each patient on danazol 800 mg/day for 3 weeks prior to the procedure. We continued the danazol for 2 weeks after the procedure with the objective of allowing healing and scar formation to occur prior to return to ovarian cyclic activity and estrogenic stimulation of the endometrium. We soon discovered that healing did not occur for prolonged periods of time, up to 4 to 5 months. Therefore, we no longer continue the danazol in the postoperative state. The atrophic endometrium, which the danazol produces, greatly facilitated the procedure and, therefore, we have continued to use it preoperatively with very satisfactory results.

There are at present several lasers whose energy can be transmitted via fiberoptics. Our selection of the Nd:YAG laser was motivated because of its high energy output, relative portability and greater degree of tissue penetration than other available lasers. We thought that tissue penetration was necessary in order to destroy the basalis layer of the endometrium. In our long experience with the diagnostic hysteroscopy, we found that dextran was a very suitable distending medium. Using dextran in the laboratory and coagulating myometrium with the laser, however, produces very large bubbles which obscured our view. These large bubbles were due to the great viscosity of the dextran solution. We are currently using 5 percent dextrose in physiologic saline as a distending medium with very satisfactory results. We investigated the potential for transmural necrosis created by the Nd:YAG laser treatment to the endometrium. This is reported fully in our initial publication.[1] We determined that with reasonable care there was little, if any, potential for transmural necrosis of the uterine wall.

Patients and Methods

Two hundred twenty-four patients were carefully selected for this procedure. All had excessive and disabling uterine bleeding and were unable or unwilling to use other methods for control. Most tissue committees would consider them as suitable candidates for hysterectomy. Patients were informed that future childbearing would not be possible. Many of the patients had had a prior tubal sterilization.

We initially sought to prevent the irrigation solution from entering the peritoneal cavity during hysteroscopic laser ablation. A Yoon ring was applied laparoscopically to the fallopian tubes of patients who had not had a prior sterilization. We believe that although destruction of the endometrium would most likely produce sterility, the serious sequelae of pregnancy in patients with Asherman's syndrome could be prevented by the use of this sterilizing technique. In subsequent follow-up, we found that there was no communication of the fallopian tube to the endometrial cavity (or what remained of it) after a period of several months. We have discontinued the application of Yoon rings. To date (over 6 years), there have been no pregnancies in any of these patients.

Initially our protocol demanded that all patients have a dilation and curettage (D&C) within 6 months of the procedure and that this D&C be unsuccessful in controlling the symptoms. Many of the patients had had multiple curettages and were still having severe menorrhagia. All patients must have a normal proliferative or secretory endometrium to enter the protocol. At this time we do not include patients with cancer precursors. We have recently come to the conclusion that D&C does not alleviate the symptoms of menorrhagia unless a polyp or submucous myoma is found and removed. At the present time, we are preoperatively doing an office hysteroscopy and suction curettage to rule out submucous myoma or endometrial polyp and to obtain endometrial samples for histologic examination.

The patients ranged in age from 12 to 53 years. One hundred three of the patients had leiomyomata of which 66 were submucous leiomyomata. Twenty-six patients were thought to have adenomyosis either by history or by hysteroscopic findings. Sixteen patients had diagnosed clotting disorders (Table 22–1). The 12-year-old in this series had Bernard-Soulier's syndrome. This is a severe platelet disorder. She had had a cerebral hemorrhage at birth due to the dyscrasia and since then has been markedly mentally retarded and severely epileptic. During

TABLE 22-1. CLOTTING DISORDERS

Symptomatic hemophilia carrier	1
von Willebrand's disease	5
ITP	1
Coumadin therapy	7
Bernard Soulier's syndrome	1
Storage-pool disease	1

her first menstrual period, she bled profusely and the hemoglobin dropped to 6 g. Attempts to control menorrhagia with hormones led to severe exacerbation of her convulsive disorder and it was decided to subject her to this procedure. She had an excellent result.

We believe that many patients with severe menorrhagia have a variant of von Willebrand's disease, however, it should be noted that in only five patients was this diagnosis actually made. This impression comes from the family history of patients with severe menorrhagia and other difficulties associated with excessive blood loss, such as dental extractions and injuries. Since the only manifestation with which we were concerned was menorrhagia, they were not investigated for a hemotologic diagnosis of von Willebrand's disease.

Procedure

We performed the operation with the patient under general or spinal anesthesia. The cervix was grasped with the tenaculum and dilated to 20 French. This is to allow the irrigating solution to pour out of the cervix around the hysteroscope and provide a constant flow of fluid at low pressure to remove blood and gas bubbles from the operative field. It is important that a free flow of fluid be obtained or we may have excessive absorption of fluid into the patient's circulation. This will be discussed more fully under Results and Complications. It may be necessary to dilate the cervix beyond 20 French to allow a free flow of this fluid.

We advanced the hysteroscope through the cervical canal into the endometrial cavity with continuous flushing of the irrigation solution. This continuous flow is maintained by an assistant who injects the solution at a rate sufficient to maintain a clear field by using 50 cc syringes. Adequate outflow around the hysteroscope is visually confirmed. In addition, a vaginal pouch is used to collect the run-off fluid and this is measured so we have an accurate determination of how much fluid the patient absorbs. If we find that the patient is absorbing excessive fluid, Lasix is given intravenously during the procedure and the cervix is further dilated to allow a free flow.

Following inspection of the endometrial cavity, the 600-μ fiberoptic is inserted through the operating channel of the hysteroscope. *A transparent protective filter is placed over the eyepiece of the hysteroscope to prevent injury to the operator's eye.* While it is unlikely that the reflected portion of the laser beam off of the endometrial surface will enter the hysteroscope, if it should the operator's macula could be permanently damaged and destroyed.

Endometrial photovaporization and photocoagulation is performed under direct vision. We use a power output of 50 W continuous wave (CW). The endometrial surface is systematically destroyed beginning in the cornual areas then across the fundus and down each sulcus to and including the isthmus. The cervix is localized by noting the mark on the hysteroscope sheath which is placed at 4 cm. The cervix is circumcised at that point to provide a future landmark. This is important because it is difficult to distinguish the endometrial surface from the endocervical surface hysteroscopically in a patient who has an atrophic endometrium. The areas between the outlines are systematically destroyed by moving the fiber tip in close approximation to the surface much as one "mows the lawn." We endeavor not to skip any endometrial surface. It is more difficult to treat the anterior endometrial surface because of the accumulation of gas bubbles. These can be removed by tipping the uterus backward and giving a rapid flush with the irrigating solution. Repeated inspection of the endometrial surface will frequently reveal areas that were skipped. Treated areas change in color from pink-white to brown-black because of carbonization of the underlying myometrium. The topography of the treated areas appears as rough channels and holes in contrast to the smooth, velvety untreated endometrial surface. Care is taken to avoid perforation in the region of the tubal ostia, which is the thinnest portion of the myometrium. The procedure takes 30 to 40 minutes in a normal-size uterus.

Results and Complications

Most patients were discharged on the day after surgery. Some patients went home the day of surgery. Many of the patients complained of uterine cramps for the first day or two which were relieved by salicylates. Patients likened the postoperative course to that following a D&C. All patients experienced various amounts of serosanguinous discharge which, in some instances, continued up to 4 or 5 weeks. Table 22–2 is a tabulation of the results. These results are for 216 patients who are more than 2 months postoperative at the time of the writing. Our definition of an excellent result is amenorrhea (about 50 percent) or hypomenorrhea (2 to 3 days of staining per month, also 50 percent). A good result is defined as

TABLE 22–2. RESULTS (IN 216[a] MORE THAN 2 MO POSTOPERATIVE PATIENTS)

Excellent	203
Good	3
Poor—retreated	4
(3 excellent afterward)	
(1 had hysterectomy)	
Hysterectomy	8
(4 adenomyosis)	
(1 ovarian cyst)	
(1 cervical bleeding)	
(2 large submucous myomas)	

[a]One patient with poor result had hysterectomy; one patient with excellent result had hysterectomy because of ovarian cyst.

improvement sufficient to have what the patient considers to be normal menstrual periods. Only three patients fell into this category. Four patients had poor results and were retreated. Following retreatment, three became amenorrheic and one had a hysterectomy due to a large submucous leiomyomata.

Eight patients had subsequent hysterectomy. Four of these had severe adenomyosis which caused both recurrent bleeding and considerable pain. We believe that endometrial regeneration may occur from the deep glands in the adenomyotic areas which probably communicate with the old endometrial surface. It is interesting that of these four patients that had adenomyosis in the hysterectomy specimen, only two were suspected of having adenomyosis at the time of the initial laser therapy of the endometrium. Therefore, we can conclude that the diagnosis of adenomyosis on both clinical and hysteroscopic basis is not without its errors. Most of the patients, however, who were thought to have adenomyosis had very good results from the laser ablation of the endometrium.

Two patients failed because of large submucous leiomyomata and had subsequent hysterectomies. In retrospect, patients with large submucous myomas are probably poor candidates for this procedure unless preoperative hysteroscopy reveals all endometrial surfaces to be accessible.

One patient had a hysterectomy for severe bleeding in the endocervix which occurred 3 weeks postoperatively. She had an artificial mitral valve and had Coumadin therapy. One must be careful when administering danazol to a patient who is on Coumadin. Coumadin dosage must be reduced during this time. Examination of the hysterectomy specimen revealed that the bleeding source was high in the endocervix. Apparently we had coagulated the endocervix which sloughed subsequently. We now mark the level of the internal os on the hysteroscope to avoid treating the endocervix. The complication has not recurred.

It can be seen that excellent results were obtained in 94 percent of the patients with one treatment. If one includes the good results and the patients that had excellent results with the second treatment, there is a 97 percent success rate.

Hysterograms were obtained 3 to 6 months following the procedure in 18 patients. All showed evidence of marked scarring and deformity of the cavity, which was often extremely contracted. The uterotubal junction was sometimes initially patent in the first hysterogram, however, on follow-up hysterogram, 1 to 1½ years later, the tubes were closed in all patients. An example is shown in Figures 22–1A, B. Figures 22–2A, B also show the continued scarring after 1 year. At that point there is no more endometrial cavity and certainly no communication with the tubes.

Biopsies of the healing surface were performed on all patients from 1 to 20 months following laser ablation of the endometrium using a Novak suction curette for the procedure. Somewhat necrotic myometrium is easily obtained up to 4 months. This tissue is histologically remarkable by the almost complete absence of inflammatory reaction other than foreign body giant cells surrounding carbon particles. Polymorphonuclear leukocytes are rare and there are very rare areas of sparse round cell infiltration. After 5 months, no muscle or scar tissue is removed and only a minute amount of normal appearing endometrial fragments can be obtained in spite of vigorous curettage.

Seven patients had a small hematometra found at the time of postoperative endometrial biopsies. These responded to dilating the cervix and did not recur.

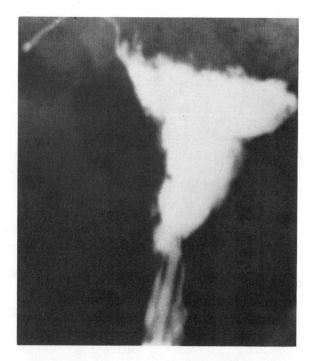

A

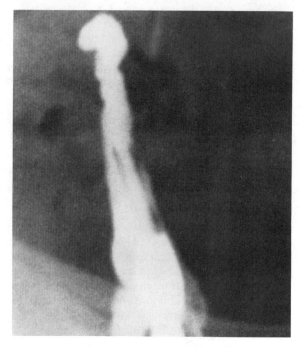

Figure 22-1. HSG 3 months (**A**) and 18 months (**B**) post laser ablation. Note patent uterotubal junction at 3 months which is no longer patent at 18 months. Beginning synechiae are seen at 3 months. Only minimal cavity at 18 months.

B

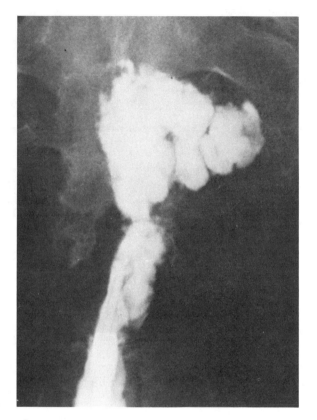

A

Figure 22-2. HSG 3 months (**A**) and 12 months (**B**) post laser ablation. Note progression of synechiae to almost complete obliteration of cavity. Note intravasation of dye characteristic of Asherman's syndrome. (*Cont.*)

Because of this complication and remembering Droegemueller's similar complication with cryosurgery, the uterus should be sounded in the postoperative healing period. Perhaps leaving a hematometra could allow regeneration of endometrial surface as a cavity would be present. In any event, by properly draining this, we should prevent the hematometra formation. One patient experienced a uterine perforation during the procedure when the endometrium was about one half treated. This occurred during manipulation of the hysteroscope when the laser was not in use. Antibiotics were started, she was discharged on the third postoperative day. Two months later she was retreated and had a very good result. It should be noted that at the second time when the procedure was almost completed, the uterus was again perforated, probably in the same location. The perforation did not occur with the laser.

Three patients had postoperative urinary tract infections. They were treated with outpatient antibiotic therapy. One patient, who had a 20-week-size myomatous uterus with a cavity only 13 cm in depth, had profuse purulent discharge

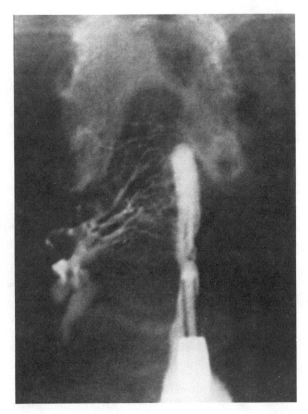

Figure 22-2.

B

approximately 1 week postoperatively. Cultures revealed many organisms, both aerobic and anaerobic. The patient was not febrile. Because she had such a large uterus, she was admitted for outpatient antibiotic therapy and the purulent discharge from the cervix subsided within 1 day of therapy. She had an uneventful posttreatment course. One patient had heavy uterine bleeding 4 weeks postoperatively, presumably because of sloughing of the treated areas. This was controlled by curettage.

Several patients had evidence of fluid overload. There was some facial edema and the patients complained of marked diuresis during the first 24 hours postoperatively. In one of these patients, in whom we had used 5 percent dextrose as an irrigating solution, serum electrolytes in the immediate postoperative period revealed a dilutional hyponatremia. This electrolyte imbalance corrected spontaneously. Since we are now using 5 percent dextrose in normal saline, this should no longer be a worrisome phenomenon. Excessive fluid absorption is worrisome if the procedure is prolonged. During the procedure of laser photovaporization and photocoagulation of the endometrium, venous channels seem to be open but the blood loss is controlled by the pressure of the irrigating fluid. There is a large raw surface and a large volume of fluid may be absorbed. We have found that wide dilation of the cervix also has reduced the intrauterine pressure by allowing the irrigating fluid to flow freely around the hysteroscope. This we believe to be most important. If there is not adequate fluid outflow, the patient can absorb a large amount of fluid rapidly. The hysteroscope should be removed and the cervix more widely dilated. If excessive fluid is absorbed, Lasix should be given intravenously. One patient developed acute pulmonary edema when we miscalculated the amount of fluid absorbed. She responded well to conservative therapy. *It is most important that an adequate fluid outflow around the hysteroscope be obtained.*

Comment

We have demonstrated an effective alternative to hysterectomy for the control of menorrhagia in patients where other treatment modalities have failed, are contraindicated, or are otherwise undesirable. The patients have minimal postoperative morbidity, discomfort, and disability. We have been performing this procedure for 6 years and believe there will be no regeneration of the endometrium. Small amounts of endometrium do survive as demonstrated by vigorous endometrial biopsy.

The seven hysterectomy specimens obtained after sufficient time for healing to have occurred show a single layer of cuboidal epithelium of typical Müllerian type with ciliated and brush borders. Cytogenic stroma is sparse and only rare endometrial glands are present. The epithelium rests directly on underlying myometrium which contains only minimum amounts of hemosiderin. Hardly any carbon particles remain. There is no inflammation. Healing is apparently complete and there is virtually no evidence of functioning endometrium. In four cases, adenomyosis was present to a marked degree.

LASER METROPLASTY

Gynecologists have long been fascinated with uterine duplication anomalies. The Strassman procedure was described for treatment of bicornuate uterus.[23] Jones and Rock have described the treatment of uterine duplication anomalies by various techniques.[24] These were all open operations requiring laparotomy. More recently, Chervenak and Neuwirth,[25] and DeCherney and Polan,[17] and March et al.,[26] have all described intrauterine surgery for removal of uterine septa and synechiae utilizing sharp scissors dissection or electrosurgery. The procedures using a scissors have been described as occasionally being very bloody. The use of high frequency cutting current is hemostatic in this situation but it does have some disadvantage in that it is impossible to determine the degree of electric spread when using this modality.

It was soon seen, while doing laser ablation of the endometrium, that several cases of septate uterus were encountered. We noted that when the laser fiber was carried across the septum, it opened very widely and we thought that it would be a very simple procedure to remove the septum in uteri where this was a clinical problem.

While we only superficially divided the septum while doing laser ablation of the endometrium, *it is important that laparoscopy be performed before or during laser metroplasty to make sure that a bicornuate uterus does not exist. Division of the septum with the laser in a patient with a bicornuate uterus would most likely result in perforation and could be catastrophic.* The procedure is a simple one. The visualization of both parts of the septum is accomplished. The tubal ostia are visualized. Beginning a suitable distance from the tubal ostia, an incision is made from one cornua down the septum, across the septum, and then beginning on the other cornua the same procedure is done. The septum immediately retracts quite widely and a visual determination is made that the septum is divided until a flat fundal area is visualized. It is noted, that occasionally, when the septum is completely divided, there will be some bleeding from the depths of the septum. This is probably where adequate blood supply exists. If this bleeding is persistent, it can be controlled by inserting a Foley catheter for tamponade.[27] As with previously described metroplasties, the patients, immediately postoperatively, were placed on large doses of estrogen and withdrawn after 2 months by the administration of progestogens. A Lippes-Loop intrauterine device (IUD) was inserted in two of the patients. The remainder of the patients had no IUD insertion. Six patients have been treated to the present time. Three had typical midtrimester pregnancy losses. Division of the septum was without difficulty. One has subsequently conceived and delivered normally. It should be noted that following this type of metroplasty vaginal delivery is feasible. It does not weaken the uterus and necessitate a cesarean section as do open operations upon the uterus. The pre- and postoperative hysterograms are seen in Figures 22–3A, B. The other two patients have not conceived as yet.

Another patient had a complete uterine septum down to the cervix. This was discovered at the time of hysterosalpingography during the course of an infertility work-up. It was decided to remove the septum prior to a tuboplasty procedure. This was done without event. Pre- and postoperative hysterograms are seen in Figures 22–4A, B. The patient had an uneventful postoperative course. She subsequently had a tuboplasty procedure, however she has not conceived. She is being considered for in vitro fertilization.

Another patient had had an intrauterine diethylstilbestrol (DES) exposure. Hysteroscopy revealed a marked uterine septum. She had had a prior myomectomy. She is considering pregnancy in the near future. It was thought advisable in view of the DES exposure, with its decreased uterine capacity, that the septum be removed prior to her undertaking a pregnancy. This was performed without incident. She has not decided to conceive to the present time.

One other patient, with a poor reproductive history consisting of an ectopic pregnancy and an early abortion, had a septum noted at the time of hysterosalpingography. She was informed of the possibility of a midtrimester pregnancy loss. She insisted upon having the septum removed prior to attempting another pregnancy. This was done without event. We are not advocating the removal of septa in anticipation of midtrimester loss except in very select circumstances.

The patients are discharged the day of surgery or the day following surgery. There is no pain. As previously stated, they were started on large doses of estrogen for 2 months and withdrawn with a progestogen. We are currently not inserting intrauterine devices as there is no evidence that synechiae will form in these patients.

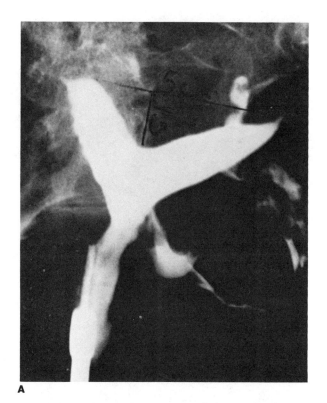

A

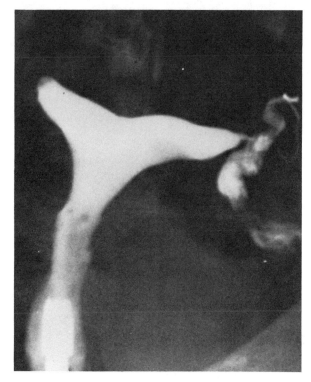

B

Figure 22-3. Preoperative (**A**) and postoperative (**B**) HSG of patient with large uterine septum. Note large capacity of uterine cavity.

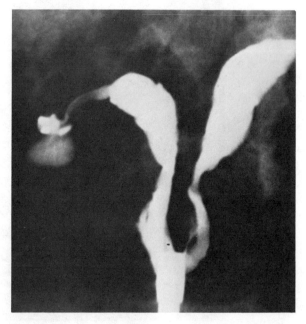

A

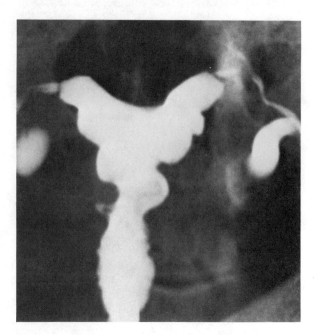

Figure 22-4. HSG preoperative (**A**) and postoperative (**B**) in patient with complete uterine septum into cervix. Variegated margins in postoperative HSG probably from effect of large doses of estrogen on endometrium. Note tubal occlusion.

B

Patients following this type metroplasty should have very little difficulty delivering vaginally. The uterine musculature should have its usual strength. This has been the experience with procedures done with electrosurgery and with scissors dissection.

We believe this is a valid procedure that is very simple, almost bloodless, and should yield excellent results. These are only preliminary studies but we foresee no disadvantage with this modality when compared to the division of the septum with the scissors or high frequency current. When compared with electrosurgical procedure, there is no danger from spread of electric current to adjacent organs. It is important that the procedure be done immediately postmenstrual or after treatment with danazol in order to work in a field with atrophic endometrium. This gives far better visualization for intrauterine hysteroscopic surgery.

Tadir has developed some very ingenious hysteroscopic instruments for utilizing the carbon dioxide laser.[28] This does not incorporate a fiber, as none is available as yet, however there is a channel through which the carbon dioxide (CO_2) laser can be utilized into the uterus. This requires a CO_2 distending medium. It perhaps holds some promise but we know of no clinical studies to the present time.

SUMMARY

The above summarizes our experience to date with intrauterine hysteroscopic laser surgery. One should always keep in mind that laser surgery, by its nature, is destructive. Tissue diagnoses cannot be obtained unless the laser is used to excise tissue. It is for this reason that we have chosen not to destroy malignant or premalignant lesions of the endometrium with the laser. It may be possible in the future to treat cancer precursors utilizing Nd:YAG laser, however, their good response to endocrine therapy at the present time would probably not warrant the risk of progression to malignancy if remnants of premalignant tissue should remain.

To the present time, we have not investigated the use of laser for sterilization purposes by destruction of the uterotubal junction. This is a possiblity, however we do not foresee enough increased advantage over laparoscopic tubal sterilization to warrant its use or testing. It does offer an intriguing possibility in that it could be done under local anesthesia and would have a minimally morbid postoperative course. It should be remembered that electrofulguration of the uterotubal junction did produce many complications and many failures. One would have to prepare a study that would preclude these poor results.

Other applications of hysteroscopic laser surgery will, most assuredly, come to mind as more gynecologists undertake this approach in the treatment of their patients. We eagerly await future development.

REFERENCES

1. Goldrath MH, Fuller TA, Segal S: Laser photovaporization of endometrium for the treatment of menorrhagia. Am J Obstet Gynecol 104:14, 1981
2. Cole P, Berlin J: Elective hysterectomy. Am J Obstet Gynecol 1-29:117–123, 1977

3. Dyck FJ, Murphy FA, Murphy JK, et al: Effect of surveillance in the number of hysterectomies in the Province of Saskatchewan. N Engl J Med 296:1326–1328, 1977
4. D'Esopo DA: Hysterectomy when the uterus is grossly normal. Am J Obstet Gynecol 83:113–122, 1962
5. Miller NF: Hysterectomy—therapeutic necessity or surgical racket? Am J Obstet Gynecol 51:804–810, 1946
6. Parrot M: Elective hysterectomy. Am J Obstet Gynecol 113:531–537, 1971
7. Nilsson L, Goran R: Treatment of menorrhagia. Am J Obstet Gynecol 110:713–720, 1971
8. Asherman JG: Amenorrhoea traumatica (atretica). J Obstet Gynecol Brit Emp 55:23–30, 1948
9. Polishuk WZ, Anteby SO, Weinstein D: Puerperal endometritis and intrauterine adhesions. Inter Surg 60:418–420, 1975
10. Evans TN: Infertility and other gynecologic problems. In Danforth (ed): Textbook of Obstetrics and Gynecology. New York, Harper and Row, 1971, p 800
11. Droegemueller W, Greer BE, Davis JR, et al: Cryocoagulation of the endometrium at the uterine cornua. Am J Obstet Gynecol 131:1–9, 1978
12. Rongy AJ: Radium therapy in benign uterine bleeding. J Mt Sinai Hosp 14:569–575, 1947
13. Crossen RJ, Crossen HS: Radiation therapy of uterine myoma. JAMA 133:593–599, 1947
14. Falconer B: The treatment of metropathia haemorrhagica: Suggestions for a therapeutic programme. Acta Obstet Gynecol Scand 27:288–296, 1947
15. Droegemueller W, Greer B, Makowski E: Cryosurgery in patients with dysfunctional uterine bleeding. Obstet Gynecol 38:256–258, 1971
16. Droegemueller W, Makowski E, Macsalka R: Destruction of the endometrium by cryosurgery. Am J Obstet Gynecol 110:467–469, 1971
17. DeCherney A, Polan ML: Hysteroscopic management of intrauterine lesions and intractable uterine bleeding. Obstet Gynecol 61:392, 1983
18. Burke L. Rubin BW, Kim I: Uterine abscess formation secondary to endometrial cryosurgery. Obstet Gynecol 41:224–226, 1973
19. Shenker JG, Polishuk WZ: Regeneration of rabbit endometrium following intrauterine instillation of chemical agents. Gynecol Invest 4:1–13, 1973
20. Polishuk WZ, Shenker JG: Induction of intrauterine adhesions in the rabbit with autogenous fibroblast implants. Am J Obstet Gynecol 115:789–794, 1973
21. Shenker JG, Nicosia SV, Polishuk WZ, Garcia CR: An in vitro fibroblast-enriched sponge preparation for induction of intrauterine adhesions. Israel J Med Sciences 11:849–851, 1975
22. Polishuk WZ: Endometrial regeneration and adhesion formation. S Afr Med J 49:440–442, 1975
23. Strassman EO: Fertility and unification of double uterus. Fertil Steril 17:165, 1966
24. Jones HW Jr, Rock JA: Reparative and Constructive Surgery of the Female Generative Tract. Baltimore, Williams & Wilkins, 1983
25. Chervenak FA, Neuwirth RS: Hysteroscopic resection of the uterine septum. Am J Obstet Gynecol 141:351, 1981
26. March CM, Israel R, March AD: Hysteroscopic management of intrauterine adhesions. Am J Obstet Gynecol 130:653, 1978
27. Goldrath MH: Uterine tamponade for the control of acute uterine bleeding. Am J Obstet Gynecol 147:869–872, 1983
28. Tadir Y, Raif J, Dagan J, et al: Hysteroscope for CO_2 laser application. Lasers Surg Med 4:153, 1984

23

Initiating a CO$_2$ Laser Program

James H. Dorsey
Michael S. Baggish

Initiating carbon dioxide (CO$_2$) laser surgery in the office or within the hospital setting entails more than just purchasing an instrument. Lasers vary in power, design, and price, and the selection of the proper instrument depends upon the intended use. Before purchasing a laser, the surgeon or the hospital laser committee must carefully plan a formal program. There are four primary questions that should be answered at the outset:

1. What operative procedures are to be done with the laser?
2. Where will the laser be located?
3. Who will use the laser?
4. Will the laser be cost-effective?

OPERATIVE PROCEDURES

The CO$_2$ laser was first used in gynecology for the treatment of cervical disease and for early neoplasia of the lower reproductive tract. These remain today the most common gynecologic applications. Most of the procedures directed to the lower reproductive tract are performed on an outpatient basis either in the office or clinic under local anesthesia; some are done in the outpatient operating rooms under general anesthesia. Gynecologists who have active colposcopy practices may well be able to justify the purchase of an office CO$_2$ laser. If there are few lasers in a practice locale, the acquisition of the instrument may itself attract new referrals. The majority of gynecologists who perform laser surgery, however, will wish to have access to the laser, but not necessarily to own it. Usually, a hospital or a group of physicians will purchase a laser and place it in an outpatient setting. This laser should be an "office type" of instrument and does not require a power output of more than 20 W. If the laser is to be moved from one examining room to another, or if it will be moved from clinic to outpatient surgery, it should be sturdy and mobile.

Certain surgical procedures in gynecology as well as operations done by specialists in other fields, such as neurosurgery, require large, more powerful lasers with articulated arms. These lasers are utilized in general operating rooms. A laser program that provides for both inpatient and outpatient laser surgery will usually require two lasers, one for office or clinic and the other for the general operating rooms. It is possible for the outpatient department to share a laser with the clinic depending upon the physical plan of the hospital. If several surgical specialities are to share the laser, a panel of qualified surgeons should be appointed to list the surgical procedures to be performed and to outline the requirements for the laser for each specific procedure. This approach should also be used for the selection of other instruments required by the laser surgeon. Many of these accessories can be used with any laser, but some require adaptation depending upon the laser model. It is important to make sure that all systems, such as colposcopes, operative microscopes, laparoscopes, and audiovisual attachments, are compatible before purchase.

Some lasers come equipped with colposcopes that are already fitted with cameras. This is somewhat confining and the most flexibility is obtained if one has a beam splitter that can be fitted with any camera or video camera.

EVALUATING THE LASER

Whether the laser be a small office type or a large surgical unit, the surgeon should have a checklist prepared before attempting to evaluate a particular model. All lasers are fascinating to use and the novice will be at a loss in trying to decide which one to purchase. There is a relatively large assortment of models available and there are also many differences that should be recognized before the decision to buy is made.

The Colposcope

Many laser manufacturers, in an effort to reduce costs, have mounted their lasers on colposcopes which provide fixed magnification, usually at a relatively high power. Colposcopes which do not have variable magnification from low to higher powers are often difficult to use for colposcopy combined with CO_2 laser surgery. It is problematic to scan the lower reproductive tract for multifocal disease with a high power magnification because it requires an inordinate amount of time, provides limited visual field, and may lead to missing lesions. It is also difficult to plan or outline the margins of a lesion without major movement of the colposcope when only a small fraction of the operative field can be seen.

Variable magnification colposcopes allow viewing at scanning powers, e.g., ×6–7, as well as operating powers, e.g., ×10–12, and high powers ×16–20 (Figs. 23–1A, 23–1B).

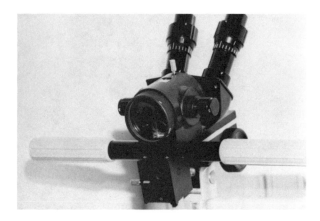

Figure 23-1A. This office model colposcope is equipped with variable magnification, interchangeable objective, and laser dovetail.

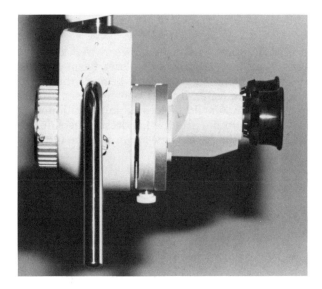

Figure 23-1B. Another office model colposcope equipped with variable magnification, but a fixed objective.

Colposcopes which cannot be fitted with beam splitters may be difficult to utilize for 35 mm photography or for videotape recording. Laser surgeons interested in recording operative procedures should make sure that the colposcope is adaptable for these techniques. It may be advantageous to have the option to select the objective lens of the colposcope and, therefore, determine the distance between this lens and the surgical target. Colposcopes equipped with objective lenses of short focal lengths may not allow enough room between patient and laser for the surgeon to insert or manipulate an instrument in the vagina. Unfortunately, every one of these options drives up the price of the equipment and may add $10,000 to $12,000 to the cost of the laser system (Fig. 23-2).

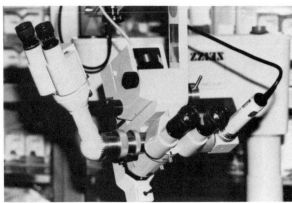

Figure 23-2. An operating room, high intensity illumination, colposcope. The optional equipment includes: A "70/30" beam splitter, a binocular teaching attachment, an iris light control, a microvideo system. Note the laser micromanipulator attached to the objective lens of the colposcope.

The Micromanipulator

The micromanipulator or "joystick" is attached to gears that move reflecting mirrors which have been placed in the path of the laser beam after it has passed through the focusing lens. These mirrors direct the beam to the target. Obviously, the micromanipulator should move easily and under the same tension in every direction. The micromanipulator should be located in a position where it is comfortable to use. While some operators prefer a handrest, others do not. Often, the surgeon must use one hand on the vaginal speculum and the other on the micro-

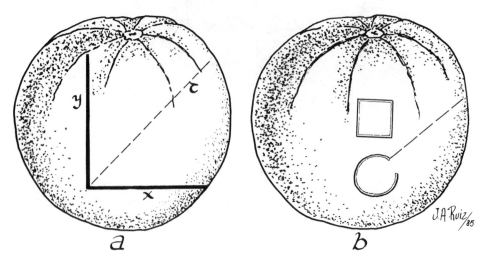

Figure 23-3A. An exercise to test the excursions of the micromanipulator demonstrated on an inanimate object, e.g., an orange. First a "Y" axis is traced from the uppermost portion of the microscopic field to the lowest extent of the field. Next an "X" axis is etched. Finally, a vector "2" is traced. **B.** In order to combine the functions in Figure 23-3A and gain a feel for the tension on the "joy stick," geometric figures simulate actual in vivo surgery.

manipulator. Laser mounting must be absolutely steady so that small motions of the micromanipulator do not jiggle the colposcope.

Unfortunately, not all micromanipulators move equally well in all directions. This can be readily evaluated by drawing some simple geometric designs, such as straight lines, circles, and squares (Figs. 23–3A, 23–3B). Using an orange for a target, measure the total excursion of the beam by constructing an X, Y, Z axis. Note the size of the operative field that is accessible without moving the laser itself. Try to draw a circle or a square and judge the response of the micromanipulator in all directions. If the lines are irregular or if the circle is difficult to draw, the design of the instrument may be faulty or adjustments may be necessary.

It is apparent that the hand-eye coordination of the surgeon enters into the evaluation of the micromanipulator, however, with a little practice, the differences become easily detectable.

The Focal Spot

Focal spot diameters may be varied on some lasers. This is a helpful option if both excisional and vaporization procedures are to be done, or if several different operators are to use the laser. For excisional laser surgery, the width of the incision is proportional to the focal spot diameter. Allowing for some additional tissue shrinkage immediately adjacent to the incision, the tissue destruction by incision alone becomes an important factor. For example, if an excisional conization is done with a laser using a focal spot diameter of 1 mm, continuous wave, the defect left in the cervix will be at least 2 mm wider in diameter than if the exact same cone is taken with a cold knife. (Figs. 23–4A, 23–4B).

This larger defect may be of no consequence in the multiparous patient with a large cervix, but in a nulliparous woman with a small cervix, a smaller defect may be more desirable. It then becomes an advantage to be able to employ a very small focal spot. By the same token, it is advantageous to have a large focal spot with which to "paint on" laser energy for vaporization producers. Again the variable spot feature may drive up the price of the laser by $2000 to $3000.

Evaluation Form

A convenient form may be used to evaluate a laser for a number of different parameters. Such a sample check list is illustrated in Figure 23–5.

CREDENTIALING FOR GYNECOLOGIC LASER SURGERY

Unfortunately, any physician with a license to practice medicine can purchase a laser and perform laser surgery in the office. Certainly, most physicians have the integrity and intelligence to recognize that suitable training is required. Hospitals have a greater problem after acquiring a laser, because with such a purchase comes the moral and medicolegal responsibility to ensure the competency of the staff physicians who wish to practice laser surgery, and to credential only those who meet acceptable standards. Although the governing body of the institution has the ultimate authority for the credentialing of staff physicians, the actual job of cre-

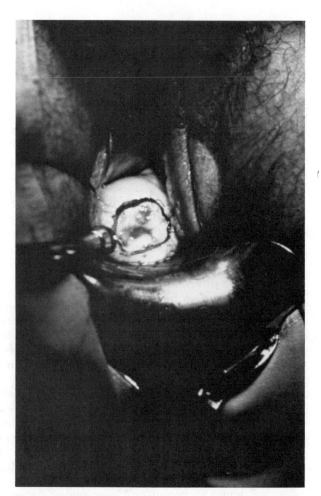

Figure 23–4A. A high power density incision is cut into the cervix; power 20 W, spot ½ mm diameter. This incision simulates a knife cut, but could be further improved by reducing the spot to ¼ mm and pulsing the laser beam at 400 p/second with 0.3×10^3 second width.

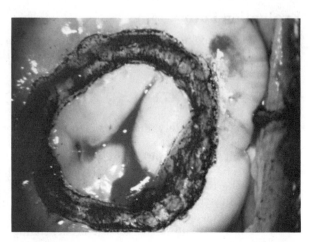

Figure 23–4B. In contrast to Figure 23–4A, this incision is cut with the same power setting, but a 1.5 mm spot. The peripheral thermal damage here is more extensive.

	1[a]	**2**[b]	**3**[c]
1. Colposcope has variable magnification	☐	☐	☐
2. Micromanipulator with variable spot	☐	☐	☐
3. Extensive laser beam excursion	☐	☐	☐
4. Comfortable configuration	☐	☐	☐
5. Colposcope with selective objectives	☐	☐	☐
6. Unit stability	☐	☐	☐
7. Ease of transportation of laser	☐	☐	☐
8. Ease of storage of laser	☐	☐	☐
9. Surgical arm mobility	☐	☐	☐
10. Photographic accessibility	☐	☐	☐
11. Low cost	☐	☐	☐

[a]Required
[b]Optional
[c]Unnecessary

Figure 23–5. A sample laser evaluation form.

dentialing is usually assigned to a committee or to the department chairman. Under the theory of "corporate negligence," hospitals that allow physicians to carry out procedures which they are not competent to perform may be held negligent in a court of law. In order to minimize liability, ensure quality care, and aid credentialing committees in making a logical decision, guidelines for credentialing in laser surgery have been developed. Hopefully, these criteria will also be followed by the office laser surgeon (Table 23–1).

Lower Reproductive Tract Surgery

1. *Colposcopic expertise.* The gynecologist who intends to treat patients for intraepithelial neoplasias with the CO₂ laser must be an experienced and competent colposcopist. Colposcopy cannot be divorced from laser surgery

TABLE 23–1. SUGGESTED GUIDELINES FOR CREDENTIALING IN GYNECOLOGIC LASER SURGERY

Lower reproductive tract surgery
    Colposcopic expertise
    Formal laser course
    Laser laboratory experience
    Laser surgical preceptorship
    Supervision by qualified laser surgeon
    Continued surgical practice to maintain competency
Intraabdominal laser surgery
    Conventional surgical experience
    Specific laser training as noted above

or, for that matter, from any outpatient therapy of the intraepithelial neoplasias.

2. *Laser course.* The laser surgeon must have a working knowledge of laser physics, safety, and laser surgical principles and techniques. This knowledge is best acquired in a well-organized laser course.

3. *Laser laboratory.* Many of the physical properties of laser are best demonstrated by simple laboratory procedures. Laser surgical procedures can be practiced and perfected on inanimate objects and surgical specimens before operating on the patient. It is absolutely mandatory that the laser surgeon develop the hand-eye coordination necessary for the proper use of the micromanipulator and this is best done in the laboratory.

4. *Laser preceptorship.* The prospective laser surgeon should acquire actual surgical experience under the tutelage of a qualified laser surgeon. The number of cases that should be thus performed will vary with the individual ability of the surgeon. Some physicians are very quick to learn laser surgery, while others have great difficulty in operating through a microscope. It is at this point that the laser surgeon must make the decision as to whether or not to continue to treat patients with this modality.

5. *Final observation.* The laser surgeon should be observed at surgery on his own patient by an experienced laser surgeon. Final credentialing is granted when the surgeon demonstrates competency.

6. *Continued practice.* Expertise should be maintained by continued practice. If clinical cases are not available, time should be spent in the laboratory for at least several hours per month.

7. *Check out on new equipment.* The surgeon should be checked out on each new laser that is to be used. Lasers vary in many features and the surgeon must be familiar with special features of every laser that he uses in actual surgery.

Intraabdominal and Endoscopic Laser Surgery

Credentialing for intraabdominal and endoscopic laser surgery follows the same guidelines as for lower reproductive tract disease, however, in this instance, the surgeon must be a capable abdominal surgeon and experienced endoscopist. For example, the laser should not be used to perform tubal surgery by anyone who is not an expert in conventional tubal surgery, nor should endometriosis be laser ablated by anyone who is not able to correctly manage this disease by conventional methods. It must also be noted that intraabdominal CO_2 laser surgery is a highly skilled technique requiring special expertise. The use of high powered CO_2 lasers, argon lasers, Nd:YAG lasers, frequency doubled Nd:YAG lasers all require special training and skills as well as suitable inservice orientation to each and every device.

SUMMARY

The purchase of a piece of equipment by an institution embarking on a laser program in either the office or hospital must be carefully considered. Lasers are powerful, precise, complex surgical instruments whose proper applications are intimately intertwined with the skill of the surgeon user. The instrument will not itself confer any mystical properties to the treatment of disease. The success or failure of an operative procedure, therefore, is the primary responsibility of the surgeon and singularly not the instrument. It is the surgeon's duty to use this excellent instrument selectively and for cases where it will be of benefit to the patient.

Glossary

ABSORPTION   The assimilation of electromagnetic energy into the body of an object.

AMPLITUDE   The magnitude of a wave.

APERTURE   An opening in a laser enclosure through which the laser radiation is emitted.

ATTENUATION   The decrease in the power of a beam of radiation as it traverses absorbing and/or scattering material.

AXIAL FLOW   The movement of gas along the length of a laser cavity.

COHERENCE   A property of electromagnetic waves that are all of the same wavelength, polarization, and precisely in phase with each other.

COLLIMATED   Lacking divergence.

DIFFRACTION   The bending of rays around the edges of obstacles.

DIVERGENCE   The angle of spread of the outer edges of a laser beam, measured in degrees or radians.

ELECTROMAGNETIC SPECTRUM   The range of electromagnetic waves classified according to wavelength or frequency; includes radio waves, microwaves, infrared light, visible light, ultraviolet light, x-rays, and gamma rays, in the order of decreasing wavelength.

EMISSION   The act of giving off radiant energy by an atom or molecule.

ENERGY   The capacity for doing work.

EXCITATION   The elevation of a particle or assemblage of particles to a higher energy state.

FOCUS   The location to which rays, after having been acted on by a lens or mirror, appear to converge.

FREQUENCY   The number of wave crests that pass a given point per unit time interval.

INTENSITY   Strictly defined as the amount of power radiated per unit solid angle (watts per steradian) but commonly used as the power incident on a unit area (the irradiance).

INTEGER   A positive or negative whole number including zero.

JOULE   A unit of energy in the metric system; 1 joule equals 1 watt expended in 1 second.

LASER   A light source which generates a highly directional, monochromatic, and coherent beam by the stimulated emission process. Laser is an acronym for *l*ight *a*mplification by *s*timulated *e*mission of *r*adiation.

LASER MEDIUM   The gas, liquid, or solid whose atoms or molecules are stimulated to emit coherent radiation.

LONGITUDINAL MODE (AXIAL)   The standing wave of a laser along the cavity length, governed by the condition that the length of the cavity between the laser mirrors must be an integral number of wavelengths of the mode.

MASER   A source of microwave energy which generates a highly directional, monochromatic, and coherent beam by the stimulated emission process. Maser is an acronym for *m*icrowave *a*mplification by *s*timulated *e*mission of *r*adiation.

METER   An instrument which measures some quantity, such as a power meter on a laser which measures the optical power in watts. Also, the unit of length in the metric (MKS) system: a meter is about 3 feet.

MODE   A standing longitudinal or transverse electromagnetic wave pattern in a laser cavity.

ORTHOGONAL   Involving right angles.

PHASE   The fractional part of a period in a wave through which time has advanced measured from some arbitrary point in time.

PHOTON   A quantum of electromagnetic energy, equal to the product of Planck's constant and the radiation frequency.

POLARIZATION (WAVE)   The alignment of the electric field vectors comprising electromagnetic radiation.

POPULATION INVERSION   A distribution of particles in which more particles are in an upper energy state than in a lower one.

PULSE DURATION   The length of time a pulse exists.

PULSE INTERVAL   The time between two consecutive pulses.

PUMPING   The process of injecting energy into a system in order to produce a population inversion.

QUANTUM   The smallest increment or parcel into which the energy of a wave may be divided.

RADIAN   A unit of angular measure equal to the angle subtended at the center of a circle by an arc length equal to the radius of the circle. One radian equals approximately 57.3 degrees.

RADIATION   In the context of optics, radiation is released electromagnetic energy or the process of releasing electromagnetic energy.

REFLECTIVE   The property of returning light rays from a surface.

REPETITION RATE   The average number of pulses per unit time.

RESONANCE   The condition of reinforcement existing in a laser cavity when the distance between the reflecting mirrors is an integral number of half-wave lengths of the laser radiation.

ROTATIONAL ENERGY   The energy an object possesses by virtue of its rotation around some axis.

SHUTTER   A device to prevent radiation from emerging from a laser, without shutting off the laser.

SUPER PULSE   A pulse that contains more instantaneous power than the output from a similar system operating in a continuous mode.

TRANSVERSE ELECTROMAGNETIC (TEM)   A TEM wave is one in which the electric and magnetic field vectors are perpendicular to the direction of propagation.

TRANSITION   For an atom or molecule to go from one energy state to another, normally with the emission or the absorption of radiant energy.

TRANSMISSION   The passage of electromagnetic radiation through a medium.

VELOCITY   The rate of change of distance with respect to time.

VIBRATIONAL ENERGY   The energy an object possesses by virtue of its back and forth motion.

WATT   A unit of power in the metric (MKS) system; 1 watt is equal to 1 joule per second.

WAVE   A progressive disturbance propagated from point to point in space or a medium.

Index